J. Ruhlmann · P. Oehr · H.-J. Biersack (Eds.)

PET in Oncology

Springer

Berlin
Heidelberg
New York
Barcelona
Hong Kong
London
Milan
Paris
Singapore
Tokyo

J. Ruhlmann · P. Oehr · H.-J. Biersack
Editors

PET in Oncology

Basics and Clinical Application

With 95 Figures, some in Color
and 58 Tables

Springer

Dr. Dr. Jürgen Ruhlmann
PD Dr. Peter Oehr

PET-Center
Münsterstraße 20
53111 Bonn, Germany

Prof. Dr. H.-J. Biersack
University Clinic Bonn
Clinic and Policlinic for Nuclear Medicine
Rheinisch-Westfälische University Bonn
Sigmund-Freud-Straße 25
53127 Bonn, Germany

Translated from German by:
Judith F. Lee, Ph.D. and Mary W. Tannert, Ph.D.

ISBN-13: 978-3-642-64220-3 e-ISBN-13: 978-3-642-60010-4
DOI: 10.1007/978-3-642-60010-4

Library of Congress Cataloging-in-Publication Data
PET in der Onkologie. English. PET in oncology : basics and clinical application / [edited by] J. Ruhlmann, P. Oehr, and H.-J. Biersack. p. cm.
Includes bibliographical references and index. ISBN 3-540-65077-6 (hardcover : alk. paper)
1. Cancer-Tomography. 2. Tomography, Emission. I. Ruhlmann, J. (Jürgen), 1955– · II. Oehr, P. (Peter), 1942– · III. Biersack, H. J. IV. Title. [DNLM: 1. Neoplasms-radionuclide imaging. 2. Tomography, Emission-Computed-methods. QZ 241 P477p 1999a]
RC270.3.T65P4613 1999 616.99'407575-dc21
DNLM/DLC for Library of Congress 99-26968

Production: PRO EDIT GmbH, D-69126 Heidelberg
Cover design: design & production, D-69121 Heidelberg
Typesetting: Mitterweger Werksatz GmbH, D-68723 Plankstadt

SPIN: 10693821 21/3135 – 5 4 3 2 1 0 – Printed on acid-free paper

Preface

Development of Positron-Emissiontomography (PET) dates back to the Mid-70ies. However, this imaging procedure gained clinical importance not before 1990. First clinical papers were published by US researchers. The patient populations were relatively small by that time, and European as well as German authors contributed results in larger patient populations. These clinical papers led to a widespread application of PET in clinical routine. The clinical relevance was documented by several PET consensus conferences. However, the National Health Service System is very reluctant to pay for PET studies. Even in Germany, PET is not yet a regular part of the reimbursement system. On the other hand, in solitary pulmonary nodules and brain tumors third party payers in United States have accepted these indications. The high popularity of PET in US will certainly lead to an improved situation with respect to reimbursement, as well as the European PET consensus conferences. Nowadays, PET is a well established routine procedure in lung and colorectal cancer as well as malignant melanoma, head and neck cancer and breast cancer. Other indications are lymphoma and pancreatic cancer. Within the next years, the diagnostic spectrum of PET will be widened, especially in the field of therapy follow-up and proof of vitality after chemotherapy.

The increased use of PET in oncology makes evident, that it is necessary to train referring physians in PET. The aim of this book is to summarize the basics and the clinical results of PET and to bring them of the attention of general medicine.

Bonn, Spring 1999

J. Ruhlmann
P. Oehr
H.-J. Biersack

Contents

Part I Principles

List of Contributors

Alexiou, C.
Department of Otorhinolaryngology
Head and Neck Surgery
Isar Right Bank Clinic, Technical University Munich
Ismaninger Straße 22, 81675 München, Germany

An, R.
Clinic and Policlinic for Nuclear Medicine
University of Bonn
Sigmund-Freud-Straße 25, 53127 Bonn
Germany

Arnold, W.
Department of Otorhinolaryngology
Head and Neck Surgery
Isar Right Bank Clinic, Technical University Munich
Ismaninger Straße 22, 81675 München, Germany

Bangard, M.
Clinic and Policlinic for Nuclear Medicine
University of Bonn
Sigmund-Freud-Straße 25, 53127 Bonn
Germany

Baum, R. P.
PET Center, Central Clinic Bad Berka GmbH
99437 Bad Berka, Germany

Biersack, H.-J.
Clinic and Policlinic for Nuclear Medicine
University of Bonn
Sigmund-Freud-Straße 25, 53127 Bonn
Germany

Bonnet, R.
PET Center, Central Clinic Bad Berka GmbH
99437 Bad Berka, Germany

Büll, U.
Clinic for Nuclear Medicine
RWTH Aachen
Pauwelsstraße 30, 52074 Aachen, Germany

Cremerius, U.
Clinic for Nuclear Medicine
RWTH Aachen
Pauwelsstraße 30, 52074 Aachen, Germany

Diederichs, C.G.
Department of Nuclear Medicine
Ulm University Clinic
Robert-Koch-Straße 8, 89070 Ulm, Germany

Grünwald, F.
Clinic and Policlinic for Nuclear Medicine
University of Bonn
Sigmund-Freud-Straße 25, 53127 Bonn, Germany

Hämisch, Y.
ADAC, Europe
Großenbaumer Weg 6, 40472 Düsseldorf, Germany

Ide, M.
HIMEDIC Imaging Center at Lake Yamanaka
Yanagihara 562-12
Hirano, Yamanashi, 401-0502, Japan

Kau, R.J.
Department of Otorhinolaryngology
Head and Neck Surgery
Isar Right Bank Clinic, Technical University Munich
Ismaninger Straße 22, 81675 München, Germany

Kaufmann, R.
Department of Dermatology, Medical Center
University of Frankfurt
Theodor-Stern-Kai 7, 60590 Frankfurt, Germany

Kozak, B.
Nuclear Medicine and Radiology Practice
Münsterstraße 20, 53111 Bonn, Germany

Laubenbacher, C.
Clinic and Policlinic for Nuclear Medicine
Isar Right Bank Clinic, Technical University Munich
Ismaninger Straße 22, 81675 München, Germany

Lowe, V.J.
PET Imaging Facility
St. Louis University Health Sciences Center
3635 Vista Avenue at Grand Blvd.
St. Louis, MO 63110-0250, USA

Menzel, C.
Clinic and Policlinic for Nuclear Medicine
University of Bonn
Sigmund-Freud-Straße 25, 53127 Bonn, Germany

Newiger, H.
Siemens AG
Medical Systems, Nuclear Medicine
Henkestraße 127, 91052 Erlangen, Germany

Oehr, P.
PET-Center
Münsterstraße 20, 53111 Bonn, Germany

Palmedo, H.
Clinic and Policlinic of Nuclear Medicine
University of Bonn
Sigmund-Freud-Straße 25, 53127 Bonn, Germany

Presselt, N.
PET Center
Central Clinic Bad Berka GmbH
99437 Bad Berka, Germany

Reul, J.
Nuclear Medicine and Radiology Practice
Münsterstraße 20, 53111 Bonn, Germany

Rinne, D.
Department of Dermatology, Medical Center
University of Frankfurt
Theodor-Stern-Kai 7, 60590 Frankfurt, Germany

Ruhlmann, J.
PET Center
Münsterstraße 20, 53111 Bonn, Germany

Shohtsu, A.
HIMEDIC Imaging Center at Lake Yamanaka
Yanagihara 562-12
Hirano, Yamanashi, 401-0502, Japan

Schwaiger, M.
Clinic and Policlinic for Nuclear Medicine
Isar Right Bank Clinic, Technical University
Ismaninger Straße 22, 81675 München
Germany

Valk, P.E.
Northern California PET Imaging Center
Sacramento, California, USA

Vollet, B.
Clinic and Policlinic for Nuclear Medicine
Westphalian Wilhelm University
Albert-Schweitzer-Straße 33, 48129 Münster
Germany

Willkomm, P.
Clinic and Policlinic for Nuclear Medicine
University of Bonn
Sigmund-Freud-Strasse 25, 53127 Bonn
Germany

Yasuda, S.
HIMEDIC Imaging Center at Lake Yamanaka
Yanagihara 562-12
Hirano, Yamanashi, 401-0502, Japan

Ziegler, S.
Clinic and Policlinic for Nuclear Medicine
Isar Right Bank Clinic, Technical University
Ismaninger Straße 22, 81675 München
Germany

Zimny, M.
Clinic for Nuclear Medicine
RWTH Aachen
Pauwelsstraße 30, 52074 Aachen, Germany

PART I

Principles

Chapter 1

Physical Principles

H. Newiger, Y. Hämisch, P. Oehr, J. Ruhlmann, B. Vollet, and S. Ziegler

1.1 PET Technology

H. Newiger

Not long after P.A.M. Dirac predicted the existence of positrons in 1927, C. Anderson was able to prove they existed (1932). Soon people began to think about medical applications for positrons, since it was recognized that they had special properties for diagnostics.

1.1.1 The Physics of Positrons

Positrons are the anti-particles of electrons. Thus they have the same physical properties. The only difference is the electric charge, which in positrons is positive. Positrons are formed during the decay of nuclides that have a large number of protons in their nuclei compared with the number of neutrons. This is true of the carbon isotope ^{11}C, for example. Since the nucleus of ^{11}C is unstable, it decays to form the boron isotope ^{11}B by emitting one positron and one neutrino (Fig. 1.1.1). While the neutrino escapes without interacting with the surrounding material, the positron is slowed down by scattering processes in the electron clouds of the surrounding materials – in the patient's tissue, for example. As soon as it has come to rest it captures an electron and together they form a positronium for a fraction of a second. Then, in a process called annihilation, the positron and electron masses are converted into 2 photons (annihilation radiation) that travel apart in exactly opposite directions (Fig. 1.1.2). Since the entire electron and positron mass is transformed, each photon has an energy of 511 keV.

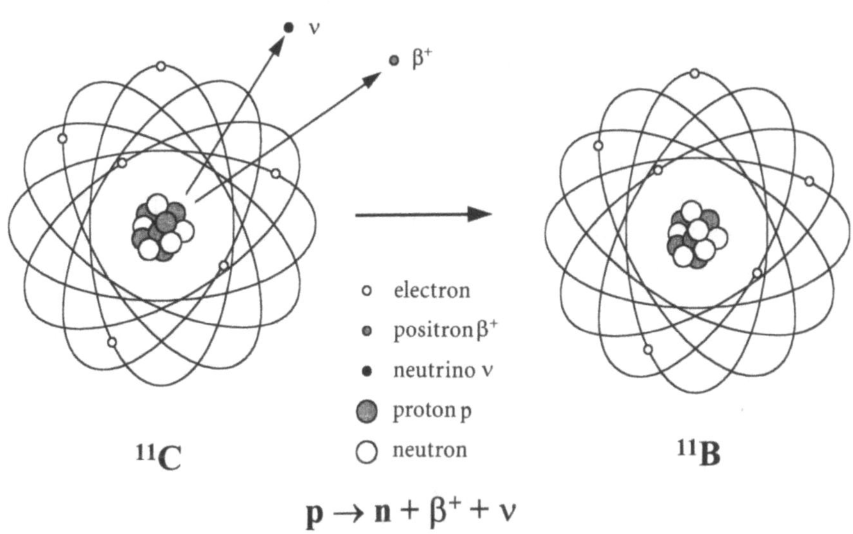

Fig. 1.1.1. Schematic diagram of positron decay

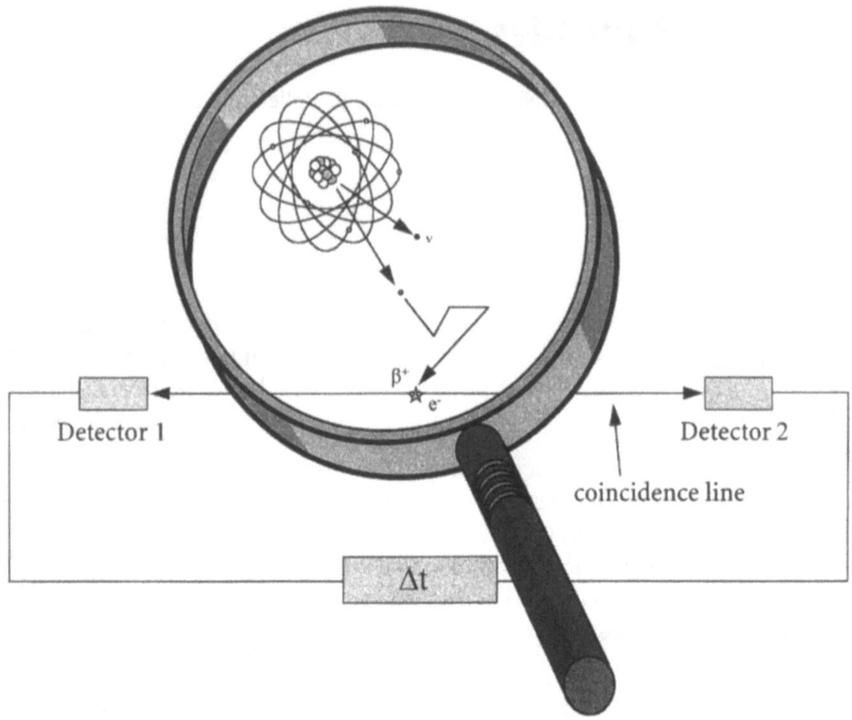

Fig. 1.1.2.
Coincidence detection of the two photons formed during annihilation

1.1.2 Measurement of Positron Radiation

When the two photons are detected by two opposite detectors (coincidence, see Fig. 1.1.2), then the site of annihilation can be located at a point on the line (coincidence line) connecting the two detectors (electronic collimation). Since the two detectors will only detect an event at precisely the same time if annihilation has occurred precisely in the middle between the two detectors, the coincidence window that is used establishes how great the time difference can be between the arrival of the two photons. Normally all events that are detected within 12 ns are recorded.

1.1.3 Advantages of PET

Because of the electronic collimation PET does not require collimators as they are necessary in single photon measurements with gamma cameras. This results in a significantly higher sensitivity of PET (factors 10–100). In addition, sensitivity is not necessarily limited by the desired resolution. The latter only depends either on the size of the individual detectors for the block detector design or the intrinsic resolution for the large area detector design. In PET sensitivity and resolution do not affect each other as much as in single photon tomography (SPECT).

Another advantage of PET involves the existing positron emitters (Table 1.1.1). Most biomolecules can be labeled using carbon (^{11}C), nitrogen (^{13}N), oxygen (^{15}O) and fluorine (^{18}F) so that their biochemical properties are not altered. In addition, the metabolism of these tracers is frequently known. This means that for ^{18}F-FDG (fluorodeoxyglucose), for example, the glucose metabolism can be calculated from the basic activity distribution (modeling, Patlak plot). Since a calculation of this type requires the input function, which is obtained using blood samples, it is frequently customary in clinical studies to limit calculations to quantification based on the standard uptake value (SUV). For this purpose the activity mea-

Table 1.1.1. Characteristics of the most common positron emitters

Positron Emitter	Half Life [min]	Product	Maximum Energy of Positron [MeV]	Maximum Linear Range [mm]	Mean Linear Range [mm]
^{11}C	20.4	^{11}B	0.96	5.0	0.3
^{13}N	9.9	^{13}C	1.19	5.4	1.4
^{15}O	2.1	^{15}N	1.72	8.2	1.5
^{18}F	110	^{18}O	0.64	2.4	0.2
^{68}Ga	68	^{68}Zn	1.89	9.1	1.9
^{82}Rb	1.3	^{82}Kr	3.35	15.6	2.6

sured in a pixel is normalized for the injected activity and the patient weight.

Today's tomographs, which have a resolution of 4–6 mm, nearly achieve the maximum resolution that is physically possible. Thus improvement below a certain value is not possible since the positrons travel a finite distance between the emission point and the site of annihilation (see mean range in Table 1.1.1). In addition, the residual pulses of the electron-positron pair prevent the two photons from traveling in precisely opposite directions. Because of these two effects, a limit resolution of 2–3 mm will apply physically to whole-body tomographs.

1.1.4 Production of Positron Emitters

As shown in Table 1.1.1, all positron emitters have a relatively short half life. Only ^{18}F, which has a half life of 110 min, can be transported over certain distances. But even in this case it has been found that in order to utilize the tracer clinically, transport times cannot exceed about one half life of the nuclide; otherwise on-site production in a cyclotron is required. This means that ^{18}F-FDG, for example, cannot be transported over distances greater than about 200 km. The shorter lived positron emitters like ^{11}C, ^{13}N or ^{15}O must

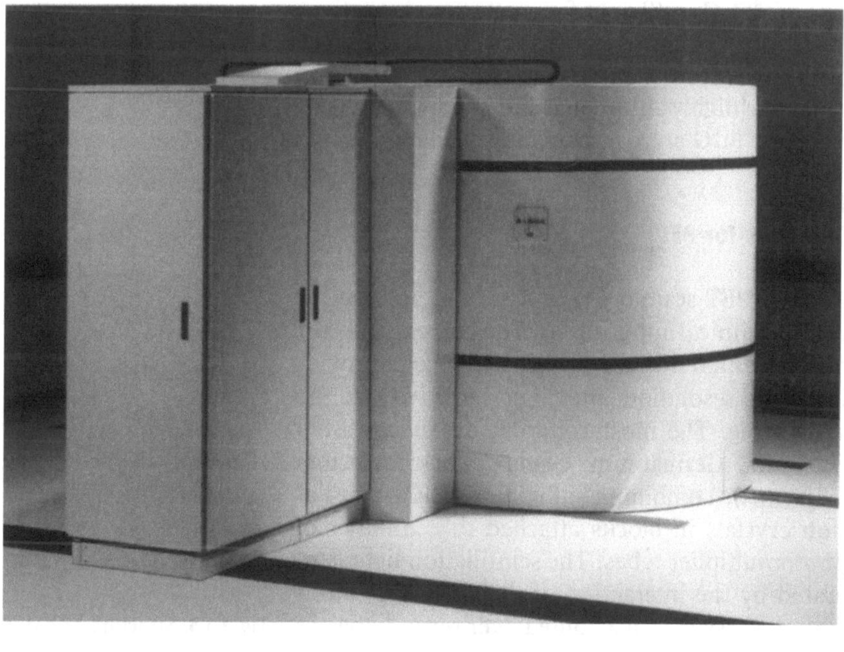

Fig. 1.1.3. The RDS111 compact cyclotron developed by CTI, Knoxville, Tennessee (USA)

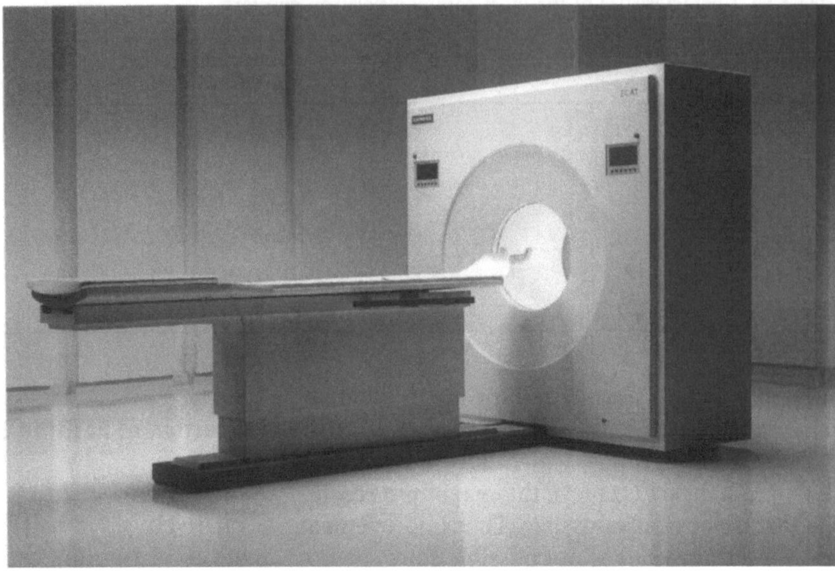

Fig. 1.1.4. The ECAT EXACT scanner marketed by Siemens, Erlangen, Germany

be produced on site or very close to their intended use.

Today this can be done with powerful and compact cyclotrons (e.g. CTI's RDS 111, Fig. 1.1.3), which even can be installed in larger diagnostic institutions. They can produce about 3 Ci of ^{18}F in an hour which can be synthesized into about 1 Ci of ^{18}FDG, sufficient for more than 20 patient investigations in various distances from the place of the cyclotron. Many of the synthesis processes today are highly automated and synthesis units as e.g. for ^{18}FDG are commercially available.

1.1.5 Detectors for PET

Today's PET scanners (Fig. 1.1.4) can be used for routine clinical applications. The current detector designs differently adress the challenge of providing high resolution and high sensitivity at the same time. The most common design are BGO (Bismuth Germanium Oxide) block detectors (Fig. 1.1.5), combining individual BGO scintillation crystals in blocks attached to a number of photomultiplier tubes. The scintillation light generated by the interaction of the 511 keV photons with the crystal is distributed over several crystals or a certain area of a larger crystal. The resulting light distribution in the attached photomultipliers indicates the crystal were the photon entered the detector system or the place on the crystal were it was hit. One of the reasons for the use of BGO in

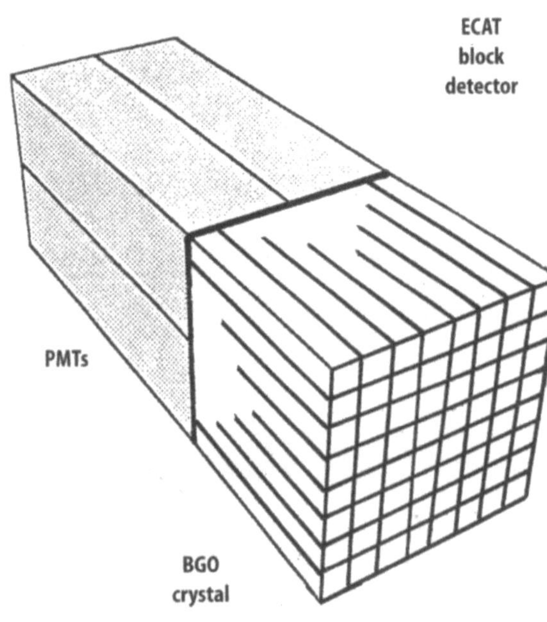

Fig. 1.1.5. Structure of block detectors

Table 1.1.2. Properties of the most important scintillators for PET

Parameter	NaI(Tl)	YSO	BGO	LSO
Density [g/cm^3]	3.67	4.54	7.13	7.4
Mean path length[a] [cm]	2.88	2.58	1.05	1.16
Hygroscopic?	Yes	No	No	No
Easy to handle?	No	Yes	Yes	Yes
Decay time [ns]	230	70	300	40
Light yield[a] [NaI(Tl)=100]	100	118	15	75
Energy resolution (%)[a]	7.8	< 7	10.1	< 10

[a] At 511 keV.

PET was it's high density leading to an almost complete absorption of all incident 511 keV photons (see table 1.1.2). Other detector materials nowadays used as NaI(Tl) (see chapter Haemisch) or under evaluation as LSO (Luthetium Orthosilikate). LSO, although more expensive, seems to be promising because it favourably combines the high stopping power of BGO with the high light output and energy resolution of NaI(Tl).

In PET scanners these blocks of detectors or the large area detectors are arranged in rings (Fig. 1.1.6) or partial rings around the patient allowing to measure the entire volume in between simultaneously. The axial field of view (AFOV) of currently available PET-scanners ranges between 15 and 25 cm. For the acquisition of larger parts of the body several of these AFOV's are measured consecutively and the data is put together into one whole-body image of the patient.

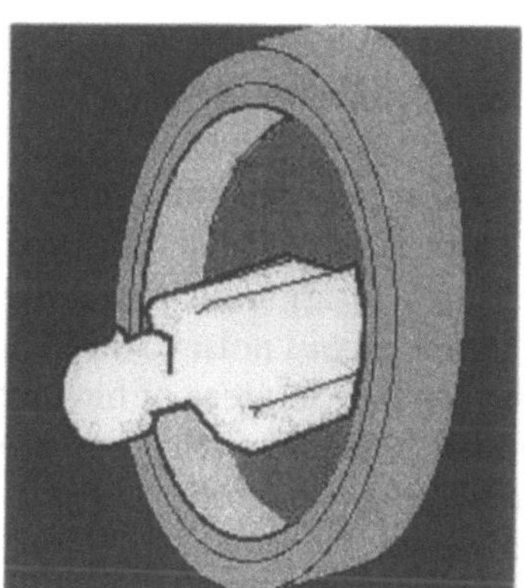

Fig. 1.1.6. Multiple detector rings permit simultaneous data acquisition for an entire body volume

1.1.6 Quantitative Imaging with PET

In order to obtain quantitative information using PET it is necessary to consider a number of parameters that will affect the accuracy of PET studies. Not only the individual detectors must be calibrated and matched, which is generally done by a normalization scan, several other factors need to be considered. These factors are listed below.

Random Coincidences

The coincidence logic of PET scanners is limited to detection of two photons within the coincidence time window. It is not possible to determine directly whether these two photons are the result of the same annihilation or whether two annihilations occurred randomly „at the same time." Therefore a certain fraction of the measured coincidences must be attributed to this type of random or accidental coincidences. These random coincidences add a homogenous noise to the image background which can be subtracted. If the countrate of each single detector and the exact coincidence timing window for each detector pair are known precisely it is principally possible to calculate the fraction of random coincidences. However, this is not practical due to the large number of parameters. There are basically two ways to correct the effect of random coincidences:

The first possibility is to use a second, delayed coincidence timing window which is afterwards corrected for real time. However, this approach has the disadvantage of adding statistical noise to the image as it is performed on an event by event basis. Therefore another method has been evaluated which estimates the amount of randoms together with the scatter from the activity which is falsely located outside the object (patient). However, this approach requires the exact knowledge of the contours of the measured object (patient) which can be provided by a transmission scan.

Dead Time Effects

Every detector system has a dead time that increases with the countrate. These effects can be corrected in PET within certain limits since true coincidences and random coincidences exhibit somewhat different dead time behavior (the count rate peak for random coincidence random line occurs at higher count rates than for true coincidences). If one also takes into account the individual count rate of the individual detectors, then dead time effects can even be corrected for high count rates.

Attenuation Correction

By measuring positron emitters in coincidence up to 80 % of the gamma radiation can be absorbed in the patient due to the longer attenuation path (both photons of an annihilation must escape). So it is obvious that not only for a quantitative determination of local activity concentrations it is essential to know accurately the effect of attenuation in the patient. Since the attenuation along a coincidence line in the patient does not depend on the depth location of the decay event the total absorption along this line can be measured using an external source of radiation. Then absorption can be taken into account during reconstruction by applying the determined correction factor along each coincidence line.

Currently most of the PET scanners are still using rod sources of ^{68}Ge, a positron emitter with a half life of 271 days, which are rotating around the patient, measuring the absorption coefficients in the object (patient) in coincidence. However, beside providing exactly the same energy of 511 keV as the emission from the patient this method suffers from its low statistics due to the coincidence mode and the limited amount of activity which can rotate within the detector ring without saturating the detectors. Furthermore the halflife of about 9 months requires an annual exchange of those sources and leads to an alternating quality of the transmission scan, depending on the age of the sources.

Therefore recent developments utilize a different nuclide, ^{137}Cs, which is a single photon emitter at 662 keV with a half life of 30 years. As ^{137}Cs emits only a single photon a collimated point source must be used in order to determine the attenuation lines through the object (patient). The use of the singles instead of the coincidence mode results in count statistics which are higher by factors of 20 compared to the coincidence mode. This leads to a drastical reduction of the acquisition time for the attenuation measurement. The long half life of the source provides a constant statistical quality of the scan and avoids replacement. A correction factor is applied in order to correct for the effects of the slightly higher energy of the transmission compared to the emission (further details see chapter "Haemisch").

Correction for Scattered Radiation

Scattering of gamma radiation occurs depending on the size and density of the measured object(s) and their relative location. Scattered coincidences add an inhomogeneous noise to a PET image, degrading the contrast in areas of high scatter (e.g. brain, bladder, liver). The effects of scattered radiation in PET can principally be reduced by two different means:

The first way is to inhibit scattered radiation to reach the detectors by using scatter shields (septa, Fig. 1.1.7) leading to the so called 2D acquisition

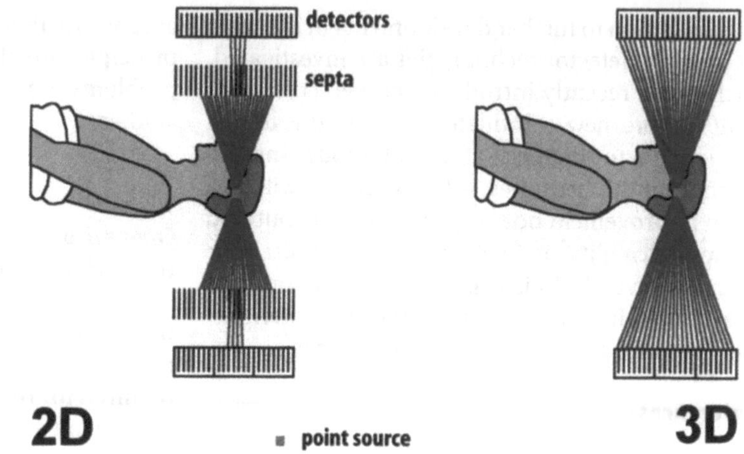

Fig. 1.1.7.
Comparison of 2D and 3D measurement

mode in PET. Since the introduction of those septa into the field of view reduces the overall sensitivity of a PET system by a factor of 4–5 one was looking for ways to avoid this. However, retracting the septa to operate in the so called 3D mode leads to a higher exposure of the detectors by scattered events. Since scattered events do have a lower energy than the unscattered ones it is possible to subtract them from the image by energy tresholding. This second approach requires a system which provides sufficient energy resolution to distinguish between scattered and non-scattered events. In addition to that mathematical correction models can be applied, determining the amount of scatter and randoms from the activity profile outside the object or from Monte-Carlo-Simulations for homogenous objects.

1.1.7
Further Development of PET Technology and Reconstruction Methods

Due to the advantage of providing higher sensitivity (and therefore shorter acquisition times) modern tomographs also offer the opportunity of 3D acquisition and reconstruction (fig. 1.1.7). Principally all possible coincidence lines between the detectors can be acquired in this mode. Due to the retracted or even omitted septa the tomograph sensitivity is increased by a factor of 4–5. However, since in this case not every slice can be reconstructed independently from the others as in 2D mode (many coincidence lines run across several slices) more sophisticated reconstruction methods are required.

Today iterative methods are more and more preferred versus the backprojection ones as they offer advantages in image quality especially in low contrast and low statistics situations as they occur in whole-body imaging. Furthermore they also improve the quality of attenuation corrected images significantly (see fig. 10 in chapter „Haemisch"). Due to the large number of coincidences acquired in 3D mode the data size of such an image can equal up to 140 MB. Therefore so called rebinning algorithms like Single Slice Rebinning (SSRB) or more recently Fourier Rebinning (FORE) are used before reconstructing the data in order to reduce the data size. After rebinning Maximum Likelihood Expectation Maximization (MLEM) or Ordered Subset Expectation Maximization (OSEM) methods are used to reconstruct the data. The rapid improvements in computer technology will enhance the feasibility of using real 3D reconstruction methods without prior rebinning of data in the near future.

The improved image quality provided by iterative reconstruction methods also helps to support the acceptance of PET as a recognized method of especially oncological diagnosis.

In addition to further developments in software alternative detector technologies are investigated, such as the recently introduced curved crystals of NaI(Tl), the new scintillator LSO or the use of semiconductor material and photodiodes instead of photomultiplier tubes. All these efforts will lead to an improvement not only of the quality but also the practicability of PET studies in clinical routine. However, in todays health care environment cost constraints are an important factor determining the introduction of new technologies.

References

Grangeat P, Amans J-L (eds) (1996) 3D image reconstruction in radiation and nuclear medicine. Kluwer, Amsterdam, pp 255–268

1.2 Dual Head Coincidence Camera

S. Ziegler

The clinical acceptance of PET, based on the imaging of fluorodeoxyglucose concentrations, has led to the development of cost-effective camera systems for positron detection. It was H. Anger (1963) who first proposed the idea of using two gamma cameras without collimators at 180° from one another for tomographic imaging of positron emitters based on electronic collimation of the annihilation photons. This principle, which was first applied primarily to focal plane tomography, was picked up again in the 1970s and 1980s (Krauss et al. 1970; Kenny 1971; Muehllehner 1975) and developed further (Paans et al. 1985). Although the systems exhibited better spatial resolution than high-energy collimators, their sensitivity and count rate performance was limited, which prevented widespread clinical application. The development of digital camera heads with fast electronics and also the improvements in electronic data processing have led to the introduction in recent years of the first commercially available, dual head coincidence cameras for clinical applications. These cameras can be used both for conventional SPECT and for positron emission tomography. In this overview we will summarize the principle involved, the specific measurement problems, and the initial results of comparative studies.

1.2.1 Comparison of the Dual Head Coincidence Camera with Other Techniques

In a coincidence camera, in contrast to dedicated ring positron tomographs, the coincidence lines required for reconstruction are not all acquired simultaneously but are imaged by rotating the heads around the patient. This type of acquisition is comparable to the type used in SPECT. However, the camera is operated without collimators, and all events detected in both detectors within a brief time window (15 ns) are assigned to one coincidence event. The exact location of the coincidence line is calculated by the coordinates of the gamma radiation detection site on the camera heads. For each angular position of the heads, therefore, coincidence events in different directions are recorded (Fig. 1.2.1), in contrast to a parallel-hole collimator, which only records the photons that appear at right angles to the camera head.

Thallium-activated sodium iodide [NaI(Tl)] is used as the scintillation material in conventional gamma cameras since this material has a very high light yield and therefore very good energy and spatial resolutions. The detectors in most ring tomographs consist of bismuth germanate (BGO) because this material has a higher sensitivity at high energies. Because a dual head coincidence camera is meant to be operated both in the coincidence mode and in the conventional SPECT mode, compromises must be made in the design since many requirements are contradictory. For example, a thin scintillation crystal (generally 0.95 cm) is required for SPECT so that the best possible spatial resolution can be achieved. Since the interaction probability for 140 keV photons in NaI(Tl) is very high, this requirement does not represent a limitation regarding detection efficiency. However, if high-energy annihilation photons are to be efficiently recorded, then thick-

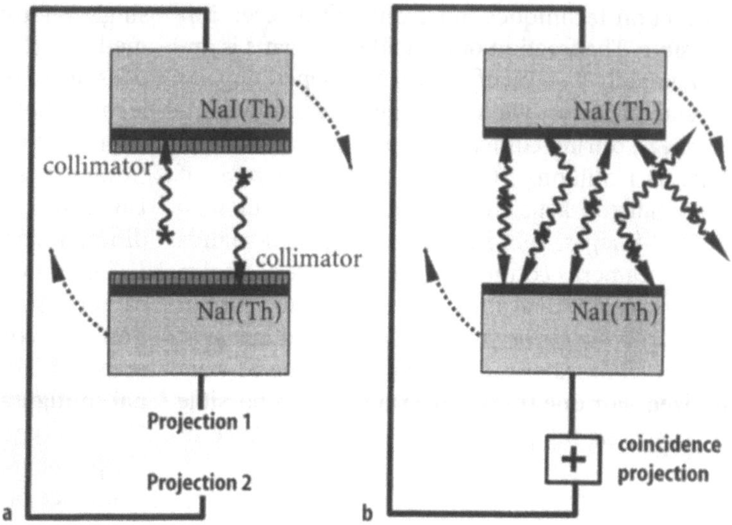

Fig. 1.2.1a,b.
Dual head coincidence camera. **a** SPECT. In single-photon tomography the incident direction of the photon is defined by the collimator. **b** Coincidence camera. In the coincidence mode without collimators the 180° emission of the annihilation photons is exploited

er crystals must be used. With a 6.4 mm thick NaI(Tl) crystal, only 7 % of the photons will deposit their entire energy (511 keV) in the crystal, and with double the crystal thickness the proportion will be 17 % (Anger and Davis 1964). Digital correction techniques are used in modern cameras so that in spite of increased crystal thickness there will be no resolution degradation in the detection of low-energy photons. In a 1.3 cm thick NaI(Tl) crystal the full energy of annihilation photons will be deposited (Events 1 and 2 in Fig. 1.2.2), but it also happens with almost the same frequency that not the total energy is deposited. The photon only participates in a scatter process and exits from the crystal (Event 3 in Fig. 1.2.2). Such events are in the low range (< 340 keV) of the cameras energy spectrum. In order to increase the number of recorded events it is thus perhaps advisable to measure not only in the photopeak window but also in a second window at lower energy. The precise location and width of the windows naturally also determines how many of the photons scattered in the patient (Event 4 in Fig. 1.2.2) are included in acquisition. Those photons have lost their original direction and contribute to an elevated background in the sectional image. A few selected events are sketched in Fig. 1.2.2 for illustration purposes.

The proportion of scattered to unscattered photons in the measuring windows depends on the type and extent of the scattering medium and is characteristic of the crystal material used. Although early studies indicated that the signal-to-noise ratio is more favorable with two appropriately selected energy windows (Thompson and Picard 1993), the issue has not yet been generally resolved for the commercial coincidence cameras currently available, particularly for images in the whole-body range. Absorber materials for low-energy photons can also reduce the fraction of scattered coincidences (Muehllehner et al. 1974).

1.2.2
Measurement Problems

Since large-area camera heads are involved, events are also detected that have their origin outside the actual field of view of the camera and increase the singles count rate in the heads (see Fig. 1.2.1). Similarly, the detectors are sensitive to photons that are scattered in the patient and reach the crystal. High singles count rates contribute to the background of random coincidences and, because of the open design, depend on the distribution outside the field of view, a fact that makes correction techniques more difficult or even impossible. The fraction of coincidence events is approximately 1–2 % of all events, depending on crystal thickness. The singles count rates in a camera head during coincidence operation can be as high as 1 million/s. Compared to count rates of less than 100 kcps, such as normally occur with SPECT images, this imposes stringent demands on the cameras count rate performance. To solve the problem of a system that is less sensitive but may nevertheless be subjected to high count rates, the possibilities of modern gamma cameras were utilized. For one thing, for example, it is possible to select the integration time for coincidence or single-photon detection using computer-assisted methods (Muehllehner et al. 1983), and it is also possible to obtain local spatial information by selecting photomultiplier subgroups and to increase count rate capacity by grouping the sampling electronics (Mankoff et al. 1990; Geagan et al. 1994). Different camera manufacturers are working on different solutions in this area.

The type of detection system in coincidence cameras permits three-dimensional data acquisition with continuous sampling. Stationary, large-area NaI(Tl) detectors are also used in a hexagonal configuration in a tomograph developed at the University of Pennsylvania (Muehllehner and Karp 1986; Karp et al. 1990). A strong position dependence of the sensitivity of the system in both the axial and transaxial directions within the field of view follows from the size of the acceptance angle that is allowed for coincidence measurement. The sensitivity profile has the shape of a pyramid or trapezoid (Fig. 1.2.3) (Clack et al. 1984). Reconstruction into transaxial slices is done either by using specific 3D algorithms or after rebinning the data (Defrise et al. 1994, 1997) using two-dimensional tomographic methods such as filtered

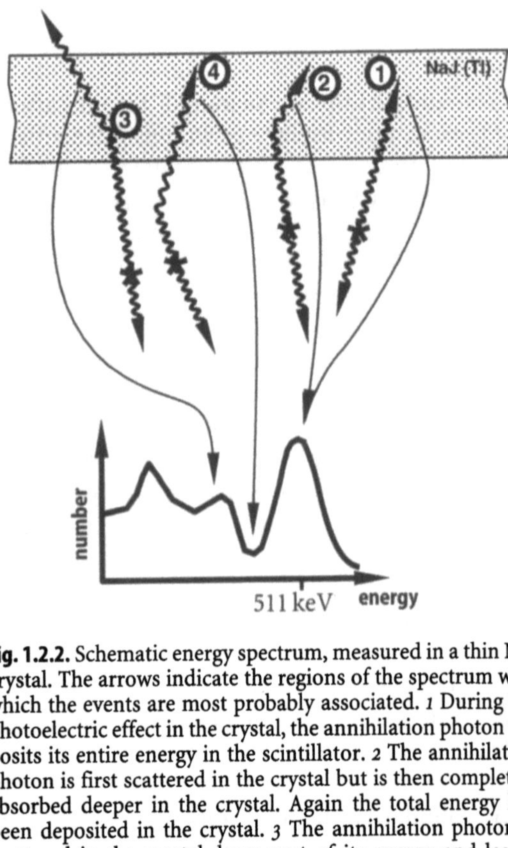

Fig. 1.2.2. Schematic energy spectrum, measured in a thin NaI crystal. The arrows indicate the regions of the spectrum with which the events are most probably associated. *1* During the photoelectric effect in the crystal, the annihilation photon deposits its entire energy in the scintillator. *2* The annihilation photon is first scattered in the crystal but is then completely absorbed deeper in the crystal. Again the total energy has been deposited in the crystal. *3* The annihilation photon is scattered in the crystal, loses part of its energy and leaves the crystal. The pulse height is in the low-energy "Compton continuum." *4* The annihilation photon is scattered outside the crystal – i.e., in the patient, loses a portion of its energy, changes its direction of travel, and is absorbed in the crystal. The pulse height is less than 511 keV

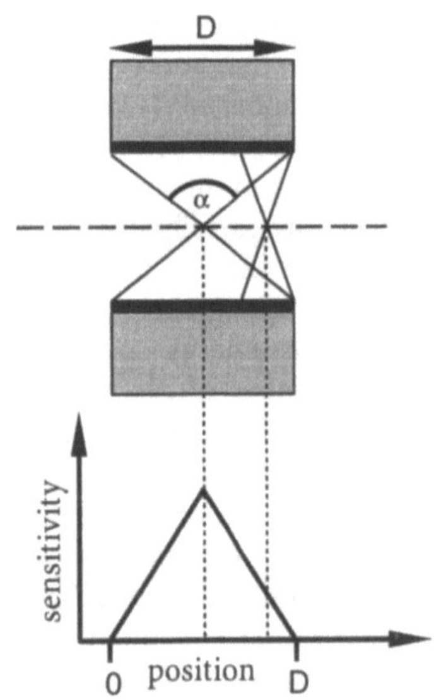

Fig. 1.2.3. In a 3D system the sensitivity is very much a function of the position within the field of view. The dependence is given by the acceptance angle *α* (*D* detector size)

Table 1.2.1. Characteristics of a ring tomograph (Siemens/CTI ECAT $EXACT_{47}$) and a coincidence camera (ADAC Vertex MCD)

	EXACT47 2D[a]	EXACT 47 3D[b]	MCD[c]
Axial field of view [cm]	16.2	16.2	38
Spatial resolution at the center:			
Transaxial FWHM [mm]	5.8	5.8	5.0
Axial FWHM [mm]	5.0	5.0	5.3
Sensitivity (s^{-1}/Bq/ml)[d]	5.8	40.5	3.2
Scatter fraction [%][d]	17	48	32

[a] With tungsten septa in the field of view, energy threshold: 250 keV (Wienhard et al. 1992).
[b] Without tungsten septa in the field of view, energy threshold: 250 keV (Wienhard et al. 1992).
[c] Acquisition in 2 energy windows (511 keV, 310 keV), each at 30 % width, detector separation: 62 cm.
[d] Measured for a cylinder (20 cm in diameter) homogeneously filled with ^{18}F.

backprojection or iterative methods (Hudson and Larkin 1994).

Table 1.2.1 compares the most important technical properties of a dual head coincidence camera (ADAC Laboratories, Vertex MCD) with those of a clinical ring tomograph (Siemens ECAT EXACT47). The most striking feature is the different sensitivities of the two systems. Different scatter fractions and contributions of random coincidences can significantly change the contrast performance, despite comparable spatial resolution in both systems. As an example, Fig. 1.2.4 shows slices of a phantom used to simulate the situation in tumor diagnostics. The phantom was filled with ^{18}F and water so that the radioactivity concentration in the spheres was three to six times as high as in the background. The absolute amount of ^{18}F and the time after filling the phantom at which the measurement was taken were selected so that the count rates in the two devices corresponded approximately to those of clinical studies. The minimum imaging time was 5 min for 2D images using the ring tomograph and 20 min for the coincidence camera. Data processing was performed in accordance with the clinical protocol either in 2D (ring tomograph) or after rebinning the 3D data (coincidence camera). At a concentration ratio of 3 : 1 the 13 mm diameter sphere was faintly visible in the PET image, whereas in the coincidence camera image the contrast was reduced, even with a longer imaging period. The smallest sphere (11 mm in diameter) was visible in the PET image at a ratio of 6 : 1, whereas it was not visible in the coincidence camera image even after a long imaging period. The external sphere was clearly delimited in the PET image,

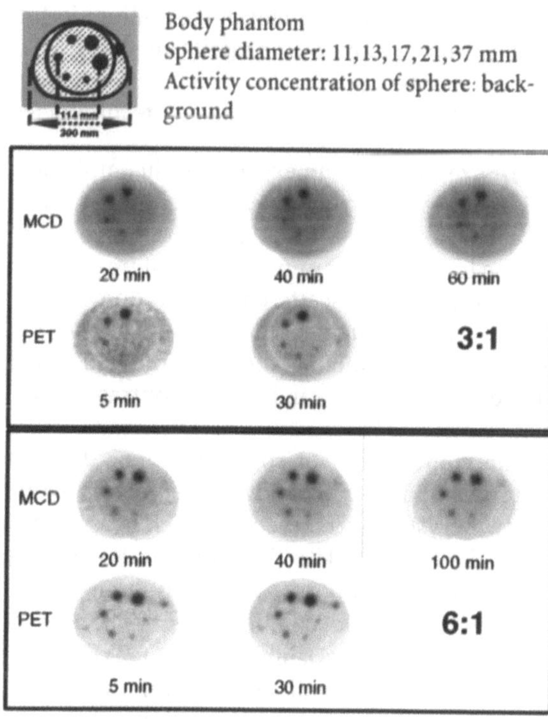

Fig. 1.2.4. Measurement using a whole-body phantom to simulate the conditions in tumor detection for two different ratios of activity concentration. The top rows in each section give data for the coincidence camera (MCD), and the bottom rows are examples of scans of the same phantom in a ring tomograph (PET). One single sphere (15 mm in diameter) was mounted externally at a larger radius

in contrast to the coincidence camera image. A probable reason for this is the decreasing resolution in the axial direction at the edge of the field of view caused by the rebinning algorithm.

Because of lower sensitivity and therefore longer scan time, the use of coincidence cameras is limited to the detection of ^{18}F-labeled substances. Initial clinical results show that the technique is promising for primary diagnosis of tumors in the lungs or in the head and neck region. Because of the fact that there is as yet no attenuation correction, studies of the myocardium are ruled out and images in the mediastinum and abdomen are only possible to a limited extent (Shreve et al. 1997).

Continued development will be especially visible in two areas:

- first, in the improvement of the sodium iodide coincidence camera, primarily in the area of data processing;
- second, in the use of new detector technologies.

For example, we can expect that the implementation of reconstruction and rebinning algorithms, as have been tested for 3D-PET, will contribute to the further improvement of image quality. Correcting for scattered and random coincidences or reducing those coincidences – possibly by optimizing the position and width of energy windows – can improve contrast performance.

The combination of completely new detector materials in a type of sandwich geometry involving two crystal layers, each of which is especially well suited for the detection either of low-energy or high-energy photons, could result in hybrid systems that would combine the advantages of different materials (Dahlbom et al. 1997).

Collection of transmission data for attenuation correction, which is normally performed in ring tomographs, is not possible in the coincidence mode because of the limited count rate capacity. On the other hand, the use of a ^{137}Cs source (energy: 662 keV) and acquisition in the single-photon transmission mode, which has been demonstrated using a scanner consisting of six NaI(Tl) crystals (Karp et al. 1995), is very promising.

Clinical indications for ring tomograph examinations cannot be applied to coincidence cameras until initial clinical studies have been completed. The current rapid development of coincidence cameras makes it necessary to continually evaluate clinical applicability.

References

Anger H (1963) Gamma-ray and positron scintillation camera. Nucleonics 21: 10–56

Anger H, Davis D (1964) Gamma-ray detection efficiency and image resolution in sodium iodide. Rev Sci Instr 35: 693–697

Clack R, zDW T, Jeavons A (1984) Increased sensitivity and field of view for a rotating positron camera. Phys Med Biol 29: 1421–1431

Dahlbom M, MacDonald L, Eriksson L, Paulus M, Andreaco M, Casey M, Moyers C (1997) Performance of a YSO/LSO detector block for use in a PET/SPECT system. IEEE Trans Nucl Sci 44: 1114–1119

Defrise M, Geissbuhler A, Townsend D (1994) A performance study of 3D reconstruction algorithms for positron emission tomography. Phys Med Biol 39: 305–320

Defrise M, Kinahan P, Townsend D, Michel C, Sibomana M, Newport D (1997) Exact and approximate rebinning algorithms for 3-D PET data. IEEE Trans Med Imag 16: 145–158

Geagan M, Chase B, Muehllehner G (1994) Correction of distortions in a discontinous image. Nucl Instr and Meth A353: 379–383

Hudson H, Larkin R (1994) Accelerated image reconstruction using ordered subsets of projection data. IEEE Trans Med Imag 13: 601–609

Karp J, Muehllehner G, Mankoff D et al. (1990) Continuous-slice PENN-PET: a positron tomograph with volume imaging capability. J Nucl Med 31: 617–627

Karp JS, Muehllehner G, Qu H, Yan X (1995) Singles transmission in volume-imaging PET with a 137 Cs source. Phys Med Biol 40: 929–944

Kenny P (1971) Spatial resolution and count rate capacity of a positron camera: some experimental and theoretical considerations. Int J appl Radiat Isotopes 22: 21–28

Krauss O, Lorenz W, Luig H, Ostertag H, Schmidlin P (1970) Imaging properties of the positron camera. Nucl Med 9: 103–119

Mankoff D, Muehllehner G, Miles G (1990) A local coincidence triggering system for PET tomographs composed of large-area positron-sensitive detectors. IEEE Trans Nucl Sci 37: 730–736

Muehllehner G (1975) Positron camera with extended counting rate capability. J Nucl Med 16: 653–657

Muehllehner G, Jaszczak R, Beck R (1974) The reduction of coincidence loss in radionuclide imaging cameras through the use of composite filters. Phys Med Biol 19: 504–510

Muehllehner G, Colsher J, Lewitt R (1983) A hexagonal bar positron camera: problems and solutions. IEEE Trans Nucl Sci 30: 652–660
Muehllehner G, Karp J (1986) A positron camera using position-sensitive detectors: PENN-PET. J Nucl Med 27: 90–98
Paans A, Vaalburg W, Woldring M (1985) A rotating double-headed positron camera. J Nucl Med 26: 1466–1471
Shreve P, Steventon R, Deters E, Gross M, Wahl R (1997) FDG imaging of neoplasms using dual head SPECT camera operated in coincidence mode. Eur J Nucl Med, p 860
Thompson C, Picard Y (1993) Two new strategies to increase the signal to noise ratio in positron volume imaging. IEEE Trans Nucl Sci 40: 956–961
Wienhard K, Eriksson L, Grootoonk S, Casey M, Pietrzyk U, Heiss W-D (1992) Performance evaluation of the positron scanner ECAT EXACT. J Comput Assist Tomogr 16: 804–813

1.3 Design Considerations of NaI(Tl) Based PET Imaging Systems Adressing the Clinical and Technical Requirements of Wholebody PET

Y. Hämisch

1.3.1 Introduction

One of the major inhibitors for the widespread use of Positron EmissionTomography (PET) in clinical environments has always been its higher costs compared to other nuclear medicine imaging procedures. These higher costs origin on one hand from the more expensive equipment and tracer, on the other hand also from the fact that there has often been required a separate infrastructure for PET investigations (rooms, staffing, equipment etc.) and that these procedures appeared to be more complicated and time consuming than other imaging techniques. Since the diagnostic value of PET investigations especially with FDG has been proven to provide significant improvements in diagnostic accuracy in many areas of clinical diagnosis and therapy control a growing interest in performing those investigations also in clinical environments arose. Industry is stimulating this increased awareness by providing lower cost PET imaging equipment such as rotating sector PET scanners with a reduced number of detectors (1) or dual headed gamma camera based PET systems (2). However, the challenge of introducing those lower cost systems is to maintain the diagnostic quality known from the established more expensive PET systems and/or to explore the appropriate fields of use of those systems by careful clinical evaluation.

The shifting focus of PET investigations towards more and more oncological applications results in a change of technical requirements associated with wholebody imaging which differ from the requirements known from neurological applications. Since wholebody or partial body investigations always require the acquisition of more than one field of view (FOV) measurement time becomes more important than it was with the single FOV in neurology. The human body is a much more inhomogenous structure than the human brain and together with the much wider variety of patients attenuation correction performed on the whole body becomes a challenge. This is not only essential for the quantitation of PET investigations, it also affects image quality and therefore the qualitative diagnosis. It will be shown how NaI-based PET systems can adress these technical requirements by delivering not only cost- but also technically efficient solutions for clinical environments.

1.3.2 Digital Detectors Improve Countrate Capability

The most significant limitation of NaI based systems for their application in positron imaging has been their limited countrate capability (3). Since the coincidence countrate is always only a fraction (0.5 – 2 % in patients) of the singles rate a tremendous enhancement in singles countrate is necessary to achieve significant improvements in coincidence performance.

Table 1.3.1 illustrates the relation between both countrates for a dueal headed system and gives an idea of the technical challenge.
The first publications on coincidence imaging by Anger (4) or Brownell (5) already indicated this

Table 1.3.1. Principal relation between coincidence countrate and detector singles countrate in a dual headed coincidence system

To achieve a coincidence rate of	Requires a singles rate (per detector) of
1 – 2 kcps	200 kcps
2 – 5 kcps	500 kcps
5 – 10 kcps	1 Mio. cps
10 – 20 kcps	2 Mio. cps

problem. The group around Muehllehner, Karp and Mankoff (6–11) has been especially working on solving these issues resulting in solutions such as flexible pulse shortening, local centroiding and multichannel triggering which have been published over the past years. They basically represent measures to limit the event detection both in time and space and therefore increase the counting capabilities of such a system. Figure 1.3.1 illustrates the principle of pulse shortening. Due to the higher light output of the 511 keV photons compared to 140 keV and due to the exponential decay of the scintillation pulse there is little information loss by shortening the integration time from about 1 μs down to 200 ns. The integration time can be made flexible depending on the arrival time

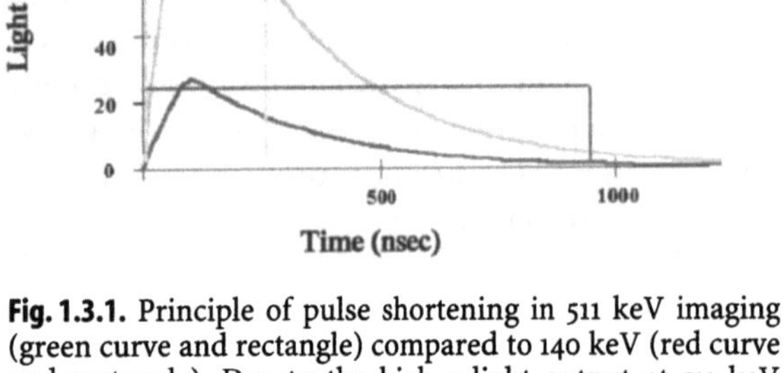

Fig. 1.3.1. Principle of pulse shortening in 511 keV imaging (green curve and rectangle) compared to 140 keV (red curve and rectangle). Due to the higher light output at 511 keV there is the same amount of light integrated in 200 ns at 511 keV as in about 1000 ns at 140 keV

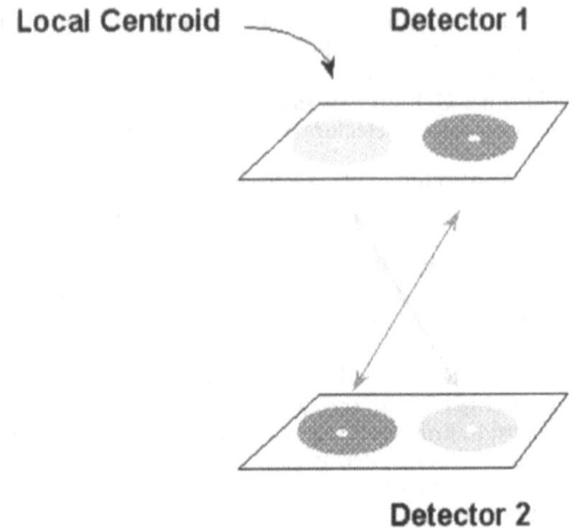

Fig. 1.3.2. The principle of local centroiding in NaI large area detectors. This enables the detectors to count more than one event per unit time

of the following pulse. Figure 1.3.2 illustrates the principle of local centroiding, an electronic division of the planar NaI detector into sections or centroids by using only a limited number of photomultiplier tubes (PMTs) for event localization around the one with the highest signal, enabling the detector to count more than one event per unit time.

These enhancements of counting capabilities of course require electronics which can handle multiple events at the same time. The design of multiple trigger channels is adressing this problem by providing parallel counting possibilities. In order to implement these measures the layout of the digital detector, principally shown in figure 1.3.3, has been developed. Each PMT is directly coupled to one A/D converter.

The principal difference in the detector design compared to the known Anger detectors leads to an improvement of singles countrate capability from about 200.000 up to a maximum of 2.5 million counts/s per detector, enabling true coincidence countrates of up to 15.000 cps for a dual headed system, one order of magnitude more than what can be achieved with conventional Anger type detectors. Later it will be shown that this significant improvement is not only essential for

Fig. 1.3.3.
Layout of the digital detector

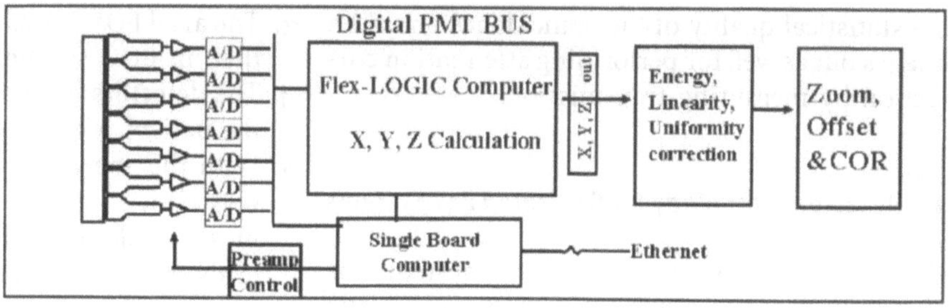

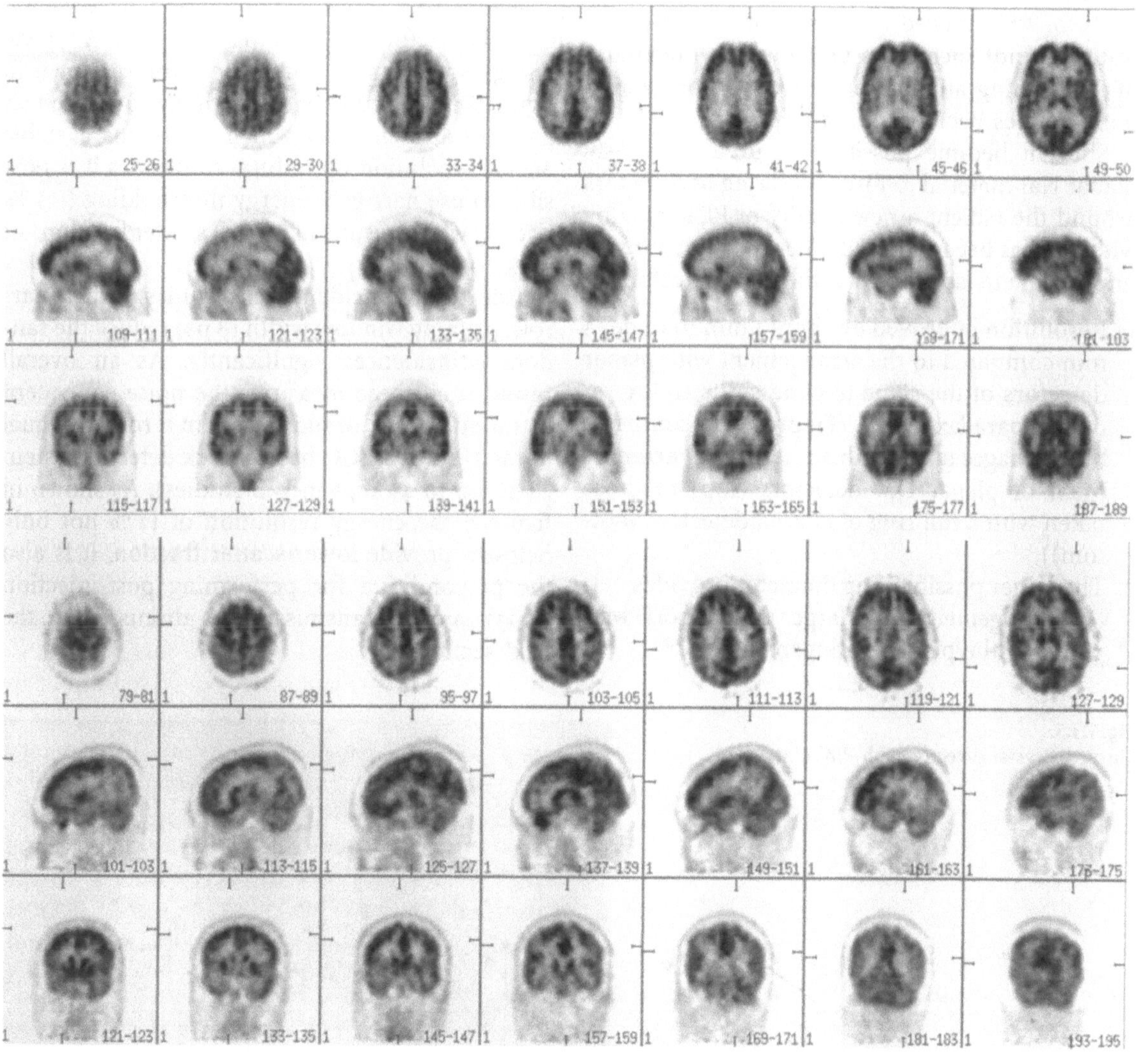

Fig. 1.3.4. Brain images of a normal volunteer taken with a hexagonal arrangement of planar NaI detectors (top three rows) compared to those taken with a full ring of curved detectors (bottom three rows). The improved resolution is remarkable especially by looking at the cortex and the nucleus caudatus

the statistical quality of the coincidence emission images but as well for performing attenuation correction by measuring transmission.

1.3.3
NaI Detector Technology for Dedicated Pet-Systems

Using NaI detectors in dedicated PET systems has some advantages since today users are especially looking at wholebody applications in oncology mainly with FDG which account for the vast majority of PET procedures. Extremely high countrates are not such an issue, however, the ability of performing attenuation correction on wholebody studies becomes more important.

Since it became possible to curve previously planar NaI material to form a full ring of detectors around the patient a new quality of PET imaging with NaI has been achieved. There are a number of improvements associated with those detectors:

1. Resolution improved by about 1 mm to under 5 mm compared to the arrangement with planar detectors of the same thickness due to the reduced parallax effect (Figure 1.3.4 compares brain images taken with an hexagonal arrangement of planar NaI detectors (top) to those taken with a full ring of curved detectors (bottom));
2. The larger possible ring diameter provides better homogeineity and a larger patient port compared to the planar arrangement;
3. The axial FOV is less limited by cost constraints than in BGO systems;
4. The detectors form a homogenous ring around the patient with very few insensitive areas;
5. With the energy resolution of NaI of 12 % (1" crystal) it is possible to operate those systems in 3D-mode also in wholebody studies. This leads to a significant improvement of the system sensitivity compared to 2D operation (factor 4–5);

Figure 1.3.5 shows a photograph of a curved crystal detector with the PMTs attached. A typical energy spectrum of such a detector is shown in figure 1.3.6. Together with an energy correction algorithm and circuitry which maintains a stable energy resolution up to high countrates it is possible to use narrower energy thresholding (-15 %, +30 %) which results in low 3D scatter fractions of $<$ 30 % (NEMA).

In addition coincidence electronics with a narrower timing window width (8 ns) reduce the random coincidences significantly. As an overall result of all these measures the noise equivalent count rate (NEC) of such a system is roughly equal to the NEC of a BGO based block detector system (NEC up to 43 kcps in WB studies). As shown in figure 6 the energy resolution of 12 % not only helps to provide lower scatter fraction, it is also the precondition for performing post-injection Cs-137 singles transmission as discussed in the next section.

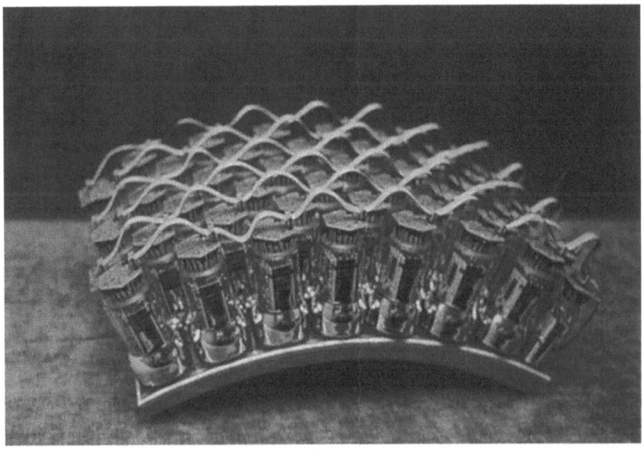

Fig. 1.3.5.
Curved Crystal detector with PMTs attached

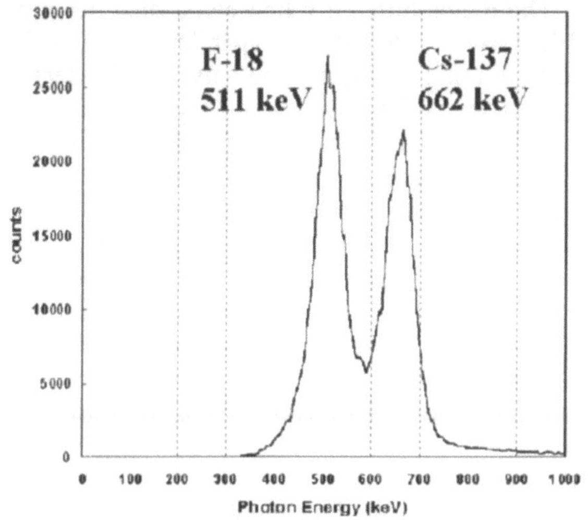

Fig. 1.3.6. Energy spectrum of curved crystal detectors showing separation of 511 keV peak from injected patient activity (*left*) and 662 keV peak from Cs-137 transmission source (*right*)

1.3.4 Post Injection CS-137 Singles Transmission Improves Clinical Image Quality, Quantitative Accuracy and Enables Flexible Clinical Operation

Due to the minimal crosstalk between the 511 keV signal of the positron emitters and the 662 keV signal of the Cs-137 transmission source(s) in NaI-detectors as shown in fig. 1.3.6 it is possible to perform both emission and transmission acquisition in an interleaved mode. Precondition for this approach is a high countrate capability of the detectors as there are external sources of radiation added to the already present emission from the patient. Figures 1.3.7a and b show the geometrical arrangement of the Cs-137 singles transmission sources for a dual headed PET-system in a 3 dimensional view (a) and a top view on one detector (b).

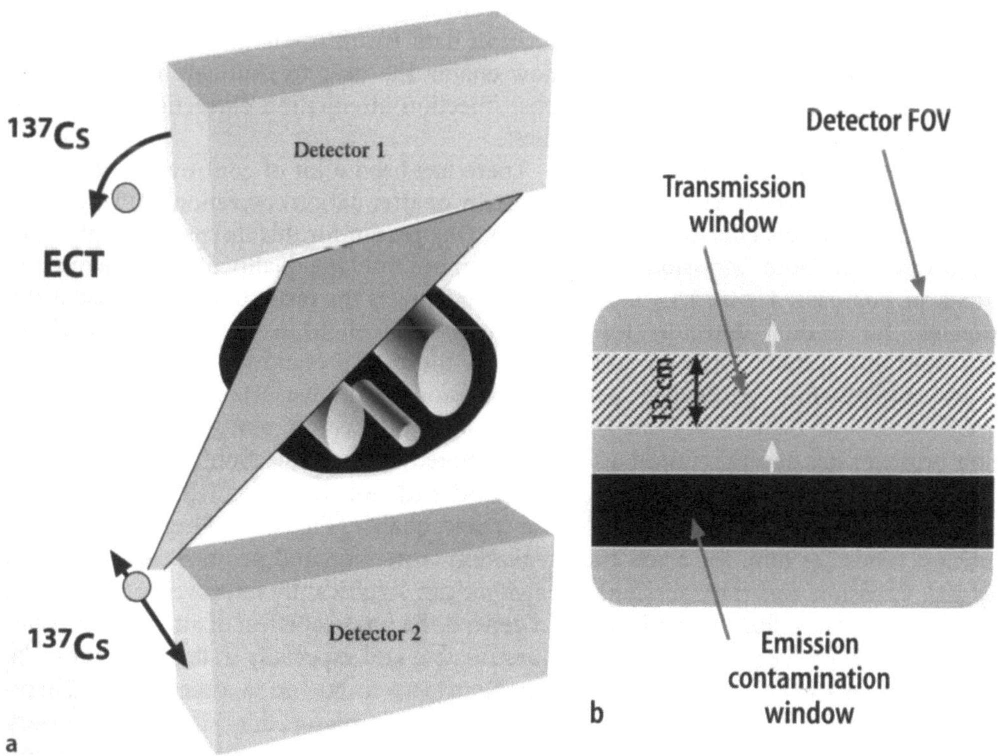

Fig. 1.3.7a,b Geometrical arrangement of the Cs-137 sources for attenuation correction on a dual detector PET system. **a** (*left*) shows the collimated sources translating along the detector sides. **b** (*right*) shows a top view on the detector surface illustrating the scanning windows for both transmission ▨ and emission contamination ■ measurements

There are two shielded and collimated transmission sources translating axially on one side of each detector. The collimated fan beam is directed to the opposing detector, scanning the volume between the detectors while the whole arrangement rotates 360 degrees. With the full 360° rotation and a lateral movement of the bed truncation is avoided. Fig. 1.3.6b shows a top view on the detector surface, illustrating the scanning windows for both transmission and emission contamination measurements. The emission contamination measurement provides a correction for the crosstalk of the 511 keV emission from the patient into the 662 keV peak of the Cs-137 transmission sources. The method is similarly performed on NaI-based dedicated PET systems as shown in fig. 1.3.8.

In the full ring system there is one Cs-137 source rotating within the stationary detector ring, which is automatically inserted for transmission scanning and housed in a shielded container in the gantry when not in use. In one turn of the source around the patient (approx. 1 min.) sufficient count statistics for a high quality transmission scan can be obtained. Due to the shape of the collimated fan beam there is no truncation. Cs-137 post injection singles transmission as described above enables NaI-based PET systems to perform interleaved acquisition of both emission and transmission data in one pass. Figure 1.3.9 illustrates the principle for a dual detector (top) and a full ring (bottom) system. Emission and transmission are subsequently performed per AFOV.

This acquisition protocol has several clinical advantages such as:

- short acquisition times (45 min. for a 100 cm whole body incl. emission and transmission)
- minimized motion artifacts due to the interleaved mode and the short acquisition time
- no repositioning of patients
- no repeated acquisition
- possibility of repeating single FOV
- ability to start reconstruction already after 1st FOV as all data is acquired

The major difference between a dual detector PET system with SPECT capability and a dedicated full ring PET system both using NaI detector technology will always remain the total acquisition time which will be about half for a dedicated system compared to a dual detector one. Current figures for a 100 cm axial scan are 45 min. for a dedicated full ring and about 90 min. for a dual detector system including emission and transmission acquisition. However, with the interleaved acquisition of both emission and transmission data and the use of the Cs-137 singles method now the relation between emission and transmission time reflects the fact that the majority of measurement time should be spent on acquiring the data whereas corrections should only need a minimal amount of time. This relation has been distorted for a long time with the conventional BGO PET systems using Ge-68 coincidence transmission. The new interleaved technique and the drastically reduced acquisition times for transmission data (from 10–15 min. down to 1 min.) now enable the user to routinely use measured post injection attenuation correction for all studies.

There has been a lot of controversy about the necessity of attenuation correction in PET studies (12,13). One reason for this discussion might have been that not only the quality of the transmission scan itself affects the result but there is also a significant impact of the reconstruction algorithm used. In the past it could have happened that a transmission scan performed in coincidence mode with low count statistics reconstructed with filtered back projection (FBP) worsened the good emission image and did not improve the image quality. Fig. 1.3.10 illustrates how attenuation correction **and** iterative reconstruction together can significantly improve image quality. In general the physical effect of attenuation is not questionable and especially in the body it can be significant (up to 80–90 % attenuation). Therefore the correction of this effect is necessary not only for performing quantitative or semi-quantitative studies but also for a qualitative improvement of the images. An example how the

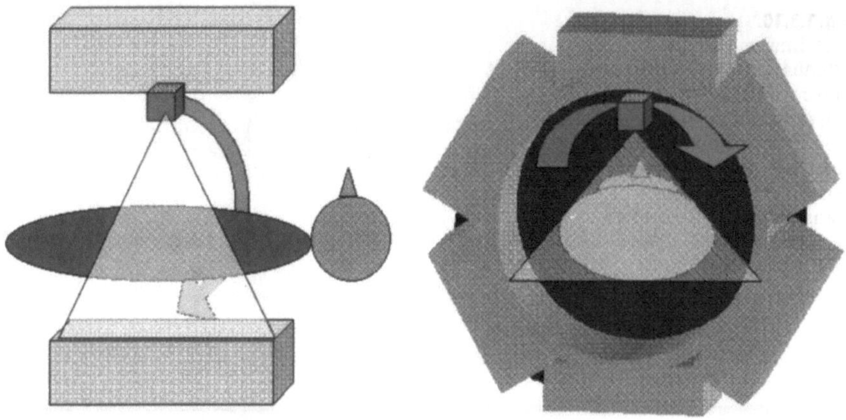

Fig. 1.3.8.
Geometrical arrangement of Cs-137 singles transmission in a NaI-based dedicated PET system, axial crossection (*left*) and transaxial crossection (*right*)

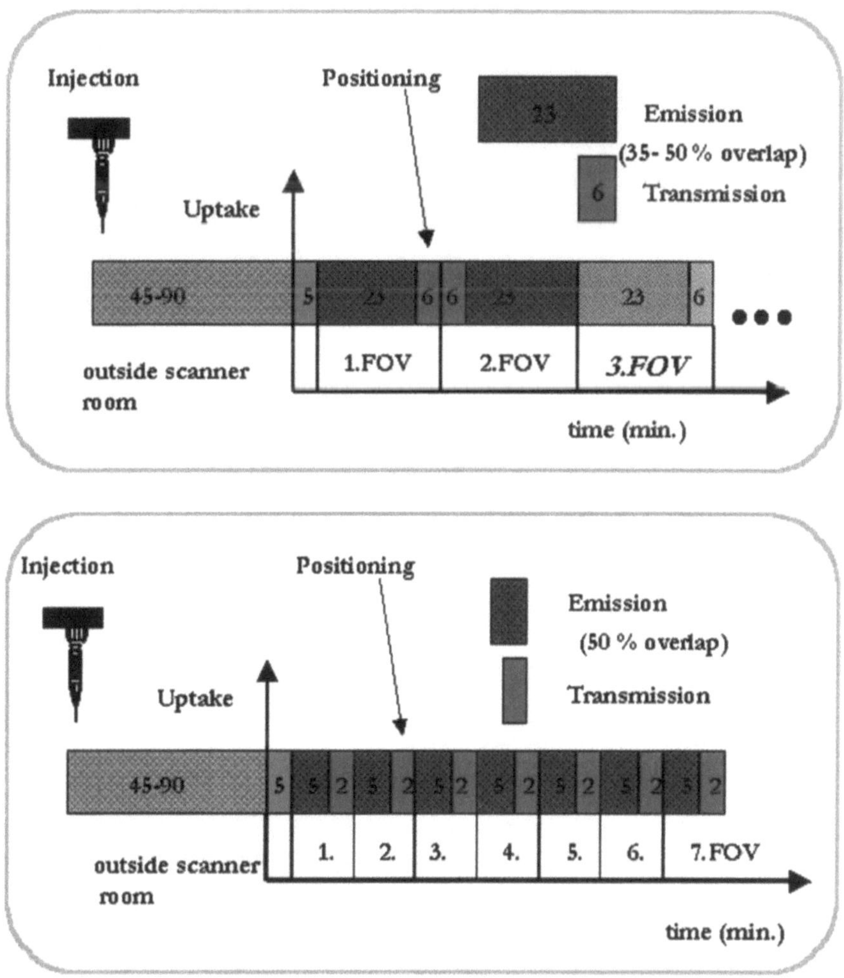

Fig. 1.3.9.
SinglePass™ acquisition protocols for dual headed PET systems (*top*) and dedicated full ring systems (*bottom*) based on NaI. Note that the axial overlap is necessary to correct for the 3D sensitivity profiles

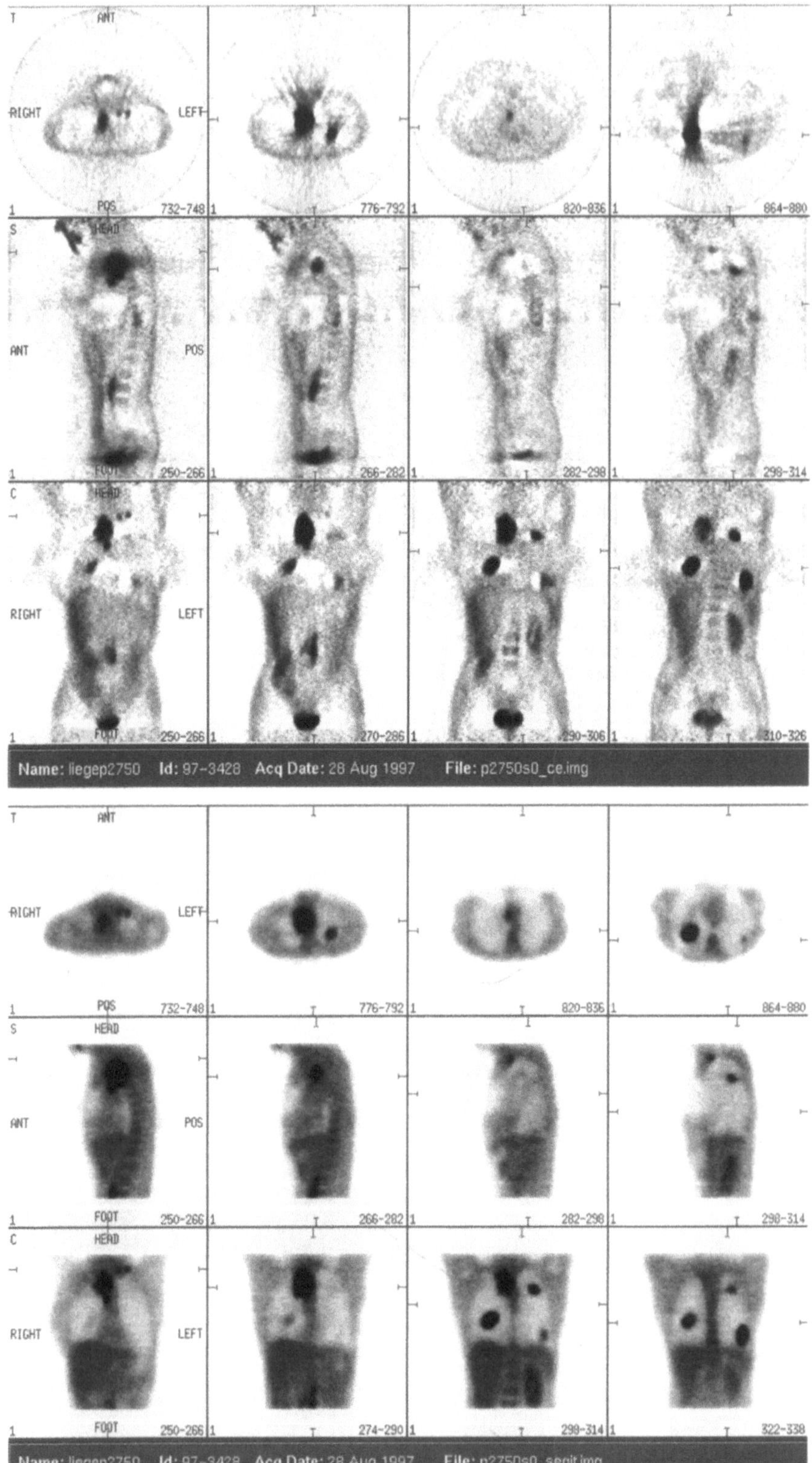

Fig. 1.3.10.
PET images without attenuation correction and reconstructed using filtered back projection (*top rows*) compared to the same data set using post injection singles transmission and iterative reconstruction (FORE/OSEM) (*bottom rows*)

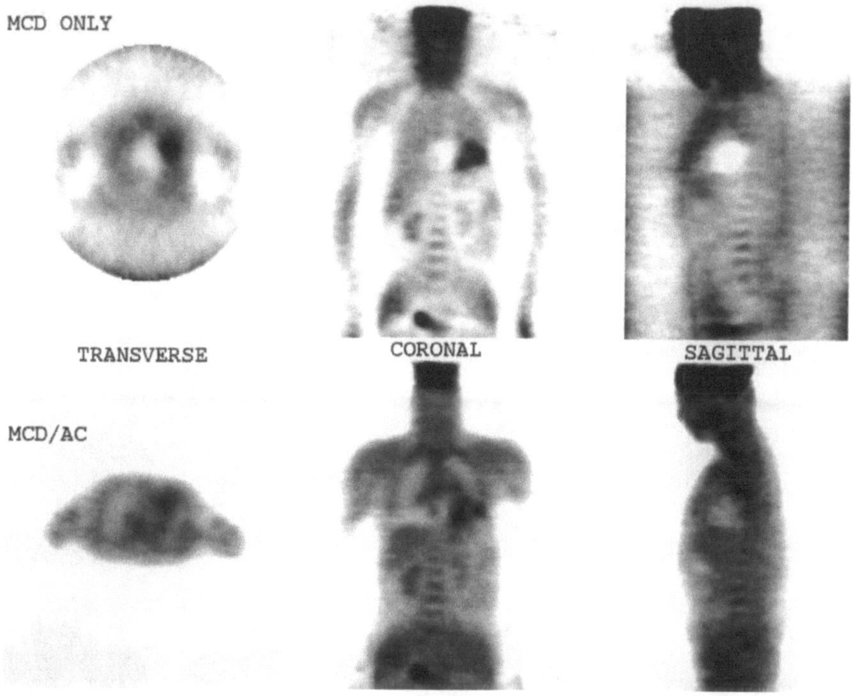

Fig. 1.3.11. Example of mediastinal lymph node involvement in lung cancer diagnosed with a dual detector PET system. The top row shows the uncorrected emission only images, bottom row the corresponding attenuation corrected ones. (images courtesy of Abdel Dajem M.D., St. Vincents hospital, N.Y.)

diagnosis of e.g. mediastinal lymph node involvement can be affected by the presence or absence of attenuation correction is shown in fig. 1.3.11. The top row displays the uncorrected transaxial, coronal and sagittal slices, the row below the corresponding attenuation corrected ones, taken with a dual detector PET system. There is a remarkable difference in the visibility of the mediastinal lymphnodes especially in the transaxial slice. Total acquisition time in this case was 90 minutes.

An example taken with a dedicated full ring NaI-based PET system is shown in fig. 1.3.12. The top row shows the uncorrected emission only images, the bottom row the transmission only images and the middle row shows the attenuation corrected images. There is a number of artifacts to be seen in the uncorrected ones, such as „hot" lungs, „cold" mediastinum, liver artifact, skin artifact and minimized uptake in the abdomen. All of these artifacts are eliminated by the attenuation correction (middle row).

Figure 1.3.13 and 1.3.14 show two more examples of attenuation corrected images from a dual detector system (fig. 1.3.12) and a dedicated full ring (fig. 1.3.13). Note the good visibility of anatomical details and the absence of artifacts caused by attenuation. The measurement time for both images was 90 minutes, but there were different scan lengths.

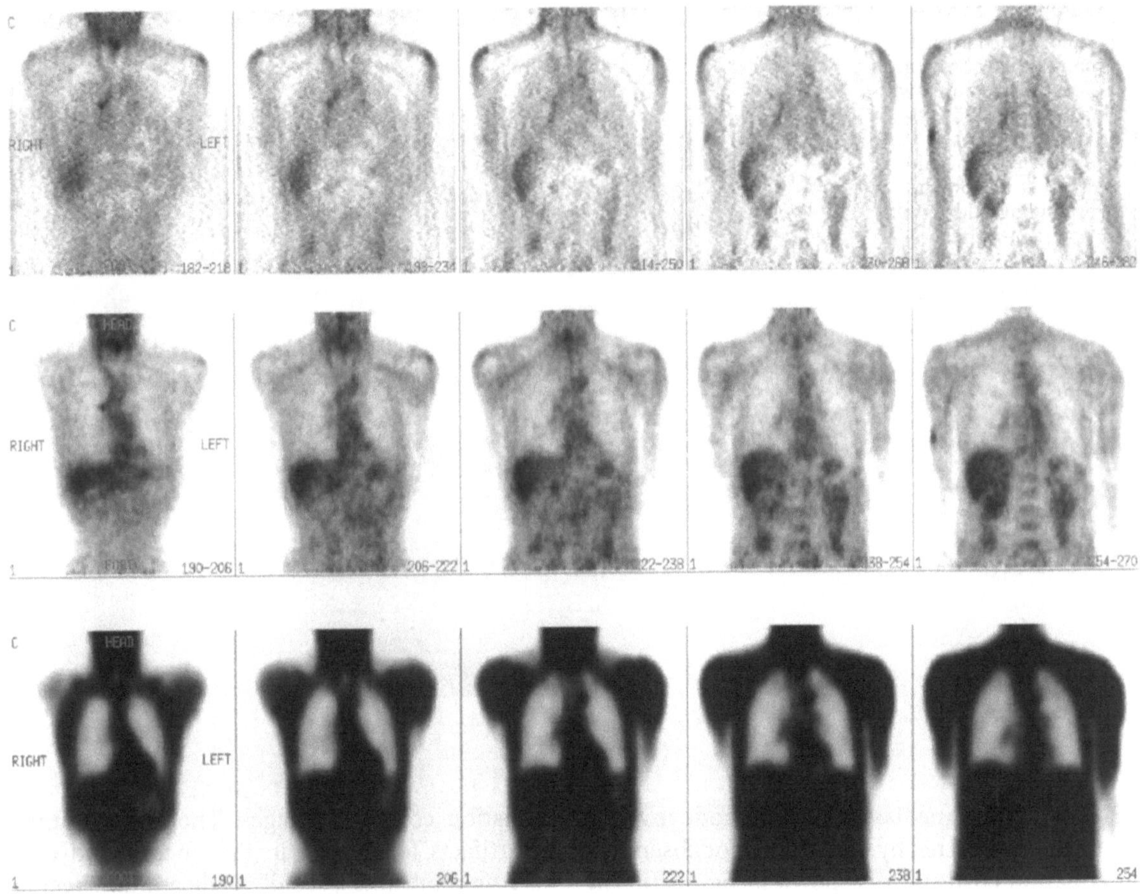

Fig. 1.3.12. Example of the effect of attenuation correction in imagestaken with a dedicated NaI full ring system: *Top row* uncorrected emission only images, *bottom row* attenuation only and *middle row* the attenuation corrected images

Summary

The above examples show that the use of NaI based detectors for positron imaging can deliver good results in todays clinical environment, provided the technical measures are taken as described above. Both the dual detector PET systems as well as the dedicated full ring systems deliver useful clinical imaging capabilities. Together with an adequate signal processing and threedimensional iterative reconstruction algorithms such as FORE/OSEM they will enable more and more clinics to use the advantages of PET and a growing number of patients to benefit from the high diagnostic value of PET investigations.

These systems now offer a choice to the user to select the PET imaging option which fits best his clinical needs and the projected patient volume. Both provide cost efficient solutions for the department as they minimize the costs of PET procedures by avoiding replacements of transmission sources, reducing tracer doses and increasing the productivity of nuclear medicine departments by shorter investigation times.

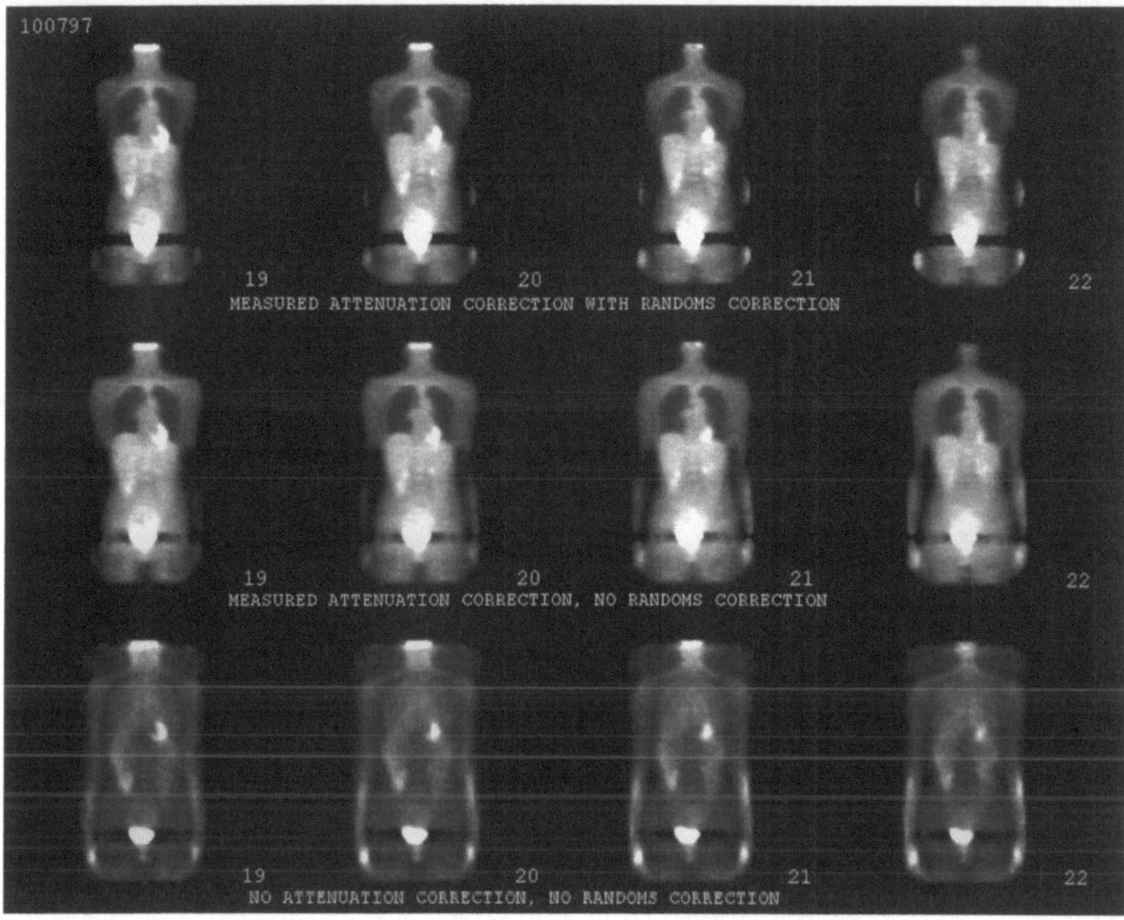

Fig. 1.3.13. Wholebody image of a normal volunteer taken with a dual detector system. Total acquisition time (emission+-transmission) was 90 minutes. (images courtesy of Abdel Dayem, St. Vincents hospital, N.Y.)

References

1. Bailey, D.L. et.al. ECAT-ART – a continuously rotating PET camera: performance characteristics, initial clinical studies and installation considerations in a nuclear medicine department. Eur. J. Nuc. med., Vol.14, No. 1, 1997
2. Nelleman, P.; Hines, H.; Braymer, W.; Muehllehner,G.; Geagan, M. Performance characteristics of a dual head SPECT scanner with PET capability. 1995 I.E.E.E. Nuclear Science Symposium and Medical Imaging Conference Record, October 21–28,1995, San Francisco
3. Phelps, M.E.; Cherry, S.R. The changing design of positron imaging systems. Clinical Positron Imaging Vol. 1, No. 1, 31–45, 1998
4. Anger, H. Gamma-ray and positron scintillation cameras. Nucleonics 21, 56–59, 1963
5. Brownell,G.; Burnham, C. A multi-crystal positron camera. I.E.E.E. Trans. Nucl. Sci. NS-19: 201–205, 1972
6. Muehllehner, G. Positron camera with extended counting rate capability, Jour. Nucl. Med. Vol. 16, No. 7, 653–657, 1975
7. Karp, J.S.; Muehllehner, G.; Beerbohm, D.; Mankoff, D.A. Event localization in a continous scintillation detector using digital processing I.E.E.E. Trans. NS-33, 550–555, 1986
8. Karp, J.S.; Mankoff, D.A.; Muehllehner, G. A position-sensitive detector for use in positron emission tomography. Nucl. Instr. Meth. A273, 891–897, 1988
9. Muehllehner, G.; Karp, J.S.; Mankoff, D.A.; Beerbohm, D.; Ordonez, C.E. Design and performance of a new positron tomograph. I.E.E.E. Trans. Vol. 35, No. 1,670–674, 1988

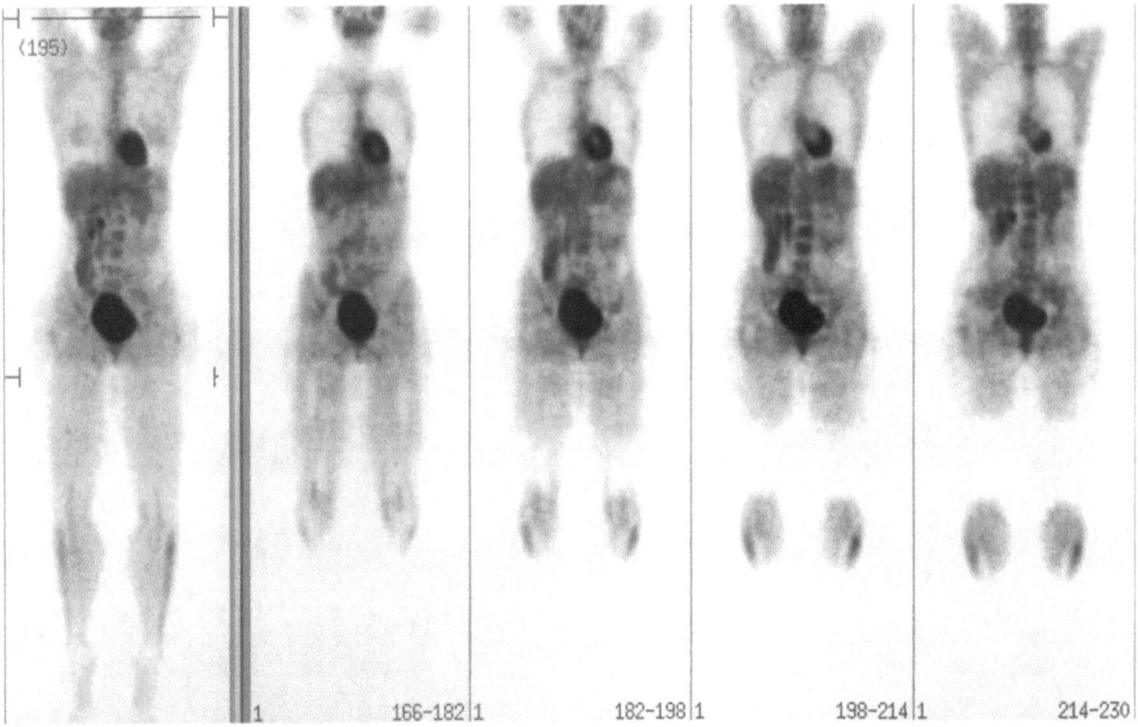

Fig. 1.3.14. Wholebody images from head to toes of a patient with negative diagnosis, taken with a dedicated NaI full ring system. Total acquisition time (emission+transmission) was 90 minutes. (images courtesy of Dr. Froehling, Karlsruhe, Germany)

10. Mankoff, D.A.; Muehllehner, G.; Karp, J.S. The high count rate performance of a two-dimensionally position-sensitive detector for positron emission tomography. Phys. Med. Biol., Vol. 34, No. 4, 437–456,
11. Mankoff, D.A.; Muehllehner, G.; Miles, G.E. A local coincidence triggering system for PET tomographs composed of large area position-sensitive detectors. I.E.E.E. Trans., Vol. 37, No. 2, 730–736, 1990
12. Bengel et. al. Europ. J. Nuc. Med. No. 24, 1091–1098, 1997
13. Imran et. al. J. Nuc. Med. No. 39, 1219–1223, 1998

1.4 Quality Control

B. Vollet

The term "quality" is defined as "the totality of features and characteristics of a product or a service that bear on its ability to satisfy stated or implied needs" [10]. Meaningful quality requirements are currently codified in various programs, standards and guidelines and are based on the goal of total quality management (TQM). Quality assurance in nuclear medicine is considered a significant requirement not only in the initiatives of the World Health Organization and the GMP, GLP and GCP regulations of the European Union but also by our national public health systems. Setting the trend in Germany, for example, are the stipulations given in Sec. 135 (2) SGB V, which is the part of the German social security code that regulates the statutory health insurance system, and the introduction of quality circles in guidelines issued by the Kassenärztliche Bundesvereinigung, the national association of health insurance system physicians [30].

In pronouncements of Germanys Federal Supreme Court regarding the implications of these quality assurance requirements, the primary concern is the safety of patient treatment [33]. Optimum patient care must also be considered in relation to economic efficiency. Rapid progress in medical technology and the acquisition of new scientific knowledge mean that differences in the quality of patient treatment will inevitably result. The implementation of standardized quality control procedures in routine clinical practice can be a powerful counterbalance to such trends. Additional personnel requirements and financial expense must be minimized, and the focus must be on practicability. The World Health Organization notes that it should be sufficient to check each nuclear medicine diagnostic system in its totality using only one or a few simple tests, since it is impossible to check a large number of individual parameters on a daily or weekly basis [29]. Every operator of a PET scanner or a gamma camera with integrated coincidence acquisition should therefore feel obligated to implement automated quality control procedures, in cooperation with the equipment manufacturer, so that the unit will be fully tested and functional when clinical work begins.

Under Sec. 42 (5) of Germanys radiation protection regulations, referred to as the "Strahlenschutzverordnung" (StrlSchV), a regular inhouse quality assurance system is required, including the obligation to keep records for 10 years. This is the basis for the specific requirements covering performance of acceptance tests and calibration checks for diagnostic instruments as specified in "Richtlinie Strahlenschutz in der Medizin" (RST-M), the German guideline for radiation protection in the medical field. With respect to nuclear medicine, only tests and calibration intervals for gamma cameras, in vivo and in vitro analyzer stations, and activity meters are covered specifically in the current version of RST-M [18]. In the formulation of test methods there are clear references to the DIN standards, which are basically recommendations [5–9, 11, 12].

There is now a DIN-IEC draft standard covering PET acceptance tests [11]. A standard for routine integrity or uniformity testing is in the development stage both in Germany (where it will be referred to as DIN 6855-4) and in Europe.

In addition, two committees of the Deutsche Gesellschaft für Nuklearmedizin (DGN) –" Clinical Quality Management" and "Science and Technology" – are also making an effort to assist equipment operators by developing recommendations [20-22, 24, 34]. Very detailed, practice-oriented quality control instructions are contained in the Procedure Guidelines of the Society of Nuclear Medicine, although the Procedure Guideline for Pet Imaging is not yet available [15, 26, 32]. The daily check procedures recommended and implemented by the manufacturers of PET systems should also be mentioned [23, 27, 28].

Diagnostic instruments for the acquisition of qualitative, semi-quantitative and quantitative PET data include not only the imaging system itself (emission and transmission) but also the invitro measuring device, the activity meter and the image documentation units. In order to check or test the condition of a diagnostic device it is of course first necessary to acquire reference data for benchmark purposes. For equipment used in nuclear medicine an acceptance test is carried out for this purpose by the operator and the equipment manufacturer during the commissioning process or when specific repairs are required. A detailed description of the acceptance tests is beyond the scope of this article. However, since integrity testing procedures are also based on the acquired reference data, some relevant terms will be discussed here in greater detail.

A basic requirement is that the acceptance test must have been performed in accordance with DIN standards.

According to DIN 6855-4, the standard that is currently being developed, quality control is defined as "integrity testing" and requires uniform system quality. The standard specifies inspection and testing procedures that are easy to carry out and also establishes sensible regular inspection intervals. The operator shall be required to integrate these into routine daily operations. It is also assumed that as long as no changes or deviations from the reference data are discove-red, proper operation of the PET system is guaranteed.

This assumption is based on two factors: first, many years of experience in the clinical application of systems of this type and second, the impossibility of carrying out quality control checks during a patient examination. However, it will never be possible to give an absolute guarantee of proper operation. For this reason the user should always review the patient data from a quality control perspective as well (artifacts, etc.) [14].

As already mentioned, appropriate rules and recommendations for PET quality control are currently being developed and written. However, in order to provide the user with a guide in the interim, we will present here the procedures recommended by specific manufacturers and also undertake to apply the provisions of RST-M (Section 6) and the DIN standards for gamma camera systems to PET systems, as appropriate.

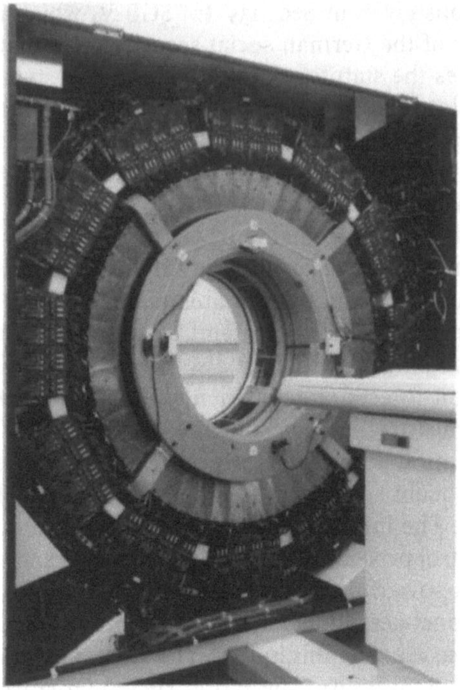

Fig. 1.4.1. When the scanner gantry is open (ECAT EXACT47, Siemens-CTI PET Systems) one can see the extreme packing density, which imposes stringent demands on temperature stabilization. Behind the first detector ring, visible in this photo, are two additional rings with similar electronic circuit boards

1.4.1 Integrity Testing for PET Scanners or Gamma Cameras with Integrated Coincidence Acquisition

The development, manufacture and final inspection of medical products is very stringently controlled by comprehensive quality assurance systems in compliance with DIN ISO 9001. The operator is therefore purchasing very high-quality, technically faultless equipment.

If this is the case, why is it then necessary to carry out routine quality checks?

In general, any process for the production of components is subject to a manufacturing tolerance that at some point in the course of the components service life may no longer be met due to wear, aging, etc. In a product as technically complex as the PET system (Fig. 1.4.1) it is important to take many different effects into account, including those listed specifically in Table 1.4.1.

The parameters described below must be determined in the standard operating mode, i.e., no changes in individual scanner settings are allowed.

Background Count Rate

Recommended interval: every work day.

The display integrated into the scanner gantry shows a total count rate [counts/s or cps] that is subject to natural statistical fluctuation. This measured value, which is a function of geographic lo-

Table 1.4.1. Unexpected events leading to changes of PET performance

Effects	Consequences or Changes
Aging of high voltage PMTs	Change in amplification performance
Cracks in the crystal-PMT bond	Decreased yield and poorer calibration factors
Temperature dependence	Change in detector efficiency [25]
Contact problems caused by corrosion and chemical reactions	Occasionally intermittent malfunctions
Drift in endurance properties (3–5 years)	Complete readjustment of the HV [16]
Abrasion of movable mechanical parts	Incorrect adjustment of the septa, bed control system and transmission sources
General thermal stress	Defects in electronic boards
Hardware updates/ upgrades	Components that are not modified are also affected
Software updates	Bugs are eliminated but other problems may be created

cation, spatial shielding and design features, provides information about any contamination that might have occurred and any general malfunction in the scanner electronics or cooling system. Supplementary information is provided by systems that continuously monitor room temperature (or water chiller temperature), humidity, and detector temperature.

Energy Window

Recommended interval: at the time of normalization or after specific repairs.

Instead of the differing peak energies of conventional radionuclides, a PET scanner discriminates events from the annihilation radiation (511 keV) of the positron reaction. This energy window is checked at the time of normalization or calibration and is permanently set digitally. This also applies to other energy windows, such as for scatter corrections (2D, 3D), if required. A daily check is therefore not necessary.

Uniformity

Recommended interval: every work day.

This check is of central importance since it is the most critical indicator of changes in system integrity [17, 25, 35].

Even manufacturers recommendations advise a daily check in the form of a blank scan (2D acquisition using transmission sources or 3D acquisition using a ^{68}Ge uniformity phantom) due to the complexity of PET scanners (Fig. 1.4.2). Generally this acquisition is done automatically before the start of the work day and should satisfy the requirements of statistical accuracy by measuring at least 20,000 counts per coincidence fan beam.

In order to determine uniformity, the efficiencies are compared with a blank scan (reference) acquired immediately after normalization.

The procedure involves the following steps:

- the differences between each detector block (or repair unit) and the mean of all blocks are calculated and deviations $> \pm 10$ %, for example, are recorded;
- the mean variance, based on a chi-square calculation, between the current blank scan and the reference blank scan is determined and deviations > 3 standard deviations, for example, are recorded as significant (Fig. 1.4.3).

However, these calculations do not make visual inspection of the blank scan sinograms (Fig. 1.4.4) superfluous, since a failure (malfunction) of individual coincidence lines is not conspicuous in the averaged statistical analysis.

Using this detailed information, the user can immediately determine if the system is ready for use and, if there are major deviations, perform a very simple fault locating procedure (simply by adjusting the energy discriminator for the specific detector module, for example, or adjusting the amplification, or even replacing a detector module). After specific repairs, however, normalization must be repeated, which is a very time-consuming procedure.

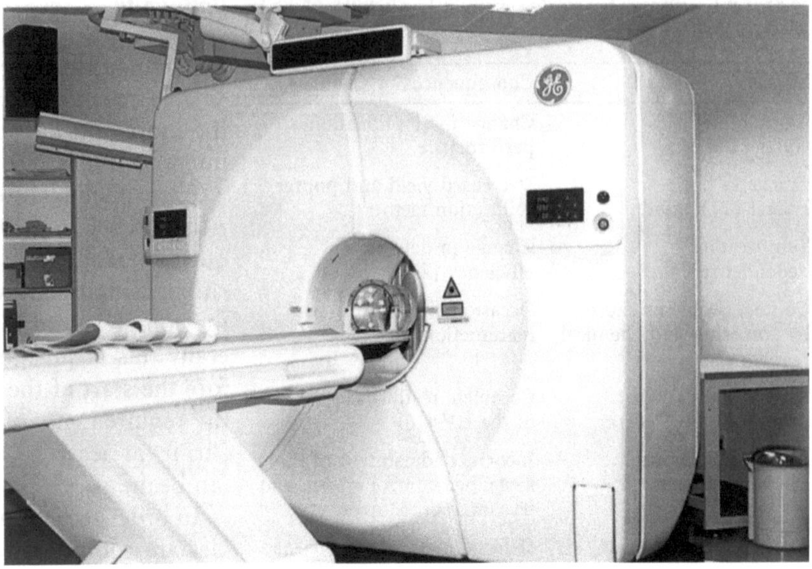

Fig. 1.4.2.
PET scanner (ADVANCE, GE Medical Systems Inc.) with a uniformity phantom, prepared for a uniformity check in the 3D mode

Yield

Recommended interval: after normalization or specific repairs.

A check of total yield or calibration factors [nCi/ml/cps/pix] should logically be a part of PET scanner quality control. Normally this measurement is performed using the uniformity phantom mentioned above with a known volume and activity concentration.

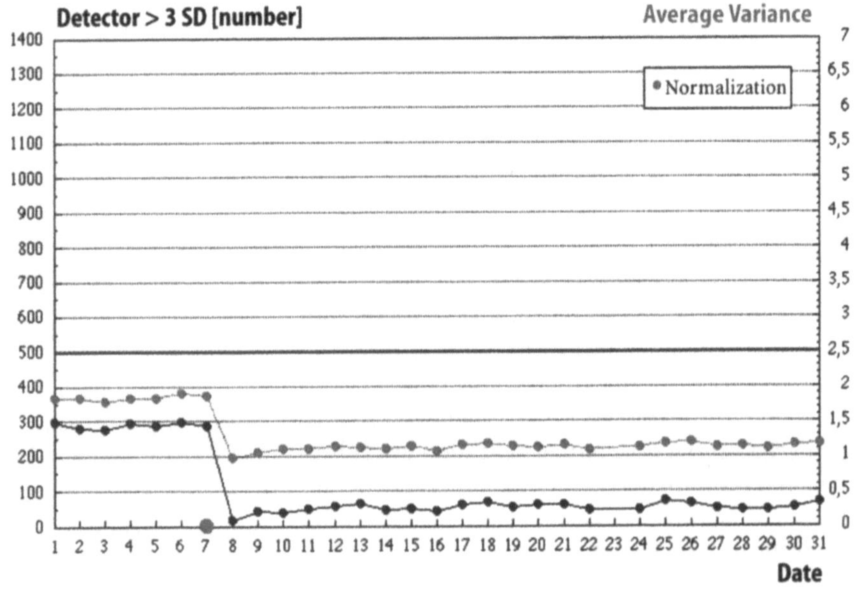

Fig. 1.4.3.
Daily check results over a period of 1 month. The two statistical parameters shown exhibit good uniformity. After re-normalization (green dot), uniformity is adjusted to an optimum value (reference value)

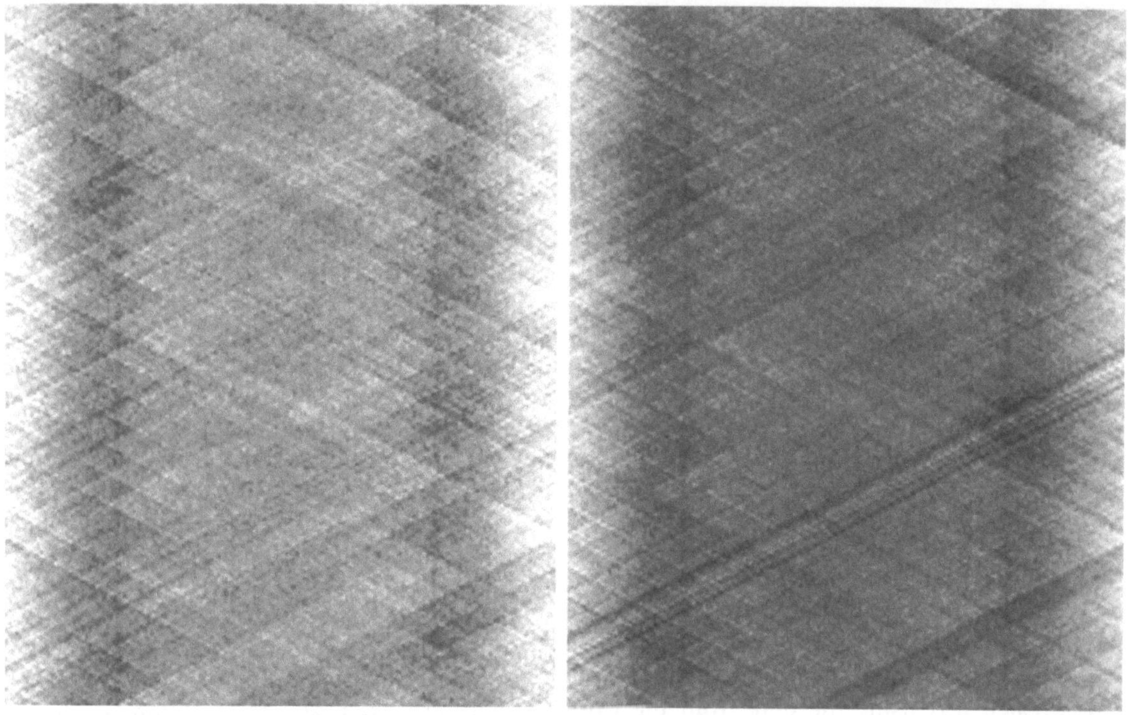

Fig. 1.4.4. Sinograms for a central slice (*left*) and a boundary slice (*right*) of a blank scan in the 2D mode. Although statistical analysis of uniformity does not reveal any peculiarities, the lack of individual coincidence lines can be detected visually

In the 2D procedure, one calibration factor per slice is calculated. Deviations from the reference value indicate decreases in detector efficiencies or faulty adjustments of the septa, etc. For statistical reasons a relatively long scan time is required, but the procedure can take place after working hours.

Imaging Scale

Recommended interval: at the time of normalization or after specific repairs.

The grid scale defined in DIN standards also applies to tomographic systems. Using these quality criteria, the user evaluates the ratio of the distance between two point sources or between two parallel line sources in the object to the "reconstructed" distance in the slice and also the matrix-dependent ratio [pixel/cm].

Both uniformity over time and spatial uniformity within the active scanned volume must be required. Suitable phantoms for checking spatial resolution and linearity are supplied by the equipment manufacturers.

System Uniformity (Correction Factors)

Recommended interval: at the time of normalization or after specific repairs.

RST-M specifies that quality assurance shall involve not only the integrity tests described above but also determination of correction factors. The goal is artifact-free quantifiable imaging of tomographic slices in the patient. This problem is discussed in detail and in exemplary fashion in the literature [14, 25].

For PET scanners a normalization is also carried out to counteract the effects already mentioned.

Recommended interval: every 1–2 months (as determined by empirical data).

The *normalization procedure* generally includes the following steps:

- Digital adjustment of amplification:
  As with coarse and fine tuning in modern SPECT systems, the same height of voltage amplitude should be achieved for all photomultipliers (PMTs) in order to generate identical energy signals "through all detectors." For this purpose the manufacturers provide an automated software routine that requires between 30 min and 2 h.
- Data acquisition using the uniformity phantom:
  This scan must be performed for the 2D and 3D modes with very high statistical accuracy and thus can require acquisition times > 6 h, but can be run automatically over night.
- Determination of the correction factors:
  In accordance with manufacturers specifications, additional data are acquired using transmission sources, and correction matrices are then calculated using the data from the two prior steps. These will be used to correct each future patient image before image reconstruction.
- Calculation of the calibration factors:
  As already described in connection with the yield parameter, one factor is calculated for each slice (differentiated for 2D and 3D modes) so that the patient image data can be represented in [Bq/ml] units.

Center of Rotation (Correction Factors)

Modern full-ring scanners are used in stationary operation (without wobble) and have a default detector orientation that is set at the factory. The same requirements that apply to SPECT cameras apply to all rotating coincidence scanning systems that have a variable radius.

Other important stability criteria are determination of the tomographic contrast [17], monitoring of the coincidence time window, and the correction technique for the "true coincidence rate." Sufficient information from manufacturers specifications regarding the last two parameters was not available for a quality control recommendation; this is presumably explained by the need to protect industrial property rights while patents are pending.

In addition, various research groups have demonstrated that quality assurance covering reconstruction techniques is becoming increasingly more important [1, 13].

1.4.2
Quality Assurance for Transmission Measurement

In a narrow sense, the transmission scan carried out for the purpose of absorption correction could be understood as a "study with enclosed radioactive substances." A clear definition would have to be included in future editions of the RST-M guideline.

The manufacturers of PET systems are also required to create quality control routines for their integrated sources. Naturally technical development in this area is also in a continuous process of change. Therefore consideration must be given both to existing transmission units involving measurement in the coincidence mode and to future systems based on much more efficient transmission options (Cs-137 sources, for example) involving measurement in the single-photon mode.

1.4.3
Integrity Testing for In Vitro Analyzers and Activity Meters

Evaluation of semi-quantitative patient data normally requires in vitro analysis (blood, urine, etc.) and measurements of injected activity. This additional information permits calculation of the standard uptake value (SUV) or similar parameters [19, 31].

Suitable measuring instruments must be equipped with adequate shielding of the measuring chamber and a sufficiently sensitive crystal (material thickness is critical), whether it be NaI(Tl) or BGO. In addition to the usual tests based on DIN 6855 Part 2, determination of the bore calibration factor should also be mentioned.

The manufacturer of uniformity phantoms also supplies a small tube (sized to fit the measuring instrument and filled with the same activity concentration) so that a simple calibration will be possible. A yield test should be performed daily.

1.4.4 Quality Assurance for Documentation of Findings

The training and clinical experience of the individual physician evaluating the findings are of critical importance for the selection of media (film, paper, monitor). Basically these types of systems must offer calibration capability in order to guarantee comparability with regard to linearity and contrast conditions for different media [2, 36]. The use of monochromatic displays (gray stages or colors) or false-color displays must be adapted to the particular biochemical and/or physiological conditions of the PET data. Quality assurance requires not only the basic image data but also specification of parameters for acquisition, reconstruction, reangulation, slice summation, etc. The standardization committee of the DGN will publish appropriate recommendations in the near future [3, 4, 22].

Conclusion

In conclusion we should note that quality control is a critical parameter for optimum nuclear medicine diagnostics. Standardization of quality control procedures should be supportive rather than restrictive for the user. Additional requirements for comparability of patient studies would also include binding protocols for acquisition and reconstruction, similar to those that have been stipulated for other imaging techniques (CT, MRI, etc.).

Regular continuing education and training of medical technologists and physicians and close ties to industry are indispensable for achieving a total quality management system.

References

1. Bailey D (1997) A comparison of reconstructions from the UK PET Centers. UK PET Special Interest Group (http://www-pet. umds. ac. uk/UKPET/) In: CTI PET Systems Inc; ECAT Technical Users Meeting, Dresden
2. Bildbeispiele zur standardisierten nuklearmedizinischen Bilddokumentation. Ergebnisse der Arbeitsgemeinschaft Standardisierung der Deutschen Gesellschaft für Nuklearmedizin. Nuklearmedizin 1997, 34, Technische Mitteilungen in Heft 7: 53–54
3. DIN 6848-1 Kennzeichnung von Darstellungen in der medizinischen Diagnostik. Beuth, Berlin 1992
4. DIN 6848-2 Kennzeichnung von Darstellungen in der medizinischen Diagnostik; Nuklearmedizinische Untersuchungen von Körperproben. Beuth, Berlin 1994
5 DIN 6855-1 Qualitätsprüfung nuklearmedizinischer Meßsysteme; In-vivo- und in vitro-Meßplätze. Beuth, Berlin 1992
6. DIN 6855-2 Qualitätsprüfung nuklearmedizinischer Meßsysteme; Meßbedingungen für die Einzelphotonen-Emissions-Tomographie mit Hilfe rotierender Meßköpfe einer Gamma-Kamera. Beuth, Berlin 1993
7. DIN 6855-11 Qualitätsprüfung nuklearmedizinischer Meßsysteme – Teil 11: Konstanzprüfung von Aktivimetern. Beuth, Berlin 1997
8. DIN 6878-1 Digitale Archivierung von Bildern in der medizinischen Radiologie – Teil 1: Allgemeine Anforderungen an die digitale Archivierung von Bildern. Beuth, Berlin 1998
9. DIN 55350-11 Begriffe zu Qualitätsmanagement und Statistik – Teil 11: Begriffe des Qualitätsmanagements. Beuth, Berlin 1995
10. DIN EN ISO 8402 und Beiblatt 1 Qualitätsmanagement – Begriffe. Beuth, Berlin 1995
11. DIN IEC 62 C/119/CDV (Norm-Entwurf) Merkmale und Prüfbedingungen für bildgebende Systeme in der Nuklearmedizin – Teil 1: Positronen-Emissions-Tomographie. Beuth, Berlin 1995
12. DIN IEC 62 C/120/CDV (Norm-Entwurf) Merkmale und Prüfbedingungen für bildgebende Systeme in der Nuklearmedizin – Teil 2: Einzelphotonen-Emissions-Tomographie. Beuth, Berlin 1996
13. Doll J, Zaers J, Trojan H, Bellemann ME, Adam LE, Haberkorn U, Brix G (1998) Optimierung der Bildqualität von PET-Aufnahmen durch 3D-Datenakquisition und iterative Bildrekonstruktion. Nuklearmedizin 37: 62–67
14. Forstrom LA, Dunn WL, O'Conner MK, Decklever TD, Hardyman TJ, Howarth DM (1996) Technical pitfalls in image acquisition, processing, and display. Semin Nucl Med 26: 278–294
15. Geworski L, Reiners C (1995) Qualitätskontrolle nuklearmedizinischer Meßsysteme. Schattauer, Stuttgart
16. Hoffmann J (1997) Extending detector life. In: CTI PET Systems Inc; ECAT Technical Users Meeting, Dresden 1997
17. Jordan K, Knoop B, Harke H (1994) Qualitätssicherung nuklearmedizinischer Meßsysteme: Was sagen die neuen Vorschriften? Nuklearmedizin 33: 49–60
18. Kemmer W, Johnke G (1992) Neufassung der Richtlinie Strahlenschutz in der Medizin, 2. Aufl. Hoffmann, Berlin

19. Keyes JW Jr (1995) SUV: Standard uptake or silly useless value? J Nucl Med 36: 1836–1839
20. Konsensus – Onko-PET. 2. Empfehlung des Arbeitsausschusses Positronen-Emissions-Tomographie der Deutschen Gesellschaft für Nuklearmedizin. Nuklearmedizin 1997, 34, DGN-Nachrichten in Heft 8: 45–46
21. Maßnahmen zur Qualitätssicherung der Meßgeräte und Radiopharmaka gemäß Richtlinie Strahlenschutz. Mitteilung des Arbeitsausschusses Leistungserfassung der Deutschen Gesellschaft für Nuklearmedizin. Nuklearmedizin 1993, 32: 273–274
22. Mester J, Bohuslavizki KH, Clausen M, Henze E (1997) Empfehlungen zur Standardisierung nuklearmedizinischer Bilddokumentationen. Nuklearmediziner 20: 197–199
23. Molecular coincidence detection quality assurance. Technical information from ADAC Laboratories GmbH, 1998
24. Müller-Schauenburg W, Bares R, Burchert W, Lietzenmayer R, Dohmen BM (1997) Prozeduren in der klinischen Nuklearmedizin – Wie ist eine Konvergenz der Methodenvielfalt über die nächsten Jahre erreichbar? Nuklearmediziner 20: 147–152
25. O'Conner MK (1996) Instrument- and computer-related problems and artifacts in nuclear medicine. Semin Nucl Med 26: 256–277
26. Parker JA, Yester MV, Daube-Witherspoon ME, Todd-Pokropek AE, Royal HJ (1996) Procedure guideline for general imaging: 1.0. J Nucl Med 37: 2087–2092
27. Performing the daily check pocedure for PET sanners. Technical information from CTI PET Systems Inc, 1998
28. Performing the daily check procedure for PET scanners. Technical information from GE Medical Systems Inc, 1998
29. Roedler HD (1993) Qualitätskontrolle nuklearmedizinischer Meßgeräte. Z Med Phys 3: 110–115
30. Ruprecht TM (1997) Gewährleistung und systematische Weiterentwicklung der Qualität im Gesundheitswesen. Entschließung der Länderkonferenz für das Gesundheitswesen am 21.11.1996 in Cottbus. QualiMed 5: 41–48
31. Sandell A, Ohlsson T, Erlandsson K, Strand SE (1998) An alternative method to normalize clinical FDG studies. J Nucl Med 39: 552–555
32. Schelbert HR, Hoh CK, Royal HD et al. (1997) Procedure guideline for tumor imaging using F-18 FDG. (http://www. snm. org/guide. html) SNM
33. Schneider A (1997) Qualitätsmanagement im Gesundheitswesen per Gesetz. QualiMed 5: 3–7
34. Schober O, Brandau W, Henze E et al. (1994) Nuklearmedizinische In-vivo-Untersuchungen. 2. Empfehlung des Arbeitsausschusses Klinische Qualitätskontrolle der Deutschen Gesellschaft für Nuklearmedizin. Schattauer, Stuttgart
35. Townsend DW (1996) Quality Control of PET Scanners. Eight Annual International PET Conference; Lake Buena Vista, Florida
36. Vollet B, Petrusch P, Sciuk J, Brandau W, Schober O (1994) Optimierung der Farb- und Grauwert-Dokumentation in der medizinischen Bildgebung mit digitaler Laser-Technologie. Zentralbl Radiol 150: 277

CHAPTER 2

Radiopharmaceutical Technology, Toxicity and Radiation Dosages

J. Ruhlmann and P. Oehr

2.1 Introduction

2-[^{18}F]fluoro-2-deoxy-D-glucose (2-[^{18}F]FDG) is the most frequently used PET radiopharmaceutical in Europe with more than 200 doses administered per week (Meyer et al. 1995). Studies described in the literature were performed with different 2-[^{18}F]FDG preparations, but the preparations do not differ significantly from one another. The differences are insignificant for the purpose of evaluating clinical data.

Over a thousand scientific reports on 2-[^{18}F]FDG were published throughout the world in the period from 1978 to 1998. Administered doses, scan parameters and evaluation protocols have generally been determined empirically and optimized based on pragmatic considerations. Initially 2-[^{18}F]FDG was used for diagnosing changes in the brain or the heart, but recently the focus of PET studies has shifted more and more to the area of oncology. This trend has not yet run its course and is also apparent in the case material of the PET Center in Bonn, Germany, for example (Fig. 2.1).

2-[^{18}F]FDG is a radioactive preparation. In Germany, radiation protection regulations (set forth in the *Strahlenschutzverordnung*) govern the use and storage of this substance, and the Guidelines for Radiation Protection in Medicine (*Richtlinien Strahlenschutz in der Medizin*) must also be followed. The specific dose rate constant for the 511 keV photons emitted by ^{18}F is 155 µSv $m^{-2}h^{-1}GBq^{-1}$. The half-value thickness in lead is 4.1 mm.

When using this pharmaceutical one must bear in mind that the half-life of 2-[^{18}F]FDG is 110 minutes. The administered volume is therefore based on the period of time between initial calibration and administration. It must be calculated using the appropriate decay correction factors and measured with a dose calibrator before injection.

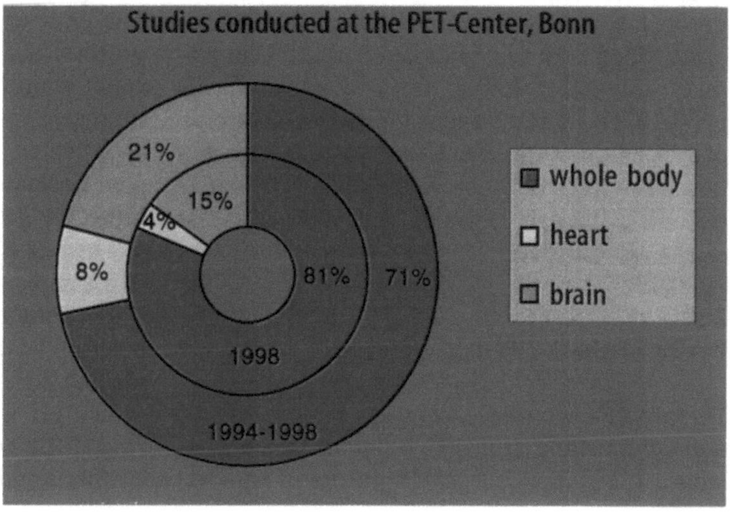

Fig. 2.1.
Changes in diagnostic focus at the PET Center in Bonn, Germany, from 1994 to 1998 (n = 3407)

2.2 The Synthesis of 2-[^{18}F]FDG

2-[^{18}F]FDG can be obtained commercially in Europe from several different centers. The production procedures differ somewhat from center to center, and only limited information is available about these procedures (Wienhard et al. 1989; Ido et al. 1977; Hamacher et al. 1986). It is therefore not possible in this report to describe all the production techniques. General guidelines are given in the literature (Meyer et al. 1993; Meyer et al. 1995; The United States Pharmacopoeia 1995; European Pharmacopoeia 1966). For this reason we will refer in general to the results of international studies, and we will describe in particular the product produced at Forschungszentrum Karlsruhe (FZK), a research center in Karlsruhe, Germany.

Biochemically, 2-[^{18}F]FDG is a non-physiological analogue of glucose. *In vivo* localization of the administered 2-[^{18}F]FDG is possible due to the emission of a positron by the ^{18}F radioisotope and the radiation resulting from the subsequent annihilation of the positron (yielding two photons of 511 keV each). ^{18}F-fluoride labeling is accomplished by nucleophilic substitution on 1,3,4,6-tetra-O-acetyl-2-trifluoromethanesulfonyl-mannopyranose in acetonitrile using a catalyst (Hamacher et al. 1986). The protective acetyl groups are split off by removal of the solvent and hydrolysis of the residue in 1N hydrochloric acid. The product is purified chromatographically in columns filled with ion-retardation resin. The primary solution resulting from synthesis has a pH between 4.5 and 6 and is ion-free. An addition of a specific amount of buffered NaCl solution followed by sterile filtration yields an approximately isotonic 2-[^{18}F]FDG solution with a pH of 7 that can be used for PET studies.

2.3 Purity of the 2-[^{18}F]FDG Solution

The product is a sterile, colorless to light-yellow, non-combustible radioactive liquid, which contains 2-[^{18}F]fluoro-2-deoxy-D-glucose in aqueous solution. The individual batch produced in the production process has a volume of 14.5 ml and a specific activity ranging between 1 and 10 GBq/µmol. The product is distributed to customers in volumes ranging from 0.05 to 10 ml.

Since 2-[^{18}F]FDG can be synthesized using different methods, there are different amounts of impurities in the products supplied by the various producers. For this reason the individual producers are also required to document the purity of their products. The 2-[^{18}F]FDG solutions that are distributed must fall within specific limits. A distinction is made between radiochemical, isomeric, radionuclidic, chemical and biological purity. General guidelines are given in the literature (Meyer et al. 1993; Meyer et al. 1995; The United States Pharmacopoeia 1995; European Pharmacopoeia 1966). The product produced by Forschungszentrum Karlsruhe (FZK) can be used as an example. Source: FZK No. SP04.01, effective Oct. 1, 1996. Radiochemical purity: $>$ 95 % of the measurable radioactivity can be attributed to 2-[^{18}F]fluoro-2-deoxy-D-glucose. Radionuclidic purity: $>$99.9 %. Impurities: Kryptofix 2.2.2 $<$100 µg/ml; acetonitrile $<$50 ppm; diethyl ether $<$500 ppm; ethanol: $<$300 ppm; bacterial endotoxins $<$17.5 EU/ml. Tonicity: 300–400 mosmol/kg.

The identity and radiochemical purity of 2-[^{18}F]FDG-FZK is determined by thin-layer chromatography (TLC) using a thin-layer scanner. The limit test for Kryptofix (from the synthesis process) is also performed using TLC and iodine vapor staining. Testing for bacterial endotoxins (pyrogens) is carried out using the Limulus test specified in *Deutsches Arzneibuch*, the German pharmacopoeia. Radionuclidic purity is determined by gamma spectroscopy.

The half-life is checked by measuring the decay of a sample.

The total molar concentration or osmolality is determined in a cryoscopic osmometer using the melting point depression method.

The pH is checked using universal indicator strips. The solvent concentration (solvent from synthesis and from equipment cleaning) is determined by gas chromatography. The activity concentration of a batch is determined during production after sterile filtration of the primary solution.

The sterility test cannot be performed before product release and shipment. The test is carried out by an outside testing laboratory using the direct feed method described in *Deutsches Arzneibuch*. Not only must routine production be sampled for sterility, it is also necessary to check the filling system using what is called a "dummy fill." Instead of the glass vials filled with bulk solution, 1 ml portions of an autoclaved buffer solution are prepared and checked for sterility.

Toxicity of the starting materials: a cryptand called Kryptofix 2.2.2 (1,10-diaza-7,7,13,16,21,24-hexaoxabicyclo[8.8.8]-hexacosan) is used as a phase-transfer catalyst to convert the ^{18}F-fluoride to a reactive form for labeling synthesis, and traces of water are removed. The LD_{50} for this cryptand in rats is 35 mg/kg (i. v.) (Baudot et al. 1977). Another reference reports that after rats had received a dose as high as 188 mg/kg they only exhibited elevated values for the liver enzymes GOT and GPT (Baumann et al. 1984). It is recommended that an upper limit of 0.22 mg/ml in a maximum of 10 ml be specified for 2-[^{18}F]FDG preparations (Meyer et al. 1995). At Forschungszentrum Karlsruhe (FZK) 26 mg of the catalyst is used to produce one batch of 2-[^{18}F]FDG, and then most of the catalyst is removed, together with the other byproducts of hydrolysis, by column chromatography. The residual concentration is specified as <100 µg/ml finished product.

Labeling is performed on a protected precursor, 1,3,4,6-tetra-O-acetyl-2-O-trifluoromethanesulfonyl-β-D-mannopyranose (TATM or triflate), in acetonitrile. Residues of the organic solvent can end up in the final product. Acetonitrile is classified as toxicologically critical (LD_{50} orally in rats: 3,800 mg/kg). The "European Pharmacopoeia" has established guidelines that specify a maximum limit of 50 ppm for acetonitrile in pharmaceutical substances for a maximum daily intake of 1.28 mg/day (Meyer et al. 1995). For drugs and pharmaceutical substances that are not administered on a long-term basis, the limit can be tripled. The allowable residual concentration of acetonitrile in 2-[^{18}F]FDG (FZK) is specified as <50 ppm, in accordance with this guideline. Toxic effects of the diagnostic agent due to the residual concentration of acetonitrile can therefore be ruled out.

Labeling is followed by an intermediate chromatographic purification process, in which the byproducts accumulated in the labeling process and any unreacted ^{18}F-fluoride are removed. Organic solvents are removed (by evaporation) from the pre-cleaned intermediate product, which is then hydrolyzed in aqueous hydrochloric acid to yield the final product, 2-[^{18}F]FDG. Complete hydrolysis of this substance, which is used for nucleophilic syntheses with ^{18}F-fluoride, yields D-glucose. Partial hydrolysis results in a mixture of partly acetylated glucose isomers, which are present as radiochemical impurities in a range of from 0.2 to 2 %. However, because only 20 mg of starting material is used for this synthesis process, these byproducts only occur in amounts in the ng to µg range. We can therefore assume that such amounts will not be toxicologically significant. 2-[^{18}F]FDG (FZK) is then purified by chromatographic elution and sterile filtration and dissolved in a buffered isotonic solution that is suitable for immediate use. Toxic doses of diethyl ether and ethanol are in the mg/kg to g/kg range. The residual concentrations of these substances in 2-[^{18}F]FDG (FZK) are <500 ppm for diethyl ether and <300 ppm for ethanol, i.e., well below the levels at which they could be considered toxicologically relevant.

2.4 2-[^{18}F]FDG Activity Dosages

2-[^{18}F]FDG is administered at the various PET centers in activity dosages ranging from 185 to 740 MBq, although the majority of centers use dosages of 185 to 370 MBq. The relationship between administered dose and cumulative concentration in the target organ and surrounding tissue (background), on the one hand, and the resulting image quality (e.g. detectability of small lesions), on the other hand, depends on the particular diagnostic system and must be determined from case to case.

Concentration Phase: Emission scans are normally begun 30–60 minutes after injection, as long as the tissue scan of 2-[^{18}F]FDG has reached an activity plateau and there is still sufficient activity for adequate count statistics.

Administered Activity: The activity administered to patients by i.v. injection normally ranges from to 185 to 370 MBq for all indications. Children receive smaller doses of 96 MBq or less. The time interval between 2 injections should be long enough to ensure that the radioactivity has decayed (physical decay) and the substance has been eliminated (biological clearance). No side effects are known that might be caused directly by one or more 2-[^{18}F]FDG injections. Emission scans should begin no sooner than 40 minutes after injection. It is also possible to wait even longer before initiating scanning. The filling volume is generally 10 ml with a fluctuation in total activity from 5.075 to 50.750 MBq, depending on synthesis technique, and a maximum specific activity of 1–100 GBq/μmol. The data given in Table 2.1 are used as the basis for determining the specific volume per administered dose.

Interactions with Other Substances: Any substance or therapeutic measure that reduces cell vitality will affect glucose metabolism indirectly. General examples are chemotherapy and external irradiation. It has been observed that a decrease in glucose utilization or 2-[^{18}F]FDG uptake during or after chemotherapy or irradiation is associated with tumor regression – whereas glucose utilization is unchanged or increases with tumor progression. This observation forms the basis for 2-[^{18}F]FDG therapy prognosis and can be used for therapy monitoring. However, chemotherapeutical agents can also result in a reduction in cellular 2-[^{18}F]FDG uptake (probably as a function of tumor vitality). Radiation therapy can cause either an increase or decrease in glucose uptake depending on the dose (Oehr 1998). Cortisone inhibits glucose utilization in lymphomas and can thus yield false-negative findings. It is therefore recommended that no cortisone be administered for a period of about 4 weeks before a 2-[^{18}F]FDG PET examination.

2.5 Radiation Exposure

^{18}F decays to ^{18}O by positron emission (97 %) and electron capture (3 %) and has a half life of 110 minutes. Positrons with an energy of 0.9 MeV are emitted primarily. The radiation detected in a PET camera is not direct positron radiation, however. Only after a positron has combined with a negatively charged electron and the

Table 2.1. Specific amounts of 2-[^{18}F]FDG per administered patient dose. Column 1 describes the case involving maximum specific activity at the lowest chemical concentration, and Column 2 shows the possible case of minimum specific activity and average chemical concentration. Column 3 shows the maximum dose of chemical concentration. Column 4 describes the case in which activity has decayed to the extent that 10 ml must be injected to reach a single dose of 370 MBq, which can result in the maximum possible chemical concentration of 652 μg per patient

	Maximum specific activity	Minimum specific activity	Activity limit	Maximum volume [10 ml]
Activity (MBq/batch in 14.5 ml)	50,750	5,075		360
Specific activity MBq (μmol)	10,000	1,000	1,000	100
Injected/patient (MBq)	180	360	450	360
μmol/patient	0.018	0.36	0.45	3.6
μg/patient (1 μmol FDG = 181.14 μg)	3.26	65.21	81.51	652.00
μg/kg patient (patient = 70 kg)	0.046	0.93	1.16	9.30

two particles are annihilated, bringing about a conversion of the combined mass to energy (2 times 511 keV), is there emission of 2 gamma quanta or photons of 511 keV each at an angle of virtually 180°.

The dosimetry for 2-[^{18}F]FDG has been estimated by various authors. The effective equivalent dose (whole-body) is 21 – 27 µSv/MBq (Meyer et al. 1995). For an activity dose of 370 MBq the total dose can be calculated as 7.8 – 10 mSv. Other publications give estimates ranging between 4 and 10 mSv. The range of natural radiation exposure in Germany is 1 – 6 mSv, and the mean value is 2.4 mSv.

The estimated radiation exposures in an adult (weighing 70 kg) after injection of 185 MBq or 370 MBq 2-[^{18}F]FDG are listed in Table 2.2. These estimates were calculated based on patient data and on 2-[^{18}F]FDG data supplied by the MIRD Commission. According to these data the bladder wall, with an equivalent dose of 120 – 170 µSv/MBq (80 – 100 mrem/mCi), must be considered as a critical organ (Dowd et al. 1991; Mejia et al. 1991; Meyer et al. 1995).

Table 2.2. Estimated radiation dose with intravenous administration of 2-[^{18}F]FDG in a patient weighing 70 kg

Organ	mGy / 185 MBq	rad / 5 mCi
Bladder wall	31.45	3.15
Bladder[a]	11.00	1.10
Bladder[b]	22.00	2.20
Heart	12.03	1.20
Brain	4.81	0.48
Kidneys	3.88	0.39
Uterus	3.70	0.37
Ovaries	2.78	0.28
Testes	2.78	0.28
Adrenal bodies	2.59	0.26
Small intestine	2.40	0.24
Gastric wall	2.22	0.22
Liver	2.22	0.22
Pancreas	2.22	0.22
Spleen	2.22	0.22
Breast	2.04	0.20
Lungs	2.04	0.20
Red bone marrow	2.04	0.20
Other tissues	2.04	0.20
Bone surface	1.85	0.18
Thyroid	1.79	0.18

[a] Bladder voided 1 h after administration.

There is no risk of non-stochastic radiation damage (such as the first clinically detectable effects of irradiation) even after multiple injections or a single accidental administration of the entire contents of a multiple-dose vial, considering that the threshold dose is 250 mSv after acute whole-body irradiation.

The risk of dying from a radiation-induced late malignancy (leukemia and carcinoma) is currently estimated to be approximately 5 – 6 to 10,000 for a radiation exposure of 10 mSv (1 rem). The mean latency period must also be considered, which for carcinomas is 20 – 25 years, for example. The life expectancy for patients with a malignancy is significantly limited, and diagnostic information is essential in choosing a treatment that might improve the quality of life and/or extend life expectancy. From this perspective radiation risk is negligible.

In patients with coronary heart disease who are known to have suffered a cardiac infarction or myocardial damage, life expectancy is also significantly limited. Here, too, diagnostic information is important for selecting a treatment that will improve quality of life or increase life expectancy. The radiation risk can therefore be considered minimal when compared with the potential benefit.

Neurological problems involve two different types of situations:

1. Pre-surgical epilepsy examination: These cases frequently involve examination of young to middle-aged patients who have a long life expectancy. Surgical implantation of electrodes and surgical removal of the epileptic focus are not without risk and are only justified if a significant

reduction in the frequency of epileptic seizures or a complete elimination of seizures can be expected. If we assume that 2-[^{18}F]FDG PET increases the probability of correctly identifying the epileptogenic focus, then the potentially increased cancer risk (normally only one 2-[^{18}F]FDG PET scan is performed) is justified by a higher quality of life and a reduction in the side-effects of long-term medication.

2. Dementia examination: Usually the patients that are examined are middle-aged to old and have a normal life expectancy. The possibility that their quality of life will be improved or maintained if suitable therapeutic measures are initiated justifies a potentially higher cancer risk.

The genetic risk after exposure to 10 mSv is estimated to be 1–2 to 100,000 for dominant mutations and 5–10 to 100,000 for recessive mutations.

2.6 Biochemical Toxicity

Several things occur when 2-[^{18}F]FDG is injected intravenously in humans (a 30 s bolus injection, for example). Non-metabolized 2-[^{18}F]FDG is eliminated by glomerular filtration without complete reabsorption into the urine. When the kidneys are functioning normally, approximately 16 % of the administered glucose is eliminated with the urine after 60 minutes, and 50 % is eliminated after 135 minutes (Gallagher et al. 1977, 1978; Woosley 1970). Cellular uptake of 2-[^{18}F]FDG is made possible by tissue-specific transport systems that are partially dependent on insulin. 2-[^{18}F]FDG reacts inside the cell with the enzyme hexokinase and is phosphorylated to form [^{18}F]FDG-6-phosphate (Gallagher et al. 1977, 1978). Because the administered concentration of 2-[^{18}F]FDG is very low (in the nmol range, see Table 2.1), it can be assumed that the normal metabolism of glucose is not affected since the glucose-plasma concentration is 1–4 mmol/l. Subsequent dephosphorylation by intracellular phosphatases is rather slow, and therefore the 2-[^{18}F]FDG-6-phosphate will be retained in the tissues for several hours.

In the animal experiments of Reivich et al. in 1979, multiple doses of FDG were administered intravenously to mice (3 injections of 14.3 mg/kg each) and to dogs (3 injections of 0.72 mg/kg each). No effects were detected either microscopically or macroscopically in the blood, urine or cerebrospinal fluid, or in tissues such as the brain, heart, spleen, liver, kidneys, lungs, ovaries or intestines. There were no signs of toxicity within a time span of 3 weeks. In humans (see Table 2.1) the administered dose of FDG is normally about 0.05–1 μg/kg and in extreme cases 9.3 μg/kg. The normal FDG dose is therefore 1000 times lower than the concentration that appeared to be harmless in animals. Similar results were reported by Som et al. in 1980. These researchers injected mice with a FDG concentration that was 1000 times the normal concentration. They were unable to detect either acute or chronic toxicity during a period of 3 weeks after injection. Even the maximum possible dose for humans (10 ml) is almost 100 times lower than this limit. Substance-related toxic side effects can be ruled out for these small doses and for this reason have not even been described in the literature.

The 2-[^{18}F]FDG dose that is administered for diagnostic purposes is therefore not expected to cause any pharmacological effects or substance-related side effects. No overdoses have been reported in the international literature to date.

2.7 Conclusions

2-[^{18}F]FDG, when administered systemically in the recommended diagnostic doses, is a substance with no apparent side effects. The estimated effective equivalent dose of approximately 10 mSv for an administered dose of 185–370 MBq is within the range of average radiation exposure when compared with other nuclear medical and radiological methods. Acute radiation damage is not expected, and the possibility of chronic radiation damage can be considered minimal.

References

Baudot P, Jaque M, Robin M (1977) Effect of a diazo-polyoxamacroobicyclic complexing agent on the urinary elimination of lead in lead-poisened rats. Toxicol Appl Pharmacol 41: 113–115

Baumann M, Schäfer E, Grein H (1984) Short term studies with the cryptating agent hexaoxa-diaza-bicyclo-hexacosane in rats. Arch Toxicol 55 [Suppl 7]: 427–429

Dowd MT, Chin-Tu C, Wendel MJ, Faulhaber PJ, Cooper MD (1991) Radiation dose to the bladder wall from 2-(^{18}F) fluoro-2-desoxy-D-glucose in adult humans. J Nucl Med 32: 707–712

European Pharmacopoeia (1996) Radiopharmaceutical preparations, pp 1424–1433

Gallagher BM, Ansari A, Atkins H et al. (1977) Radiopharmaceuticals XXVII. 18F-labeled 2-desoxy-2-fluoro-D-glucose as a radiopharmaceutical for measuring regional myocardial glucose metabolism in vivo: tissue distribution and imaging studies in animals. J Nucl Med 18: 990–996

Gallagher BM, Fowler JS, Gutterson NI, MacGregor RR, Wan CN, Wolf AP (1978). Metabolic trapping as a principle of radiopharmaceutical design: some factors responsible for the biodistribution of 2-Deoxy-2-[^{18}F]fluoro-D-glucose. J Nucl Med 19: 1154–1161

Hamacher K, Coenen HH, Stöcklin G (1986) Efficient stereospecific synthesis of no-carrier-added 2-[^{18}F] fluoro-2-deoxy-D-glucose using aminopolyether supported nucleophilic substitution. J Nucl Med 27: 235–238

Mejia AA, Nakamura T, Mastoshi I, Hatazawa J, Masaki M, Shoichi W (1991) Estimation of absorbed doses in humans due to intravenous administration of fluorine-^{18}F-fluorodeoxyglucose in PET studies. J Nucl Med 32: 699–706

Meyer G-J, Coenen HH, Waters SL et al. (1993) Quality assurance and quality control of short-lived radiopharmaceutikals for PET. In: Stöcklin and Pike (eds) Radiopharmaceuticals for PET. Kluwer, Amsterdam, pp 91–150

Meyer GJ, Waters SL, Coenen H H., Luxen A, Maziere B, Langström B (1995) PET radiopharmaceuticals in Europe: current use and data relevant for the formulation of summaries of product characteristics (SPCs). Eur J Nucl Med 22/12: 1420–1432

Oehr P, Ruhlmann J, Rink H (1989) 18F-FDG Transport: Abhängigkeit von Glucosekonzentration und Strahlendosis. Nuklearmedizin 37: A68

Reivich M, Kuhl D, Wolf A et al. (1979). The [^{18}F] fluorodeoxyglucose method for the measurement of local cerebral glucose utilization in man. Circ Res 44: 127–137

Som P, Atkins HL, Bandoypadhyay D, Fowler JS et al. (1980) A fluorinated glucose analog, 2-fluoro-2-deoxy-D-glucose (F-18): nontoxic tracer for rapid tumor detection. J Nucl Med 21: 670–675

United States Pharmacopeia, USP (1995) Fludeoxyglucose F18 Injections. USP 23: 674

Woosley RL, Kim YS, Huang KC (1970) Renal tubular transport of 2-deoxy-D-glucose in dogs and rats. J Pharmacol Exp Ther 173: 13–20

CHAPTER 3

Metabolism and Transport of Glucose and FDG

P. Oehr

The kinetics of the radiopharmaceutical 2-[^{18}F]fluoro-2-deoxy-D-glucose (2-[^{18}F]FDG), a glucose derivative, are determined by its distribution in the blood stream and tissues and by its metabolism.

In principle, only the distribution of the radionuclide ^{18}F is measured, although 2-[^{18}F]FDG is the pharmaceutical that is originally administered. Metabolic processes in the body can convert 2-[^{18}F]FDG into a different chemical form that has a different biological behavior. In order to develop a biokinetic model it is therefore necessary to know the possible chemical reactions that this radiopharmaceutical can undergo – including reactions under pathological conditions. The physiological determinants that are significant for tracer kinetics will be described in the following sections, and the possibilities for measuring those factors will be discussed.

3.1 Biological Functions of Carbohydrate Metabolism

3.1.1 Carbohydrate Requirements & Supply

The adult human organism has a minimum glucose requirement of 180 g per day. This amount of glucose is necessary in order to supply energy to those cells and organs that absolutely depend on glucose, namely the nervous system (144 g glucose per 24 h) and the red blood cells (36 g glucose per 24 h). The daily supply should even exceed 180 g of glucose-providing carbohydrates so that the other organs that have a minimum glucose requirement can also be supplied.

After all carbohydrate building blocks have been reabsorbed from the intestine, the glycogen supply (and later glucogenesis) is needed to provide glucose.

The monosaccharides glucose, fructose and galactose are the essential building blocks of our carbohydrate diet. With respect to glucose, the carbohydrate diet should not be formed by the direct supply of monosaccharides but by the supply and splitting of polysaccharides. In addition to the hexoses mentioned above, the pentoses (xylose, ribose, arabinose and xylitol) are of secondary importance quantitatively since they are present in food only in very small quantities. In diabetics the sugar substitutes fructose, sorbitol and xylitol can be of critical importance since they are utilized independently of insulin and are therefore used in the diet. The most important monosaccharide in the blood is glucose. The glucose pool in humans is approximately 0.11 mol and is distributed throughout a volume of about 28 liters. This corresponds to an average postprandial concentration of 5 mmol glucose per liter (90 mg/dl). Glucose is absorbed into the cells from the glucose pool by facilitated diffusion with the assistance of specific carrier types (Glut 1–5).

3.1.2 Regulation Mechanisms

Glucose is broken down by the metabolic pathway called glycolysis (Fig. 3.1). This degradative pathway is present in all organs and cell systems. The breakdown of fructose, mannose, sorbitol and xylitol also involves glycolysis. Glycolysis can be fol-

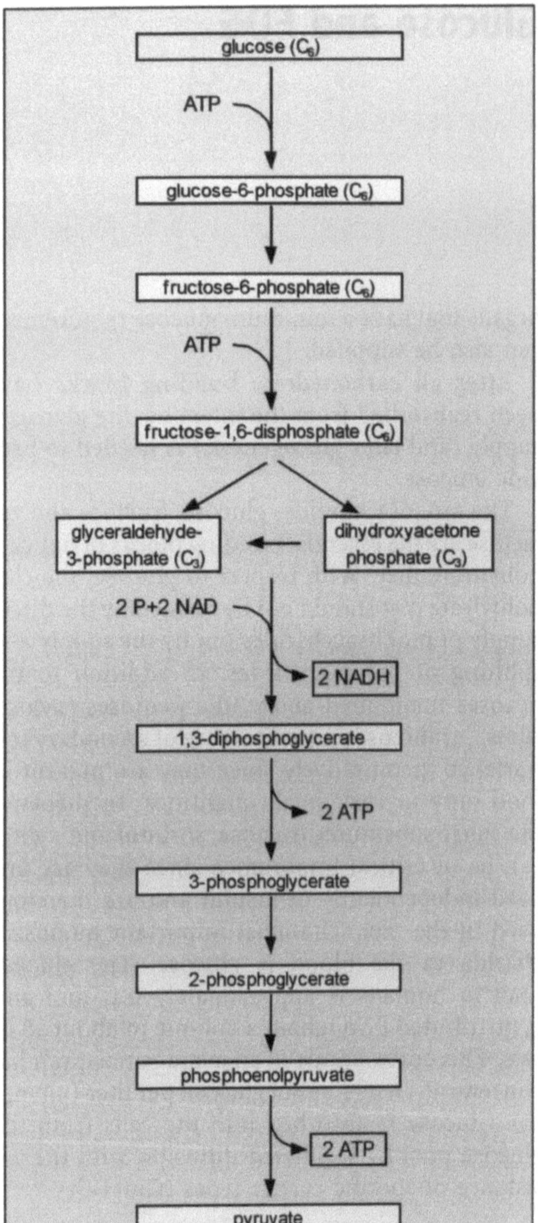

Fig. 3.1. Metabolism of glucose

lowed by the pentose phosphate pathway, by glycogen synthesis, or by the formation of heteroglycanes, as required.

The relative proportion of glycogen synthesis and pentose phosphate pathway differs from one cell type to another. Glycogen (see Fig. 3.1) is basically only formed in the liver and in muscle tissue. The throughput through the pentose phosphate pathway varies significantly (lactating mammary gland 60 %, liver 40 %, muscle tissue 5 %). The chief role of the pentose phosphate pathway is to provide NADPH for various metabolic pathways (reduced glutathione, synthesis of fatty acid, etc.) and also pentoses for the synthesis of nucleotides and nucleic acids. The glycogen concentration in the liver is 5–8 % on average, and in non-exercised muscle tissue it is generally less than 1 %. Only the glycogen in the liver is available for regulating blood sugar; the glycogen in the muscle is only able to satisfy the organs own glucose requirements.

Gluconeogenesis occurs only in the liver and kidney. Synthesis of 1 mol glucose from 2 mol pyruvate requires 6 mol ATP and 2 mol NADH. The gluconeogenesis metabolic pathway represents a reversal of glycolysis, except for the fact that "gluconeogenetic enzymes" are involved instead of the enzymes hexokinase, phosphofructokinase and pyruvate kinase. Provision of a substrate for gluconeogenesis and control of the activity of the gluconeogenetic enzymes is affected by hormones.

3.1.3 Factors in Glucose Homeostasis

A precisely balanced system of hormones, enzymes and substrate streams is required in order to maintain homeostasis. Determination of the glucose concentration in peripheral blood relates only to the concentration in the extracellular glucose pool and does not provide any direct information about the rate of intracellular breakdown or of gluconeogenesis. The glucose flow rate or glucose conversion rate can be determined approximately under defined conditions by using the clamp technique. More accurate analyses can only be obtained by means of radioactively or non-radioactively labeled glucose molecules (tracer method).

An increase in glucose concentration in excess of 130 mg/dl in individuals with an empty stomach is referred to as hyperglycemia and is one of the primary symptoms of diabetes mellitus. A drop in glucose concentration below 50 mg/dl in combination with clinical symptoms is referred to as hypoglycemia. Serious cases of hypoglycemia have a negative effect on physical and mental performance and eventually lead to unconsciousness.

Euglycemia in individuals with an empty stomach is maintained when the consumption of 2 to 2.4 mg glucose/kg/min (132–170 mg/kg/h) is balanced out by an equally high rate of glucose production in the liver (glycogenolysis, gluconeogenesis). Fasting states that last for long periods of time result in an increase in gluconeogenesis in the liver and a decrease in glucose consumption in peripheral tissues. In chronic fasting states ketone bodies can compensate for some of the glucose consumption in the brain. The limitation of glucose utilization and reduced responsiveness to insulin that can be observed in longer-lasting fasting states, in Type II diabetes, and in the post-aggression state is referred to as insulin resistance. Insulin resistance can stem from reduced insulin sensitivity or a reduced metabolic response (unresponsiveness). An increase in glucogenesis and glycogenolysis with reduced consumption in the muscles and fatty tissue leads to an increase in the extracellular glucose pool and thus to hyperglycemia. Conversely, peripheral consumption in hyperinsulinism (insulinoma) can be increased so sharply that hypoglycemic metabolic conditions involving unconsciousness can occur if there is simultaneous inhibition of gluconeogenesis.

Insulin plays the key role in regulating glucose homeostasis. Because of its inhibiting effect on gluconeogenesis in the liver and the fact that it increases glucose uptake in skeletal and cardiac muscles and fatty tissue, dangerous reductions in the actual glucose concentration in the blood can result. Conversely, a lack of this hormone and consequently a predominance of catabolic hormones (adrenaline, cortisol, and glucagon) bring about an increase in hepatic glucose release and a decrease in peripheral glucose uptake in muscles and fat. In the post-aggression state and in Type II diabetes, an imbalance develops between hepatic glucose production and peripheral consumption, allowing hyperglycemic metabolic conditions to arise. The carbohydrate metabolism in the kidney is only of secondary importance for glucose homeostasis. The gluconeogenesis of the proximal tubule is again balanced out by insulin-independent glucose uptake in other sections of the nephron. Renal glucose production is only significant for lactic acidosis and for decompensation of gluconeogenesis in the liver.

Under hyperglycemic metabolic conditions the kidney has an important function as regards the elimination of glucose from the cardiovascular system. Normally 0.05 % of the glomerular-filtered glucose volume is eliminated. If the reabsorption capacity of the tubules is exceeded (renal threshold), glycosuria is observed. Determination of glucose in the urine is an important diagnostic tool for monitoring hypoglycemia.

3.2 Metabolism of Glucose, 2-DG, 2-FDG and 3-FDG

3.2.1 Glucose

The metabolic process by which glucose is converted to pyruvate is referred to as glycolysis. In aerobic organisms glycolysis is a preliminary stage of the citric acid cycle and the respiratory chain, processes in which most of the free energy of glucose is released. The ten glycolysis reactions (see Fig. 3.1) take place in the cytosol. In the first stage glucose is converted to fructose-1,6-diphosphate by means of phosphorylation, isomerization, and then a second phosphorylation process. In these reactions two molecules of ATP are consumed for each glucose molecule, and then, in subsequent steps, net synthesis of ATP is initiated. In the second stage fructose-1,6-diphosphate is split by aldolase into dihydroxyacetone phosphate and glyceraldehyde-3-phosphate, which can easily be interconverted. Glyceraldehyde-3-phosphate is then oxidized and phosphorylated, yielding 1,3-diphosphoglycerate, an acylphosphate with a high phosphoryl group transfer potential. This is followed by the formation of 3-phosphoglycerate with simultaneous generation of ATP. Phosphoenol pyruvate, a second intermediate product with a high phosphoryl group transfer potential, is produced in the last stage of glycolysis through rearrangement of the 3-phosphoryl group and elimination of water. An additional ATP is formed during conversion of the phosphoenolpyruvate into pyruvate. This means that a total of 2 molecules of ATP are obtained through the formation of two pyruvate molecules from one glucose molecule. The electron acceptor in the oxidation of the glyceraldehyde-3-phosphate is NAD^+, which must be regenerated for continuation of glycolysis.

Glycolysis has 2 functions: it breaks down glucose for the purpose of ATP generation, and it provides building blocks for the synthesis of cell constituents. The rate of conversion of glucose to pyruvate is controlled so that these two chief cell requirements are taken into account. The glycolysis reactions are reversible under physiological conditions with the exception of the reactions that are catalyzed by hexokinase, phosphofructokinase and pyruvate kinase. Phosphofructokinase, the most important glycolysis control element, is inhibited by high ATP and citrate levels and activated by AMP and fructose-2,6-diphosphate. In the liver this diphosphate signals that there is an abundant amount of glucose. Phosphofructokinase is also active if either energy or building blocks are required. Hexokinase is inhibited by glucose-6-phosphate, which accumulates when phosphofructokinase is inactive. Pyruvate kinase, the other control point, is inhibited allosterically by ATP and alanine. Pyruvate kinase has its maximum activity therefore when the energy charge is low and intermediate glycolysis products accumulate. Pyruvate kinase is regulated by reversible phosphorylation, just like the tandem enzyme that controls the fructose-2,6-diphosphate level. A low glucose level in the blood promotes phosphorylation of liver pyruvate kinase, which reduces its activity and thus reduces glucose consumption in the liver.

3.2.2 Metabolism of 2-DG, 2-FDG and 3-FDG

As shown in Fig. 3.2, metabolism of the glucose derivatives described in this section, namely 2-deoxy-D-glucose (2-DG), 2-fluoro-deoxy-D-glucose (2-FDG) and 3-fluoro-deoxy-D-glucose (3-FDG), decreases in the order in which they are named. Phosphorylation of these molecules – with the exception of 3-FDG – takes place when the sugars are absorbed by the cell. One phosphate molecule with the alcohol group is added to the 6th carbon atom of a glucose or 2-FDG molecule. This requires the enzyme hexokinase, which is contained in the cells. In this case glucose, 2-DG and 2-FDG compete for the enzyme binding site. Glucose-6-phosphate and 2-DG-6-phosphate are metabolized further, but 2-FDG undergoes a reverse reaction to a limited extent by way of the enzyme glucose-6-phosphatase (see Fig. 3.3). Thus it can be transported out of the cell again. PET examinations take place 1-2 hours after injection of the tracer. Within this period it is still possible to disregard the reverse reaction. 3-FDG is not phosphorylated (see Fig. 3.2). Therefore it is not subject to the trapping mechanism and is eliminated more rapidly from the cells. Because of these different metabolic properties, the kinetics for accumulation in the cell are therefore very different for glucose, 2-DG, 2-FDG and 3-FDG (see below).

3.3 FDG Uptake

3.3.1 Glucose Transport Systems

A group of transport proteins makes it possible for glucose to enter or leave animal cells. Two principal mechanisms for glucose entry into tumor cells have been described (Table 3.1)

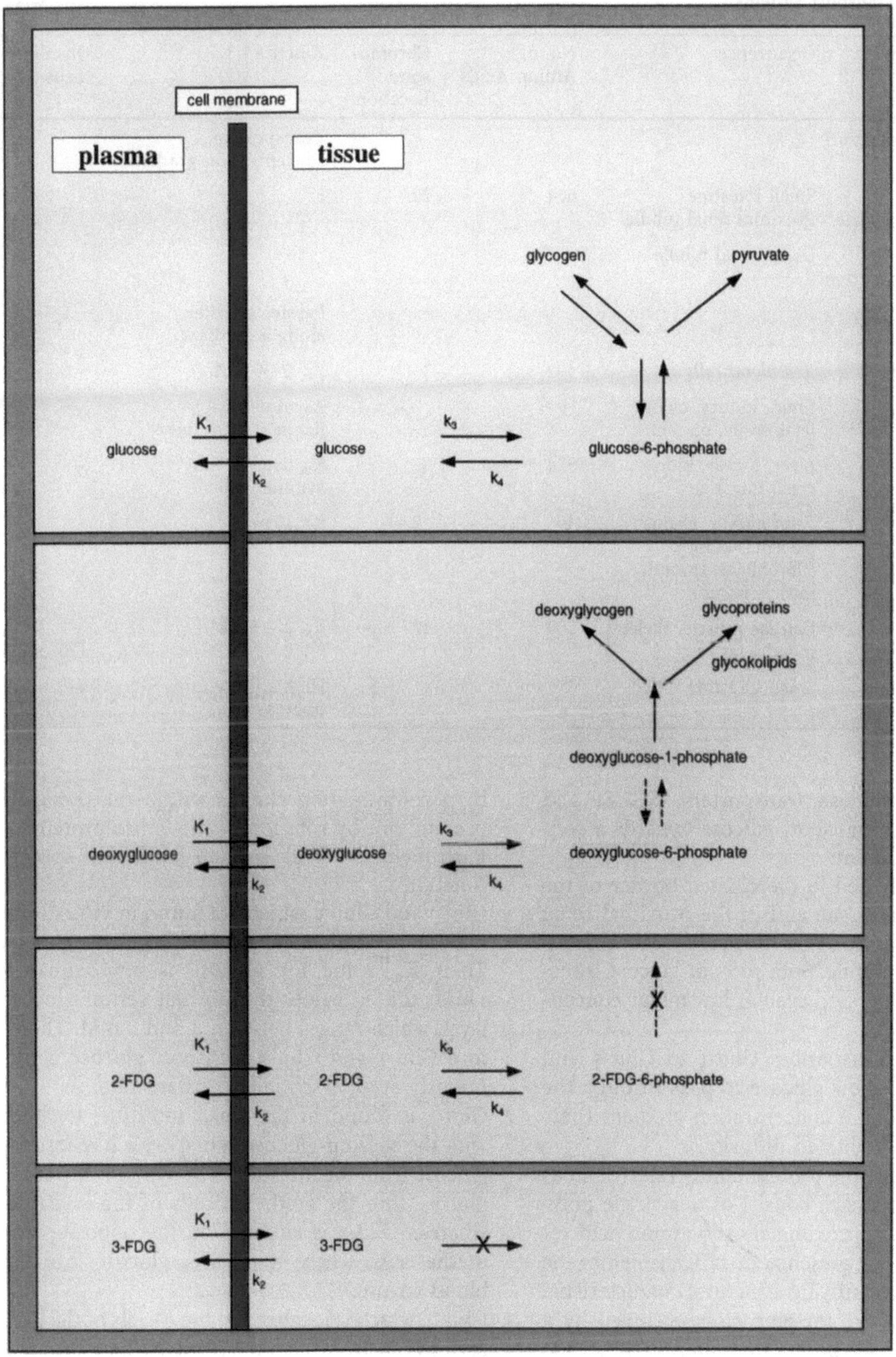

Fig. 3.2. Metabolism of glucose, 2-DG, 2-FDG and 3-FDG

Table 3.1. Glucose Transport Systems

Transporter System	Occurrence	No. of Amino Acids	Chromosome Location	Kinetics	Insulin-Sensitive
I. Na^+-glucose cotransport or symport				**Transport to concentration gradient**	
SGLT 1 Na^+/glucose cotransporter	Small intestine Proximal renal tubule	664	22		
SGLT-2 Na^+/glucose cotransporter	Distal renal tubule				
II. Facilitated diffusion				**Passive transfer along a gradient**	
	Red blood cells	492	1	K_m 5–30 mM	–
Glut-1	Brain, kidney, colon, fetal tissue, placenta			Asymmetrical K_m in <<Km out	–
Glut-2	*Liver*, β-cells, kidney, small intestine	524	3	K_m liver 60 mM Symmetrical	–
Glut-3	*Fetal muscle*, brain, placenta, kidney (fibroblasts, smooth muscle tissue)	496	12	K_m 10 mM	–
Glut-4	Cardiac muscle, skeletal muscle, fat cells	509	17	K_m 2 – 5 mM	+ (20–30)
Glut-5	Small intestine	501	1	High affinity for fructose	–

I. The sodium-glucose transporters (SGLT1 and SGLT2), which transport glucose towards a concentration gradient:
SGLT1 is expressed in the ciliated border of the small intestine tissue and in the proximal renal tubule, whereas SGLT2 is normally located distally in the renal tubule. Both sodium-glucose transporters are expressed even at low molar concentrations.

II. The glucose transporters Glut-1 to Glut-5 and Glut-7, which allow glucose to pass through the membrane along a concentration gradient (passive transfer, facilitated diffusion):
The members of the protein family referred to as Glut-1 to Glut-5 each consist of one single polypeptide chain approximately 500 amino acid residues long. The presence of 12 transmembrane segments is the unifying structural characteristic. If the binding site for glucose is occupied by a sugar, then the site points alternately to the inside and outside of the cell. This inversion is achieved by a conformation change within the transport protein, not by rotation of the entire protein.
Each member of this protein family has specific functions:

1. Glut-1 and Glut-3, which are found in virtually all mammalian cells, ensure the basic glucose supply. Their K_m value for glucose is approximately 1 mM; this is below the normal serum glucose level, which ranges between 4 and 8 mM. Therefore Glut-1 and Glut-3 transport glucose continuously at an essentially constant rate.
2. Glut-5 is found in the small intestine; together with the sodium-glucose transporter it reabsorbs glucose from the intestine. The symporter pumps glucose into the epithelial cells of the intestine, whereas Glut-5 is situated on the opposite side of the cells, where it releases glucose into the blood stream.
3. Glut-2, which is localized in the β-cells of the liver and pancreas, is characterized by an especially high K_m value for glucose (15–20 mM). This

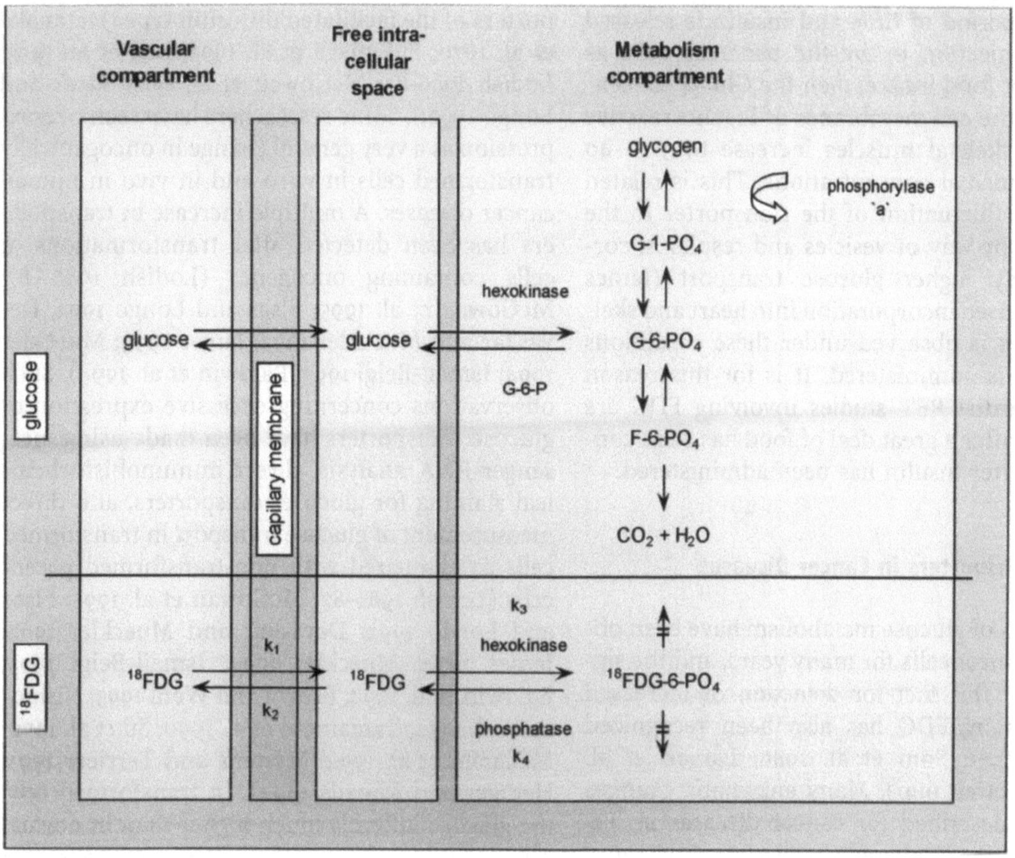

Fig. 3.3. Three-compartment model for calculating glucose metabolism using the [^{18}F]FDG method (after Sokoloff 1977)

means that the rate of glucose entry into these tissues is proportional to the blood glucose level. Thus the pancreas is able to measure the glucose level and adjust the rate of insulin secretion accordingly. The high K_m value of Glut-2 also guarantees that glucose will only enter the liver cells during periods of abundance. If the blood glucose level is low, however, glucose will tend preferentially to enter the brain and other tissues whose glucose transport proteins have a lower K_m value than the transport proteins in the liver.

4. Glut-4 has a K_m value of 5 mM and facilitates the entry of glucose into muscle and fat cells. Insulin, which signals the saturation state, brings about a rapid increase in the number of Glut-4 transporters in the plasma membrane. Insulin promotes glucose uptake in muscles and fat tissue.

This family of transport proteins shows how isomeric forms of a single protein can have a lasting effect on the metabolic characteristics of cells and contribute to their variety and functional specialization. Because this family of transport proteins has different K_m values and different regulation modes, they influence the metabolic characteristics of cells in different organs.

Glucose processing in mammals is complex due to the fact that many enzymes are involved. In many human tissues with physiological blood concentrations, transport through the cell membrane is the limiting factor (Baldwin et al. 1994) wherever the insulin concentration in tissues is low and wherever there are high-affinity transporters (low K_m value). When individuals have fasted for a long period of time and insulin is released either by injection or by the pancreas cells as the result of food intake, then the Glut-4 concentrations in the cell membranes of insulin-reactive heart and skeletal muscles increase to 5 to 40 times the normal concentrations. This is related to the transfluctuation of the transporter to the membrane by way of vesicles and results in correspondingly higher glucose transport (James 1994). Increased incorporation into heart and skeletal muscles is observed under these conditions when FDG is administered. It is for this reason that myocardial PET studies involving FDG are performed after a great deal of food has been consumed or after insulin has been administered.

3.3.2 Glucose Transporters in Cancer Diseases

Higher rates of glucose metabolism have been observed in cancer cells for many years, and the significance of this fact for detection of increased metabolism by FDG has also been recognized (Warburg 1931; Som et al. 1980; Larson et al. 1981; Wahl et al. 1991). Many enzymatic changes have been described for cancer diseases in humans, including increased glucose transport rates, higher rates of glucose phosphorylation and generally very low rates of glucose-6-phosphate dephosphorylation (Weber et al. 1961; Monakhov et al. 1978; Hatanaka et al. 1970; Flier et al. 1987; Fukunaga et al. 1993; Graham et al. 1989). There are also a number of published papers that deal with the different changes in cell metabolism (Flier et al. 1987; Fukunaga et al. 1993; Graham et al. 1989).

However, we should note that when FDG is used as an indicator for glucose metabolism, it cannot be handled by the cells in the same way as glucose because the affinity of the membrane transporters and the hexokinase and phosphatase enzymes for FDG and glucose may vary (Graham et al. 1989; Bell et al. 1993). Moreover, FDG is a poor substrate for phosphoglucoisomerase and other glycolytic enzymes.

In current cancer research great attention is being paid to the overexpression of glucose transporters of the facilitated diffusion type (Hatanaka et al. 1970; Fukunaga et al. 1993; Bell et al. 1993; Lodish 1986-87; McGowan et al. 1995; Elsas and Longo 1992;). Some researchers have seen overexpression as a very general change in oncogenically transformed cells in vitro and in vivo in human cancer diseases. A multiple increase in transporters has been detected after transformations of cells containing oncogenes (Lodish 1986–87; McGowan et al. 1995; Elsas and Longo 1992; Devaskar and Mueckler 1992; James 1994; Mueckler 1994; Ismail-Beigi 1993; Baldwin et al. 1994). Such observations concerning excessive expression of glucose transporters have been made using messenger-RNA analysis, direct immunohistochemical staining for glucose transporters, and direct measurement of glucose transport in transformed cells as compared with non-transformed parent cells (Lodish 1986-87; McGowan et al. 1995; Elsas and Longo 1992; Devaskar and Mueckler 1992; James 1994; Mueckler 1994; Ismail-Beigi 1993; Baldwin et al. 1994; Brown and Wahl 1993; Nishioka et al. 1992; Yamamoto et al. 1990; Su et al. 1990; Mellanen et al. 1994; Mertens and Terriere 1993; Hediger and Rhoads 1994). In transformed cells the glucose influx is much higher than in normal cells. The membrane of transformed cells also contains a glucose transporter that has a higher affinity for glucose (i.e. a low K_m value); this transporter normally only occurs in brain cells and red blood cells. The rapid and high-affinity glucose uptake by the glucose transporter correlates with the high glucolytic activity of tumor cells. A typical overexpression of the glucose transporter Glut-1 was detected recently in tissues of primary human mammary carcinomas as compared with normal mammary tissue (Brown and Wahl 1993). An overexpression of Glut-1 was also detected by Reske et al. 1997 in pancreas carcinoma. Overexpressions of the high-affinity transporters in cancer, namely Glut-1 and Glut-3, are typical in very different types of cancers, and the literature dealing with this phenomenon is rapidly increasing (Brown and Wahl 1993; Nishioka et al. 1992; Yamamoto et al. 1990; Su et al. 1990; Mellanen 1994). It is also logical to develop radiopharmaceutical substances that can detect overexpressed glucose transporters (Mertens and Terriere 1993).

Not much has been published regarding the relationship between SGLT transport systems and cancer. SGLT1 has been detected in colon cancer tissues. However, there is also the opinion that this does not play a big role in tumor-specific glucose transport (Hediger and Rhoads 1994).

3.3.3
Kinetics of Glucose Transport

The simplest substrates for transport measurements are those that are converted to phosphorylated compounds immediately after entry into the cell. The cell membrane is impermeable for intermediate phosphorylated products, and the substrate thus remains trapped inside the cell (trapping mechanism, see Fig. 3.3). D-glucose, 2-DG and 2-FDG fall into this category, since they are phosphorylated by hexokinase and ATP (Hatanaka et al. 1970; Renner 1972; Gallagher et al. 1978; Minn et al. 1991). Of course they are transformed or broken down by further metabolic steps and can then leave the cell in different ways. Thus the path of glucose breakdown does not end with the third compartment.

2-FDG exhibits relatively limited reabsorption in the kidney in vivo compared with glucose and is therefore discharged into the urine virtually unchanged. 2-FDG is therefore concentrated in vivo with the simultaneous clearance of non-phosphorylated 2-FDG. This provides a good contrast for the PET imaging technique (Gallagher et al. 1978). Because of the trapping mechanism the cell can concentrate the absorbed substrate in phosphorylated form in a substantially greater concentration than occurs in the surrounding milieu. This makes it possible to measure the accumulation over a certain time period within a constant transport rate and thus to determine the initial transport rates. The initial incorporation of the substrate by the cells follows normal Michaelis-Menten kinetics (see below). In the case of transport measurements over a longer period of time it is possible to determine that the incorporation rate decreases sharply and is even reversed. There are several reasons for this: 2-DG transport into the cell is faster than phosphorylation, for example, and a portion of the non-phosphorylated substrate is transported out again, i.e., flows out of the cell. A second reason may be that the metabolism of 2-DG does not provide new ATP for the phosphorylation reaction (as shown in Fig. 3.1). This is to be expected for the transport of 2-FDG alone, since later the substrate no longer appears to be metabolized (Gallagher et al. 1987; Minn et al. 1991). While high glucose concentrations retard 2-FDG transport in cell cultures, small glucose concentrations can stimulate transport. This indicates the necessity of an energy source (Oehr et al. 1998, in preparation). Measurements of the substrate transport from the cell can be determined using substances that are not metabolized by the cells. Substrate transport from the cell, like transport into the cell, is a process that is subject to saturation. 3-O-methyl-D-glucose, which is transported by the same carrier as glucose but is neither phosphorylated nor metabolized, has approximately the same K_m and V_{max} values for transport both into the cell and out of the cell (Renner et al. 1972). The same is probably true for 3-FDG (see Fig. 3.2). The K_m values for the various transport systems detected in humans are listed in Table 5.1. With facilitated diffusion there are considerable differences ranging from 2 to 60 mM. In addition to this variation, the number of carriers per cell may also vary, and one cell may be provided with one or more carriers (see Table 5.1). This makes it difficult to attribute kinetics specifically to one or more transport systems. Given this situation, the only way to determine the kinetics of the process absolutely is to carry out specific inhibition experiments with carrier-specific antibodies or other chemical inhibitors such as cytochalasin and phloretin (facilitated diffusion) or phlorizine and ouabain (Na^+/glucose symport) (Tetaud et al. 1997; Bissonnette et al. 1996). Furthermore it has been shown that after an irradiation dose of 10 Gy the tumor cells in cell cultures exhibit as much as a five-fold increase in 2-FDG uptake within one week, whereas uptake increases for up to 2 days after an irradiation dose of 50 or 100 Gy and then decreases again (Oehr et al. 1998).

3.3.4 Quantification of PET Measurements

Compartment Models for [^{18}F]FDG

Radioactively labeled molecules such as [^{18}F]FDG can be traced in the living organism from the outside. In order to determine the relevant quantity (such as rate of metabolism) from the measured activity distributions and their course over time, it is necessary to use models to simplify complicated processes so that they can be described by simple mathematical equations. Linear compartment models have been used most widely. A compartment model consists of a number of spaces or regions; the labeled compound is distributed among these compartments in accordance with the constants that describe the kinetics ("rate constants"). It is assumed that the labeled compound is uniformly distributed within a compartment. It is further assumed that the amount of tracer that is transported per time unit from one compartment to an adjacent compartment is proportional to the total amount present in the compartment and can be described by a transport constant or "rate constant" having the dimension 1/time. The model is represented schematically by a number of sequentially numbered rectangles that are linked by arrows, beside which are written the transport constants k (see Fig. 3.2 and 3.3).

Most tissues can be divided into 4 compartments as regards FDG distribution:

1. FDG in the blood plasma
2. FDG in the interstitial tissue
3. FDG in the cell
4. FDG-6-P in the cell

The biochemical nature of radiopharmaceuticals can change in each of these compartments, whether by metabolism or unspecific bonding – to proteins, for example – or by specific bonding to enzymes. All diffusion and transport processes must also be analyzed bidirectionally. Major simplifications are necessary in order to model experimental data. Sokoloff et al., for example, developed a three-compartment model for calculating glucose metabolism using the [^{18}F]FDG method (Fig. 3.3).

When appropriately labeled substrate analogues are used it is not just the flow of blood or plasma that determines the amount of radioactivity that reaches the tissue but also (and more significantly) the cellular transport and/or intracellular metabolic reactions (e.g. transport and phosphorylation in the case of 2-FDG). The factors that determine the rates of transport and metabolism will be described below.

Passive Diffusion

Passive diffusion, such as through the capillary wall, is basically a symmetrical bidirectional process. It affects small molecules in particular – such as H_2O, O_2, CO_2, NH_3, ethanol, and similar nondissociated molecules. Since radioactive indicators are generally injected by intravasation, the initial retention of a labeled endogenous substance in the section of tissue under examination is determined by the influx (in the direction of the substrate concentration gradient through the membrane). The influx (unidirectional diffusion rate) is described by the following equation (after Henze et al. 1994):

$$N_i = F\ c_p(1 - e^{PS/F}) \qquad (1),$$

where N_i is the substrate, P is capillary permeability, S is the capillary surface per tissue mass, F is the blood flow per tissue mass, and c_p is the intraarterial concentration of the substrate in the plasma. The influx of activity is obtained from the relation (generally time-independent) between the intravascular activity concentration (the labeled endogenous substance) and c_p.

The exponential term in Equation 1 should be disregarded with very high permeability. In such a case the influx rate becomes a linear function of perfusion. Perfusion thus becomes the limiting factor governing substrate uptake by the tissue. Diffusion between extra- and intracellular space can also be analyzed in analogy to Equation 1.

Carrier-Supported Transport

Michaelis-Menten Constant

Carrier-supported transport (facilitated diffusion) is also a process that is passive (i.e., independent of metabolic energy) and bidirectional and is determined by the direction of the concentration gradient through the membrane. Of course the transport rate is a function of the properties of the carrier in the membrane. This type of transport system can be saturated and inhibited just like active transport (with consumption of metabolic energy in the direction of an electrochemical gradient). The molecular process that takes place in a transport system is similar to that of an enzyme-catalyzed chemical reaction and can therefore be described in accordance with the theory of Michaelis and Menten:

$$N_i = (v_{max} \cdot c_p)/(K_m+c_p) \quad (2),$$

where N_i is again the substrate uptake rate, v_{max} is the maximum transport rate, and K_m is the Michaelis-Menten constant; c_p is the concentration of the free substrate in the plasma. Equation 2 expresses the fact that the transport system must be saturated by high substrate concentrations. The chemical kinetics must be described in similar fashion, i.e., the dependence of the reaction rate v (metabolic rate) on substrate concentration in the case of constant enzyme concentration

$$v = (v_{max} \cdot c_s)/(K_m+c_s) \quad (3).$$

Here v_{max} is the maximum reaction rate reached at saturation and c_s is the substrate concentration (Fig. 3.4); K_m is the substrate concentration at which $v = 1/2\, v_{max}$ (Michaelis-Menten constant).

Lineweaver-Burk Diagram

In order to determine the Michaelis-Menten constant experimentally, the reciprocals of v and c_s are plotted (Lineweaver-Burk diagram, Fig. 3.5). This diagram permits simple graphic determination of the quantities that characterize the kinetics, K_m and v_{max}.

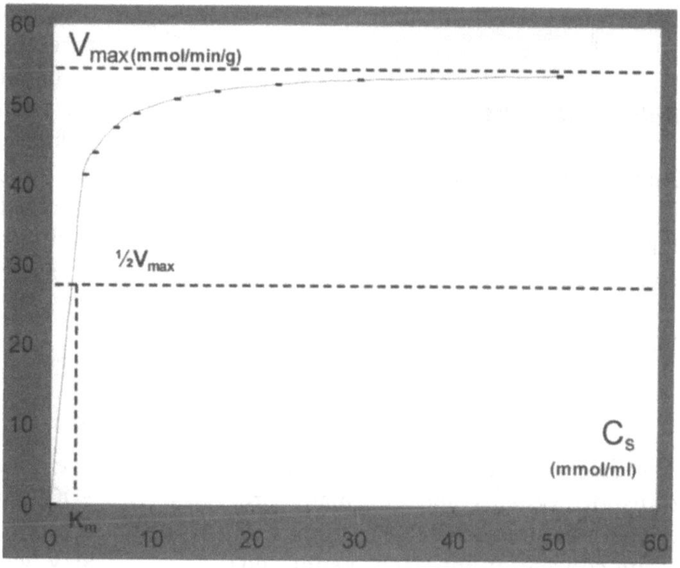

Fig. 3.4. Reaction rate v as a function of substrate concentration c_s in an enzyme-catalyzed chemical reaction. v_{max} = maximum rate (with saturation), K_m = Michaelis-Menten constant

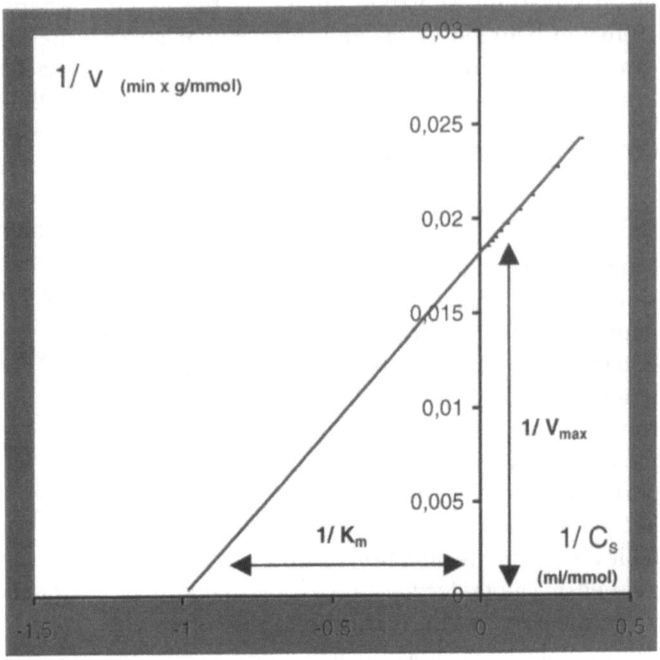

Fig. 3.5. Lineweaver-Burk diagram. The coordinates show the reciprocals of the variables in Fig. 3-4. 1/v is plotted as a function of $1/c_s$

The reciprocal of the Michaelis-Menten constant indicates to what extent the dynamic reaction equilibrium is on the side of the reaction product. v_{max} is a measure of the amount of the enzyme required for the reaction or – analogous to carrier-supported transport – for the number of carriers per volume unit (Henze et al. 1994).

Eadie-Hofstee Plot

Another form of linear representation of Michaelis-Menten kinetics is the Eadie-Hofstee plot, Fig. 3.6. It indicates the presence of various system components better than the Lineweaver-Burk plot by deviating from linearity. It is obtained from the following equation:

$$v = K_m \cdot v/c_s + v_{max} \quad (4).$$

The diagram shows that the characterization of transport systems and enzymatic processes requires measurements at a minimum of two substrate concentrations (Henze et al. 1994).

Tumor-Standardized Uptake Value

Visual qualitative representation of PET studies is normally sufficient for evaluation. However, in many cases a quantitative evaluation is advantageous. This is the case with carcinoma of the breast, for example. In order to be able to compare the PET images of different patients, the PET data calibrated to activity concentration are normalized for image analysis with respect to injected activity and patient weight. The resulting transversal parametric slices represent a standardized measure of the regional tracer concentration at the point of uptake. This is referred to as the "standardized uptake value" (SUV) (Strauss et al. 1991).

$$SUV = \frac{\text{activity concentration in the tissue } [Bq/g]}{\text{administered activity } [Bq/\text{body weight } (g)]}$$

These data are used for both visual and quantitative evaluation. SUV-normalized diagrams of FDG distribution are recorded on X-ray film for the purpose of visual evaluation of PET scans. SUV values from zero to five for examination

Fig. 3.6.
Eadie-Hofstee plot

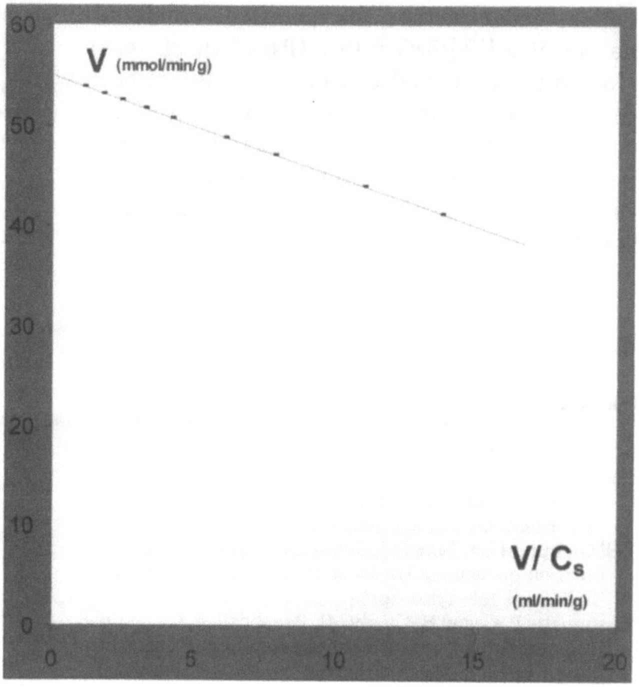

of the mammary glands or from zero to four for images of the axillae are represented by a linear gray-value display (Römer et al. 1997).

Positron emission tomography permits absolute activity measurement in vivo and therefore quantification of tracer concentration in addition to qualitative evaluation of the distribution of glucose in the body. The regional FDG image (SUV value) is determined using the "region of interest" (ROI) technique. The average SUV value within a ROI is used for evaluation. Quantitative image analysis is also affected by tumor size. Because of partial volume effects, tumors less than 2 cm in diameter yield a SUV value that is too low. However, partial volume correction is possible using the "recovery coefficient," a correction factor determined by phantom measurements (Römer et al. 1997; Sokoloff et al. 1977; Patlak et al. 1985). Although the idea is simple, the SUV method is difficult to use because it involves many corrections (Lowe et al. 1994; Zasadny et al. 1993; Fischmann et al. 1993; Minn et al. 1995; Gatenby 1995). It is also difficult to standardize since many variable factors such as glucose concentration, body weight, time after injection, ROI size, and the resolution capability of the PET unit play a role (Lindholm et al. 1994; Minn et al. 1994; Keyes et al. 1995). It is hardly possible to compare SUV values from different institutes using different PET systems and different working protocols.

Complex Compartment Models and the Lumped Constant

Relatively complex compartment models designed to determine glucose consumption are available for measurements of the transport of glucose and different FDG derivatives (Patlak et al. 1985; Sokoloff et al. 1977; Phelps et al. 1979; Huang et al. 1986; Becker et al. 1998). Here we should also mention the term "lumped constant." This constant functions as a calibration factor between 2-FDG and glucose and hardly changes at the local level. The lumped constant is used in the

Patlak-Gjedde method for quantitative determination of 2-[^{18}F]FDG influx (Patlak et al. 1985). However, the lumped constant has not yet been determined for tumors. The heterogeneity of glucose uptake in tumors, among other things, makes it difficult to determine this value. In conclusion it can be noted that the scientific development of complex compartment models is still an open area of research.

References

Baldwin SA, Kan O, Whetton AD et al. (1994) Regulation of the glucose transporter Glut-1 in mammalian cells. Biochem Soc Trans 22: 814–817

Becker G, Piert M, Bares R, Machulla HJ (1998) Konzentrationsabhängigkeit des Transports von 3-[^{18}F] FDG in der Schweineleber. Nuklearmedizin 37: 68

Bell GI, Burant CF, Takeda J, Gould GW (1993) Structure and function of mammalian facilitative sugar transporters. J Biol Chem 268: 19161–19164

Bissonnette P, Gagné H, Coady MJ, Benabdallah K, Lapointe JY, Berteloot A (1996) Kinetic separation and characterization of three sugar transport modes in Caco-2 cells. American J Physiol 270: G833–G843

Brown RS, Fisher SJ, Wahl RL (1993) Autoradiographic evaluation of the intra-tumoral distribution of 2-deoxy-D-glucose and monoclonal antibodies in xenografts of human ovarian adenocarcinoma. J Nucl Med 34: 75–82

Brown RS, Wahl RL (1993) Overexpression of glut-1 glucose transporter in human breast cancer. Cancer 72: 2979–2985

Devaskar SU, Mueckler MM (1992) The mammalian glucose transporters. Pediatr Res 31: 1–13

Elsas LJ, Longo N (1992) Glucose transporters. Ann Rev Med 43: 377–393

Fischmann AJ, Alpert NM (1993) FDG-PET in oncology: there's more to it than looking at pictures. J Nucl Med 34: 6–11

Flier JS, Mueckler MM, Usher P, Lodish HF (1987) Elevated levels of glucose transport and transporter messenger RNA are induced by *ras* or *src* oncogenes. Science 235: 1492–1495

Fukunaga T, Enomoto K, Okazumi S, Isono K (1993) Analysis of glucose metabolism in patients with esophageal cancer by FDG-PET: estimation of hexokinase activity in the tumor and prediction of prognosis: clinical PET in oncology. Proceedings 2nd Intl Symposium on PET in Oncology, Singapore, World Scientific, pp 87–90

Gallagher BM, Fowler JS, Gutterson NI, MacGregor RR, Wan CN, Wolf AP (1978) Metabolic trapping as a principle of radiopharmaceutical design: some factors responsible for the biodistribution of [^{18}F] 2-deoxy-2-fluoro-D-glucose. J Nucl Med 19: 1154–1161

Graham MM, Spence AM, Muzi M, Abbott GL (1989) Deoxyglucose kinetics in a rat brain tumor. J Cereb Blood Flow Metab 9: 315–322

Gatenby RA (1995) Potential role of FDG-Pet imaging in understanding tumor-host interaction. J Nucl Med 36: 839–899

Hatanaka M, Augl C, Gilden RV (1970) Evidence for a functional change in the plasma membrane of murine sarcoma virus-infected mouse embryo cells. Transport and transport-associated phosphorylation of ^{14}C-2-deoxy-D-glucose. J Biol Chem 245: 714–717

Hediger MA, Rhoads DB (1994) Molecular physiology of sodium-glucose cotransporters. Physiol Rev 74: 993–1026

Henze E, Knapp H, Meyer GJ, Müller S (1994) 5: Prinzipien der Diagnostik. In: Büll U, Schicha H, Biersack HJ, Knapp WH, Reiners C, Schober O (Hrsg) Nuklearmedizin. Thieme, Stuttgart New York, S 114–138

Huang SC, Phelps ME (1986) Principles of tracer kinetic modeling in positron emission tomography and autoradiography. In: Phelps ME, Maziotta JC, Schelbert HR (eds) Positron emision tomography and autoradiography: principles and applications for the brain and heart. Raven, New York

Ismail-Beigi F (1993) Metabolic regulation of glucose transport. J Membr Biol 135: 1–10

James DE (1994) Targeting of the insulin-regulatable glucose transporter (GLUT-4). Biochem Soc Trans 22: 668–670

Keys JW Jr (1995) SUV: standard uptake or silly useless value? J Nucl Med 36: 1836–1839

Larson SM, Weiden PL, Grunbaum Z et al. (1981) Positron imaging feasibility studies. II: Characteristic of deoxyglucose uptake in rodent and canine neoplasms: concise communication. J Nucl Med 22: 875–879

Lindholm P, Leskinen-Kallio S, Kirvela O et al. (1994) Head and neck cancer: effect of food ingestion on uptake of C-11 methionine. Radiology 193: 863–867

Lowe VJ, Hoffmann JM, DeLong DM et al. (1994) Semiquantitativ and visual analysis of FDG-PET images in pulmonary abnormalities. J Nucl Med 35: 1771–1776

Lodish HF (1986–87) Anion-exchange and glucose transport proteins: structure, function and distribution. Harvey Lect 82: 19–46

Lowe VJ, Hoffmann JM, DeLong DM et al. (1994) Semiquantitativ and visual analysis of FDG-PET images in pulmonary abnormalities. J Nucl Med 35: 1771–1776

McGowan KM, Long SD, Pekala PH (1995) Glucose transporter gene expression: regulation of transcription and mRNA stability. Pharmacol Ther 66: 465–505

Mellanen P, Minn H, Grénman R, Härkönen P (1994) Expression of glucose transporters in head-and-neck tumors. Int J Cancer 56: 622–629

Mertens J, Terriere D (1993) 3-radioiodo-phloretin – a new potential radioligand for in vivo measurement of glut proteins: a SPECT alternative for [^{18}F]FDG. J Nucl Biol Med 37: 158–159

Minn H, Zasadny KR, Quint LE et al. (1995) Lung cancer: reproducibility of quantitative measurements for evaluating 2-[F-18]-fluoro-2-deoxy-D-glucose uptake at PET. Radiology 196: 167–173

Minn H, Nuutila P, Lindholm P et al. (1994) In vivo effect of insulin on tumor and skeletal muscle glucose metabolism in patients with lymphoma. Cancer 73: 1490–1498

Minn H, Kangas L, Knuutila V, Paul R, Sipilä H (1991) Determination of 2-fluoro-2-deoxy-D-glucose uptake and

ATP level for evaluating drug effects in neoplastic cells. Res Exp Med 191: 27–35
Monakhov NK, Neistadt EL, Shavlovskii MM et al. (1978) Physicochemical properties and isoenzyme composition of hexokinase from normal and malignant human tissues. J Natl Cancer Inst 61: 27–34
Mueckler M (1994) Facilitative glucose transporters. Int J Biochem 219: 713–725
Nishioka T, Oda Y, Seino Y et al. (1992) Distribution of the glucose transporters in human brain tumors. Cancer Res 52: 3972–3979
Oehr P, Ruhlmann J, Rink H (1998) 18F-FDG Transport: Abhängigkeit von Glucosekonzentration und Strahlendosis. Nuklearmedizin 37: 68
Patlak CS, Blasberg RG (1985) Graphical evaluation of blood-to-brain transfer constants from multiple-time uptake data. Generalisations. J Cereb Blood Flow Metab 5: 584–590
Phelps ME, Huang SC, Hoffmann EJ (1979) Tomographic measurement of local cerebral glucose metabolic rate in humans with (F-18) 2-fluoro-2-deoxy-D-glucose: validation of method. Ann Neurol 6: 371–388
Römer W, Avril N, Schwaiger M (1997) Einsatzmöglichkeiten der Positronen-Emissions-Tomographie beim Mammakarzinom. Acta Med Austriaca 24: 60–62
Sokoloff L, Reivich M, Kennedy C et al. (1977) The [^{14}C]-deoxyglucose method for the measurement of local cerebral glucose utilization: theory, procedure, and normal values in the conscious and anesthetized albino rat. J Neurochem 28: 897–916
Som P, Atkins HL, Bandoypadhyay D et al. (1980) A fluorinated glucose analog, 2-fluoro-2-deoxy-D-glucose (^{18}F): nontoxic tracer for rapid tumor detection. J Nucl Med 21: 670–675
Strauss LG, Conti PS (1991) The applications of PET in clinical oncology. J Nucl Med 32: 623– 648
Su, TS, Tsai TF, Chi CW, Han SH, Chou CK (1990) Elevation of facilitated glucose-transporter messenger RNA in human hepatocellular carcinoma. Hepatology 11: 118–122
Tetaud E, Barrett MP, Bringaud F, Baltz T (1997) Kinetoplastid glucose transporters. Biochem J 325: 569–580
Wahl RL, Hutchins GD, Buchsbaum DJ, Liebert M, Grossman HB, Fisher S (1991) 18F-2-deoxy-2-fluoro-D-glucose uptake into human tumor xenografts: feasibility studies for cancer imaging with PET. Cancer 67: 1544–1550
Warburg O (1931) The metabolism of tumors. Richard R Smith, New York, pp 129–169
Weber G, Banerjee G, Morris HP (1961) Comparative biochemistry of hepatomas. I. Carbohydrate enzymes in Morris hepatoma 5123. Cancer Res 21: 933–937
Yamamoto T, Seino Y, Fukumoto H et al. (1990) Overexpression of facilitative glucose transporter genes in human cancer. Biochem Biophy Res Commun 170: 223–230
Zasadny KR, Wahl RL (1993) Standardized uptake values of normal tissues at PET with 2-(fluorine-18)-fluoro-2-deoxy-D-glucose: variations with body weight and a method for correction. Radiology 189: 847–850

PART II

Clinical Applications

Chapter 4

Patient Preparation

B. Kozak

4.1 PET Scanning Technique

PET is a logistically complicated diagnostic technique. Given the desire for optimal cost-effectiveness, it places high demands on medical and technical personnel in terms of planning and performing a diagnostic scan. The complexity of a particular clinical problem, when viewed from the same perspective, also requires that the diagnostician performing the examination have extensive experience in the area of indications as well as sound clinical and technical knowledge of the method. Given the conditions that are technically feasible today, the need to adjust the patient or the scan in a particular case to the conditions that are technically possible is in many cases unavoidable – more than would otherwise be desirable (consider, for example, the factor of external nuclide supply). However, this is done solely to ensure that it will be possible to obtain physiological information from the measured data in as comprehensive and accurate a manner as possible. Another requirement – in addition to routine quality control, reproducible measurement checks, and acquisition of all clinically relevant data – is to explain the procedure thoroughly to the patient. A patient who understands the procedure will be much more willing and able to cooperate, and this will guarantee that scanning will proceed as optimally as possible.

It is important, therefore, to inform the patient well in advance of the PET scan about the scanning procedure, the duration of the scan, and especially about any delays or wait time that might occur. This is important in order to avoid unnecessary misunderstandings regarding the day's schedule and to allay the patient's anxiety. Planning should begin even before the PET appointment is made. In addition to the acquisition of fundamental clinical data, questions such as the patient's body size and weight (both factors can have an effect on scanning time) and relevant metabolic diseases (e.g. diabetes mellitus) are of central importance. The patient is ordered to fast before the actual scan. The patient is allowed to drink unsweetened beverages on the morning of the scan, but the last meal should have been consumed the evening before. For oncological problems that require afternoon appointments, a light breakfast before 8 o'clock in the morning is acceptable in certain cases. However, the patient must not eat after that point. Special medications can continue to be administered, of course. Patients with manifest diabetes mellitus are excepted from these rules since they must continue to eat their standard snacks between meals and receive insulin injections or infusions before undergoing oncological scans.

The most important data are generally obtained from the medical history taken on the date of the scan. In the case of oncological problems, questions should be asked about all aspects of every previous treatment either before or in conjunction with surgery, about radio- and chemotherapies (including even non-traditional treatment methods), and about times and dosages and any local consequences that might have resulted. Central factors include the basic disease, the therapy to date, and how that therapy correlates with diagnostic results already obtained. This is followed by a physical examination in which the patient is examined with regard to local postoperative wound conditions, horizontal drainage, or similar changes. Other points that should be documented are the current blood sugar level, the time of injection, the time in the scanner, patient size and weight, and amount of radioactive substance administered. Normal blood-glucose levels are best for scanning purposes. Latent diabetes is not a reason to forego oncological scanning. Patients with low blood-glucose levels should perhaps be examined on another day under more stable conditions and while taking their regular standard medication.

The scanning protocol to be followed depends on the type of disease. It may be advisable, depending on the case, to perform secondary scans between the base of the skull and the proximal femural region and also additional scans of the brain or the distal extremities. The reason a brain scan is performed is normally to rule out existing cerebral metastases since PET can only offer morphological information and is otherwise inferior to MRI in this situation. However, since PET is available as a whole-body diagnostic method, it is certainly advisable in particular cases to include the scan of the cerebrum so that any major metastases can be immediately detected.

The appendix to this chapter offers a list of the scanning techniques customarily used for various specific diseases.

After the patient's medical history has been taken, the patient is positioned on the patient bed or pallet – e.g. in a supine position with the head in the gantry. The next step is to mark the patient's skin to indicate the scan starting point – at the pelvis, for example. An upper and a lower mark for the first position should be made on the patient's skin using a waterproof marker. The side and the center should also be marked. These marks must be made from the neck to the proximal upper thighs for all bed positions. The number of bed positions must be determined before the scan and will depend on the examination protocol and the size of the patient.

The transmission scan begins after the patient is marked. Currently it takes 7 minutes per bed position (9 minutes for overweight patients). The patient is covered with a blanket or cover because of the low temperatures in the examination room. If desired, the patient may listen to music through earphones. Five (5) bed positions are required for a normal whole-body scan from the base of the skull to the proximal upper thigh region. This means that a scanning time of 35 minutes will be needed for the transmission scan. This should be explained to the patient before starting the scan.

The transmission scan is generally followed by a break of about 1–2 hours during which the patient must continue to fast but is allowed to drink water, tea, or coffee without sugar or milk.

Table 4.1 gives an overview of a typical daily schedule at the PET Center in Bonn. Before injection of the radioactive tracer, capillary blood

Table 4.1. Daily schedule including scanning and injection times for 6 patients (example). 124 mCi must be ordered = 4588 MBq; 4600 MBq are ordered. Delivery: 9:30 AM

Time since delivery [h]	MCi	Pat. No.	Inj. Time	Start	End	Scan
0.0	8	1	9:30 AM	10:00 AM	10:30 AM	Brain
0.5	9	2	9:45 AM	10:30 AM	11:30 AM	Whole-body 1
1.0	11	3	10:45 AM	11:30 AM	12:30 PM	Whole-body 2
2.5	20	4	11:45 AM	12:30 PM	1:30 PM	Whole-body 3
3.0	24	5	12:45 PM	1:30 PM	2:30 PM	Whole-body 4
					3:05 PM	TR 35 min
5.0	52	6	2:15 PM	3:05 PM	4:05 PM	Whole-body 5
					4:40 PM	TR 35 min

Table 4.2. Activity decay as a function of transport time

Time since production [h]	Required initial activity mCi	mBq
0.0	8	296
0.5	9	333
1.0	11	407
1.5	14	518
2.0	17	629
2.5	20	740
3.0	24	888
3.5	30	1110
4.0	36	1332
4.5	43	1591
5.0	52	1924

sugar is determined in blood drawn from the finger pad. ^{18}F-fluorodeoxyglucose, the radiotracer used for the whole-body PET scan, is injected into the supine patient through a three-way catheter. This should always be followed by isotonic saline irrigation. Strictly intravenous administration is required in order to rule out the risk of paravenous injection, if possible, and the associated imaging of the regional lymph nodes. The injection should be administered under standardized conditions in a darkened room, and the patient should ideally close his or her eyes and should not speak.

After the injection it is advisable to have the patient lie in a relaxed position for at least 5–10 minutes in order to prevent the injection solution from concentrating in the muscle. Then the patient is asked to go into the waiting room. After an incubation period of approximately 45 minutes and voiding of the bladder, the patient is then repositioned on the bed in accordance with the transmission scan markings. If tumor screening in the pelvic region is involved, then forced diuresis is advisable during the 45-minute incubation period (by i. v. injection of 20 mg Lasix, for example) in order to prevent any bladder activity that might disturb the scan.

The emission scan is performed with the identical positioning in accordance with the transmission scan markings. For 5 bed positions, for example, it will take 50 minutes. This may be followed, if necessary, by additional "fast" emission scans of the legs lasting 3 minutes for each leg. In the event of additional scans of the brain. a 5-minute transmission scan is followed by a 10-minute emission scan. Approximately 8 mCi ^{18}F-FDG is normally injected per patient. Table 4.2 gives an overview of the tracer decay time as a function of the required transport time from the production site to the application site.

Appendix

An overview of the practical procedure for the most important oncological scans, including scanning parameters and documentation, is given below.

The emission scans and attenuation-corrected scans for each completed examination should always be analyzed and documented. The findings should always be evaluated on the monitor, in addition to evaluating printouts. This provides additional information, particularly as regards evaluation of any intestinal activity or ureteral activity concentration, and dynamic processes can be differentiated from focal regions. Quantitative measurements of the activity distribution in a specific "region of interest" can also be carried out. This information can also be stored electronically and will then be available for follow-up purposes.

1. Thyroid Cancer

- Transmission scan:
  - Duration: 7 min/bed position (depending on the age of the germanium sources and patient weight)
  - Bed positions: n = 4–5 from parotid to pelvis
  - Move-in (thorax → pelvis)
- Emission scans:
  - Duration: 10 min/bed position
  - Start: 45–60 min after injection
  - Bed positions: n = 4–6 (similar to transmission scan)

- Documentation:
  - Emission scans:
    coronal, sagittal, transverse
  - Attenuation-corrected tomograms:
    coronal, sagittal, transverse

2. *Malignant Melanoma*

- Transmission scan:
  - Duration: 7 min/bed position (depending on the age of the germanium sources and patient weight)
  - Bed positions: n = 4–6 from mid-neck region to bottom of pelvis
  - Move-in (thorax → pelvis) for lesions in thorax region or higher
  - Move-out (pelvis → thorax) for lesions in abdominal region or lower
  - Administration of liquid (mineral water or water, 1 bottle minimum); for abdominal lesions and lesions located caudally to the abdomen administration of Lasix with FDG (inguinal and parailiac lymph nodes)
- Emission scans:
  - Duration: 10 min/bed position
  - Start: 45–60 min after injection
  - Bed positions: n = 4–6
    (similar to transmission scan)
- Additional scans:
  - Brain (always: 15 min/scan)
  - Feet (from lesion to bottom of pelvis): 3 min/bed position
- Documentation:
  - Emission scans: coronal, sagittal, transverse
  - Attenuation-corrected tomograms:
    coronal, sagittal, transverse

3. *Colorectal Cancer*

- Transmission scan:
  - Duration: 7 min/bed position
  - Bed positions: n = 4–6 from bottom of pelvis to mid-neck region
  - Move-out (pelvis → thorax) for lesions in abdominal region or lower
  - Administration of liquid (mineral water or water, 1 bottle minimum); administration of Lasix with FDG (inguinal and parailiac lymph nodes, perivesical environment)
- Emission scans:
  - Duration: 10 min/bed position
  - Start: 45–60 min after injection
  - Bed positions: n = 4–6 (similar to transmission scan)
- Documentation:
  - Emission scans:
    coronal, sagittal, transverse
  - Attenuation-corrected tomograms:
    coronal, sagittal, transverse

4. *Head and Neck Tumors*

- Transmission scan:
  - Duration: 7 min/bed position
  - Bed positions: n = 3–4 from base of skull to bottom of lung
  - Move-in (thorax → pelvis)
- Emission scans:
  - Duration: 10 min/bed position
  - Start: 45–60 min after injection
  - Bed positions: n = 3–4 (similar to transmission scan)
- Additional scans:
  - 2 bed positions, 3 min each; bottom of lung to pelvis
- Documentation:
  - Emission scans: coronal, sagittal, transverse
  - Attenuation-corrected tomograms:
    coronal, sagittal, transverse

5. *Ovarian Cancer (and Other Gynecological Tumors)*

- Transmission scan:
  - Duration: 7 min/bed position
  - Bed positions: n = 4–6 from bottom of pelvis to mid-neck region
  - Move-out (pelvis → thorax) for lesions in abdominal region or lower
  - Administration of liquid (mineral water or water, 1 bottle minimum); and Lasix with FDG (inguinal and parailiac lymph nodes, perivesical environment)
- Emission scans:
  - Duration: 10 min/bed position
  - Start: 45–60 min after injection

- Documentation:
  - Emission scans:
    coronal, sagittal, transverse
  - Attenuation-corrected tomograms:
    coronal, sagittal, transverse

6. Pulmonary Nodules

- Transmission scan:
  - Duration: 7 min/bed position
  - Bed positions: n = 3 from mid-neck region to bottom of lungs
  - Move-in (thorax → pelvis)
- Emission scans:
  - Duration: 10 min/bed position
  - Start: 45 – 60 min after injection
  - Bed positions:
    n = 3 (similar to transmission scanning)
- Additional scans:
  - 2 bed positions, 3 min each; bottom of lung to pelvis
- Documentation:
  - Emission scans:
    coronal, sagittal, transverse
  - Attenuation-corrected tomograms:
    coronal, sagittal, transverse

7a. Breast Cancer (Whole-Body Scan) for Tumor Screening After Breast Cancer and Surgery

- Transmission scan:
  - Duration: 7 min/bed position
  - Bed positions: n = 4 – 6 from mid-neck region to bottom of pelvis
  - Move-in (thorax → pelvis)
  - Administration of liquid (mineral water or water, 1 bottle minimum); and Lasix with FDG
- Emission scans:
  - Duration: 10 min/bed position
  - Start: 45 – 60 min after injection
  - Bed positions:
    n = 4 – 6 (similar to transmission scanning)
- Documentation:
  - Emission scans:
    coronal, sagittal, transverse
  - Attenuation-corrected tomograms:
    coronal, sagittal, transverse

7b. Suspected Breast Cancer

Problem: status of a suspicious node Examination of patient in prone position on special pillow (cutout for breasts)

- Transmission scan:
  - Duration: 15 min/bed position
  - Bed positions: n = 1 – 2
  - Move-in (thorax → pelvis)
- Emission scans:
  - Duration: 20 min/bed position
  - Start: 45 – 60 min after injection
  - Bed positions:
    n = 1 – 2 (similar to transmission scanning)
- Documentation:
  - Emission scans:
    coronal, sagittal, transverse
  - Attenuation-corrected tomograms:
    coronal, sagittal, transverse

8. Lymphoma

- Transmission scan:
  - Duration: 7 min/bed position
  - Bed positions:
    n = 5 – 6 from parotid to pelvis
  - Move-in (thorax → pelvis) for lesions in thorax region or higher
  - Move-out (pelvis → thorax) for lesions in abdominal region or lower
  - Administration of liquid (mineral water or water, 1 bottle minimum); and Lasix with FDG
- Emission scans:
  - Duration: 10 min/bed position
  - Start: 45 – 60 min after injection
  - Bed positions:
    n = 5 – 6 (similar to transmission scanning)
- Documentation:
  - Emission scans:
    coronal, sagittal, transverse
  - Attenuation-corrected tomograms:
    coronal, sagittal, transverse

Reference

James DE (1994) Targeting of the insulin-regulatable glucose transporter (glut-4). Bioch Soc Trans 22: 668 – 670

CHAPTER 5

Clinical Indications

C. Alexiou, R. An, W. Arnold, M. Bangard, R. P. Baum, H.-J. Biersack, R. Bonnet, U. Büll, U. Cremerius, C. G. Diederichs, F. Grünwald, R. J. Kau, R. Kaufmann, C. Laubenbacher C. Menzel, P. Oehr, H. Palmedo, N. Presselt, J. Reul, D. Rinne, J. Ruhlmann, M. Schwaiger, P. Willkomm, and M. Zimny

5.1 Malignant Melanoma

D. Rinne, R. Kaufmann, and R. P. Baum

5.1.1 Epidemiology

The incidence of malignant melanoma is increasing more rapidly than any other kind of cancer; since 1973 it has risen by 4–6 % per year in the United States. While in 1935 the risk of an American developing malignant melanoma during his lifetime was 1:1,500, by 1991 the risk was 1:105, and it is estimated that it will be 1:75 by the year 2000 (Boring et al. 1994; Harris et al. 1995). Among women between the ages of 20 and 29 it is the most frequent type of tumor (Friedman et al. 1991; Katsambas and Nicolaidou 1996; Kof 1991; Johnson et al. 1994; and Schneider et al. 1994).

In the U.S. today, approximately 32,000 people suffer from malignant melanoma annually, and 6,500 people die of it. Although it comprises only 5 % of all skin tumors, more than 75 % of all deaths caused by skin cancer can be attributed to malignant melanoma.

5.1.2 Histology and Staging

Clinically and histologically, 4 types of malignant melanoma can be differentiated:

1. superficial spreading melanoma (SSM, approximately 60 %);
2. nodular melanoma (NM, approximately 20 %);
3. lentigo maligna melanoma (LMM, approximately 10 %);
4. acral lentiginous melanoma (ALM, approximately 5 %).

The remaining 5 % is distributed among atypical types and unclassifiable melanomas.

Malignant melanoma can metastasize primarily via the lymphatic or haematogenic system and involve any organ. Most common are cutaneous metastases and those of the lymph nodes, lungs, liver, cerebrum and bone. Early detection of malignant melanoma (ABCD rule, epiluminescence microscopy) and its surgical removal are decisive for the prognosis.

TNM classification subdivides 4 categories: primary tumor (stage I and II), locoregional spread (stage III) and systemic spread (Stage IV).

5.1.3 Prognosis

Concerning the primary tumor, the most important prognostic factors are:

1. Vertical tumor thickness according to Breslow (10-year survival rate > 95 % for thin (< 0.75 mm) melanomas and < 70 % for those thicker than 4 mm).
2. Invasion level according to Clark (especially the distinction between Clark Level II and Level III)
3. Ulceration

In addition, the location of the primary tumor and the patient's sex seem to have a certain prognostic relevance. Patients with a melanoma on the extremities enjoy a better prognosis than those with localizations on the torso, head, or neck (Breslow 1970; Koh 1991; Rogers et al. 1983; Vollmer 1989). Women have a better chance of survival than men; in women melanomas are localized more frequently on the extremities and are thinner and less often ulcerated (Breslow 1970; Kopf et al. 1987; Rogers et al. 1983; Vollmer 1989). Other criteria as tumor type or mitotic rate are of minor importance (Koh 1991). Metastatic lymph node involvement decreases the survival tremendously; therefore, additional methods for lymph node staging, e.g. the sentinel node biopsy, are currently investigated, while elective lymph node dissection is not recommended as routine procedure.

5.1.4 Malignant Melanoma Therapy

Treatment of the primary tumor consists of its complete surgical removal with a variable safety margin (1–3 cm) depending on the tumor thickness. In stage III, the removal of regional lymph node metastases can lead to recovery. The value of elective procedures is controversial and cannot yet be conclusively evaluated (Balch 1988; Godellas et al. 1995; Lyons and Cockrell 1994). In stage IV, the surgical removal of isolated metastases can be curative in single cases. In disseminated metastases therapy is always palliative and must respect patients' life quality. Since monotherapies with dacarbazine and more toxic drugs (e.g. cisplatin) are of limited benefit, they are combined with diverse other chemotherapeutics as well as immunotherapy.

5.1.5 Staging and Follow-Up

Conventional Diagnostics (CD)

A complete diagnostic work-up is performed for exclusion or early detection of potentially curable tumor spread. For this purpose, a number of standard imaging techniques are currently combined, including ultrasound, magnetic resonance imaging (MRI), X-ray computed tomography (CT) and conventional x-ray. As these methods are all indicative only of morphological alterations at suspected secondary tumor sites, they mostly rely on active metastatic growth. Additional efforts have focused on earlier detection of metastatic spread. Gallium-67 scintigraphy and immunoscintigraphy using monoclonal antibodies could not dramatically improve in diagnostic sensitivity. (Böni et al. 1995a; Divigi and Larson 1989; Horgan and Hughes 1993; Huzaid et al. 1993; and Kagan et al. 1988).

Positron Emisson Tomography

As conventional diagnostics showed disappointing results in early detection of tumor spread, more recent interest was focused on metabolic imaging by positron emission tomography (PET).

In contrast to conventional imaging techniques, PET is not based on morphological changes but rather on the increased metabolism of tumor cells. As those changes precede morphological alterations, PET has been shown to be superior in the early detection of melanoma metastases and for staging melanoma patients demonstrating a very high sensitivity and specificity (Gritters et al. 1993; Steinert et al. 1995, Rinne et al. 1998).

PET Technique

After a fasting time of 12 hours, 370 MBq F18–FDG (2-Fluor-2-Deoxy-D-Glucose) per 75 kg body weight were injected strictly intravenously. After immobilization for 45–60 minutes, furosemide (40 mg) was injected for rapid renal washout of the tracer. PET studies were acquired on an Ecat Exact 47 whole-body tomograph (Siemens-CTI, Knoxville,TN) with a transaxial field of view of 16.2 cm (slice thickness 3.4 mm; resolution approximately 4 mm) in whole-body technique. Five to nine bed positions were taken. Standardized uptake values (SUV) were calculated to obtain quantitative information on the FDG uptake. Only strong focal hypermetabolic lesions (SUV > 2.5) were considered as malignant.

Results were recorded on x-ray film and as color printouts (for further detailed information, see Chapter 5.4.)

5.1.6 Indications

At the Frankfurt University Medical Center, Germany, 100 melanoma patients were prospectively investigated by PET. PET was performed in addition to conventional diagnostics (CT, MRI, radiography, sonography) in 52 high-risk melanoma patients for primary staging (Group A), and in 48 patients suspicious for recurrence (Group B). The patients' age was 50.8 years in average (23–83 years of age).

All findings had to be confirmed by histology and/or clinical follow-up.

Sensitivity and specificity were calculated as follows:

$$\%\,\text{Sensitivity} = \frac{\text{TP}}{\text{TP} + \text{FN}} \times 100 \quad \%\,\text{Specificity} = \frac{\text{TN}}{\text{TN} + \text{FP}} \times 100$$

Primary Staging

In Group A (primary tumor staging for high-risk melanoma, tumor thickness at least 1.5 mm), PET and conventional imaging revealed no pathological finding in 37 of 52 patients.

PET detected 9 lymph node metastases in 4 patients; these had not been revealed by conventional imaging. All lesions were histologically identified (Fig. 5.1.1).

Three lesions were described as metastases by PET, but no malignant involvement was shown in follow-up. These three foci (SUV $> 2.5 < 3$) were located in a cervical lymph node, in the para-aortic/infrahepatic region, and in an inguinal lymph node (reactive alteration after surgery).

Using conventional diagnostics, ten foci were described as possible metastases, of which four were in lymph nodes, three intrapulmonary, and three in the liver (all false positives).

Sensitivity for PET was therefore 100 % for single lesions (9/9 metastases) and for patients (4/4), whereas the sensitivity of conventional imaging was 0 %. PET specificity was 94 % for metastases and 93.8 % on a patients basis. In comparison, conventional diagnostics achieved a specificity of 80 % for metastases and 83.3 % for patients respectively. The diagnostic accuracy of PET was 94.9 % (metastases) and 94.2 % (patients) respectively, whereas the accuracy of conventional imaging was 67.8 % for metastases and 76.9 % for patients, respectively.

Re-Staging

In Group B (suspected recurrence), PET detected 112 lesions (Fig. 5.1.2 and 5.1.3), whereas 79 focal abnormalities (suspected metastases) were described by conventional imaging. In 13 of 48 patients no metastases were found by either imaging technique. The sites of the detected lesions are shown in Table 5.1.1.

Overall, a total of 121 metastases were found in 48 patients. PET provided only one false positive finding (abdomen), whereas conventional diagnostics revealed ten false positive findings (mediastinum 2, liver 2, abdomen 4, lymph nodes 1, bone 1), as proven by clinical outcome (except for lymph node lesions, which were all histologically examined). PET was false negative for 10 metastases (lung 7, mediastinum/hilum 2, peripheral lymph nodes 1), while conventional diagnostics were false negative for 51 metastases (neck lymph nodes 4, lung 3, mediastinum 4, liver 2, abdomen 11, abdominal lymph nodes 1, peripheral lymph nodes 17, bone 1, skin 8). Sensitvity, specificity and diagnostic accuracy as calculated for the number of patients and lesion by lesion are listed in Table 5.1.2. In addition, the results are given for different body regions (Table 5.1.3).

5.1.7 Summary

In malignant melanoma staging, one major objective is the earliest possible detection of metastases at a potentially curable stage. For this purpose, several imaging techniques are currently combined. As conventional diagnostics (ultrasound,

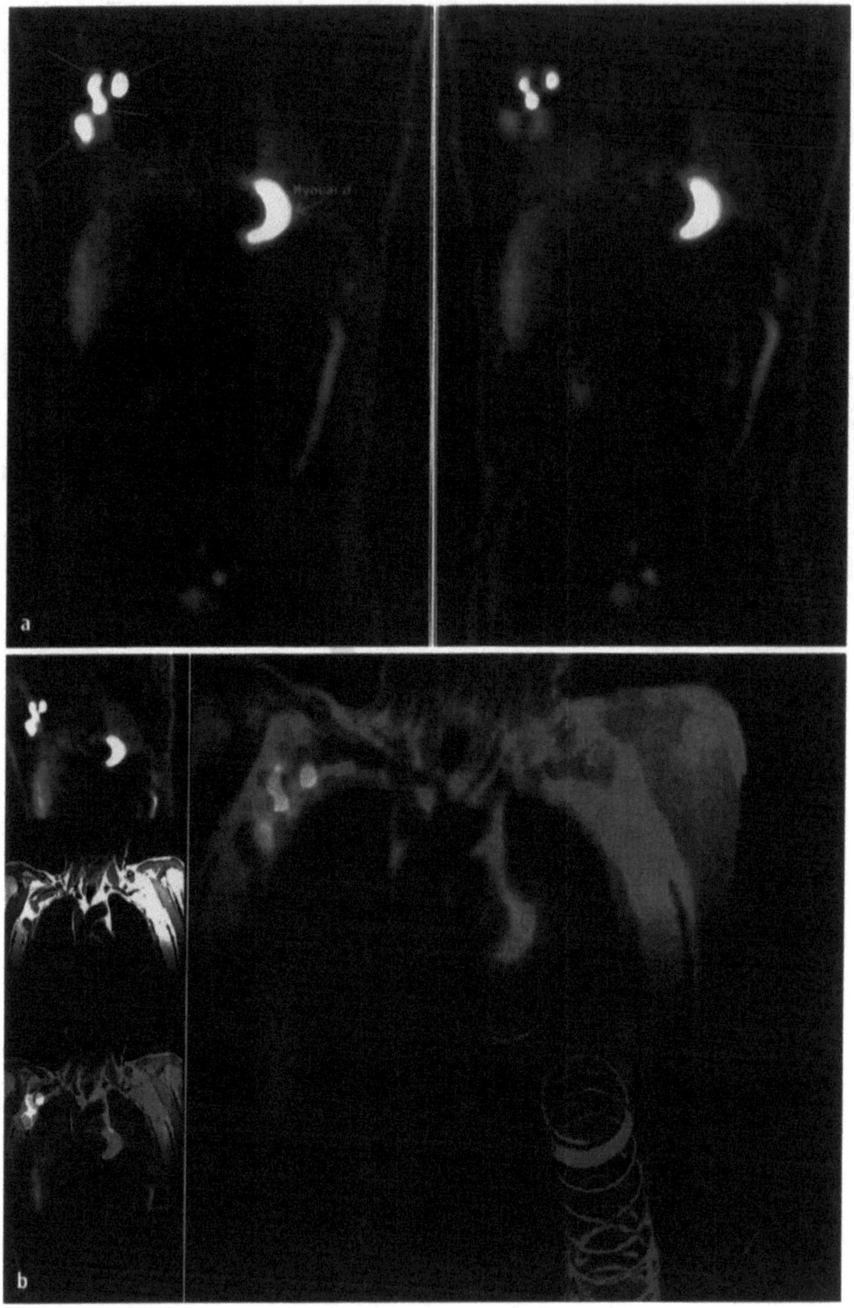

Fig. 5.1.1.
a Primary staging shortly after excision of a para-umbilical nodular melanoma (Clark level IV, pT4a, tumor thickness 5 mm). Conventional diagnostics, including high-resolution lymph node sonography, were normal. Whole-body PET detected multiple hypermetabolic metastases in right axillary lymph nodes. **b** Image fusion of PET and MRI, showing several lymph node metastases, > 2 cm in diameter, along the axillary artery and vein, as well as multiple smaller lymph nodes (approximately 5 mm in size). All lesions were completely removed and histologically confirmed as metastases. Distant metastases have not appeared since that time (observation period: 26 months). Another single lymph node metastasis in the supraclavicular area (also detected by PET in the routine follow-up) was resected > 2 years later

computed tomography, magnetic resonance imaging) are indicative for morphologic alterations, they mostly rely on active tumor growth. Although sonography generally yields anatomic details with high accuracy, imaging of retroperitoneal and para-aortal lymph nodes in obese patients might become difficult (Blessing et al. 1995; Fornage and Lorigan 1989). Moreover, the results

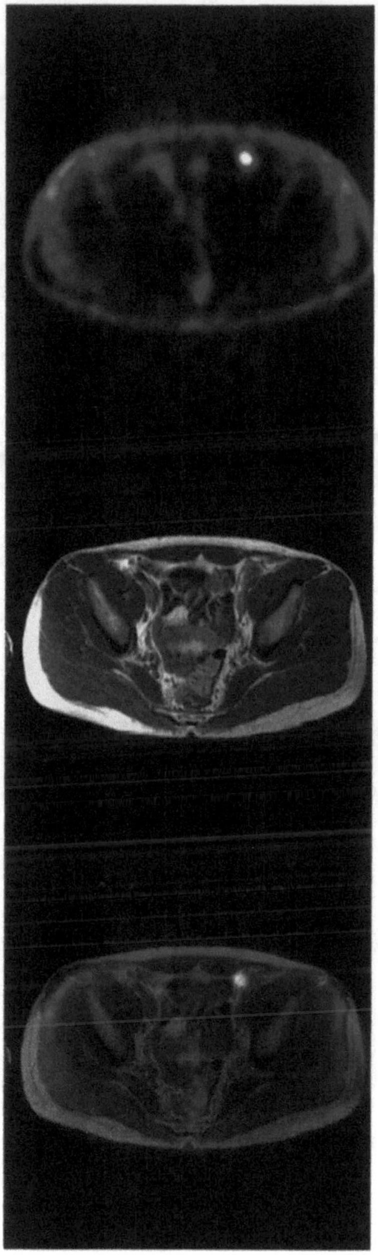

◀ **Fig. 5.1.2.** Re-staging with FDG-PET after two excisions of left inguinal lymph node metastases of a malignant melanoma (unknown primary localization). Abdominal and lymph node sonography – performed just a few days before the PET examination – had revealed no pathological findings. The FDG-PET (transverse slice, top image, without transmission correction) revealed an intense hypermetabolic focus suspicious for a new lymph node metastasis (in projection upon the left external iliac lymph node). MRI of this region demonstrated no pathological findings (middle image). Image fusion of PET with MRI (bottom image) shows the exact anatomic localization; the lymph node metastasis (histologically confirmed) was again surgically removed. Additional metastases have not appeared in this region to date (observation period: 26 months)

depend on the investigators' experience. Bone scintigraphy is a very sensitive method, but it is not tumor-specific and small osteolytic metastases or lesions limited to the bone marrow might be missed (Haubold-Reuter et al., 1993). CT is exceptionally reliable for detecting small lung metastases, but morphologic changes smaller than 10 mm in the mediastinum and in the hilar regions can not be judged (Buzaid et al. 1993; Sasaki et al. 1996; Scott et al. 1996). Abdominal CT detects liver metastases with high sensitivity, but abscesses or other benign lesions might mimick metastatic spread. Again, for abdominal lymph node metastases, the size is a limiting factor. Due to these disadvantages of conventional imaging techniques, recent interest has focused on the usefulness of PET in tumor staging (Adler et al. 1993; Blessing et al. 1995; Böni 1996; Böni et al. 1995b and 1996; Chin et al. 1995; Gritters et al. 1993; Grünwald et al. 1996; Shreve et al. 1996; and Steinert et al. 1995). Early results revealed a sensitivity of 92 % and a specificity of 100 % in the detection of malignant melanoma metastases (Steinert et al.1995). One major advantage of PET is the possibility of whole-body scanning and the evaluation of different organs and structures. Furthermore, PET combines metabolic tumor characterization with quantitation of glucose uptake, which might be important for evaluating therapy response.

These results and those of other groups indicate clearly that PET is superior to conventional diagnostics in sensitivity, specificity, and diagnostic accuracy, especially in the mediastinum and hilus (PET sensitivity 71.4 % vs. CD 20 %) and in the abdomen (PET 100 % vs. CD 26.6 %). In our prospective study (Rinne et al., 1998), CT was superior to PET in the detection of small lung metastases (PET 69.6 % vs. CT 87 % based

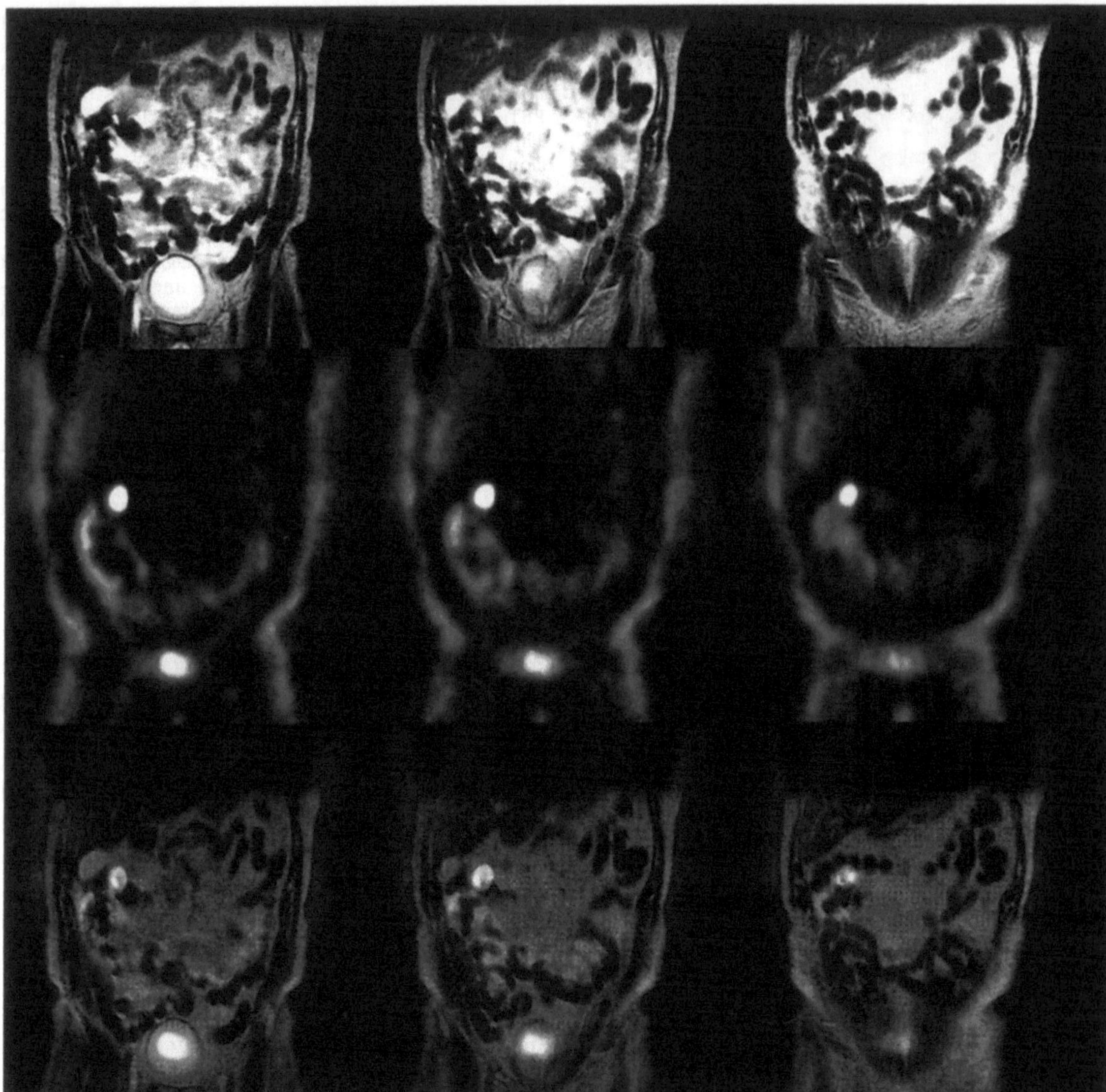

Fig. 5.1.3. Follow-up investigation of a SSM (Level III), primary tumor excision July 1992 in the region of the left upper abdomen. Resection of an infraclavicular lymph node metastasis (5 cm in size) in April 1994, and of a very large pleural metastasis (inferior pulmonary lobe resection) in December 1996. Interim interferon and DTIC chemotherapy. Patient clinically free of complaints. FDG PET (middle row, coronal view) shows a hypermetabolic lesion in the right paracolic area (diameter approximately 3.2 cm). Abdominal CT showed subsequently no pathological findings. MRI (with contrast) showed no pathological findings. The PET/MRI fusion image confirms the location described above. A tumor, 3.5 cm in size, which had started to infiltrate the ileum, was completely removed by surgery in March 1997 (histologically a melanoma metastasis). A follow-up PET, performed one year later in March 1998, showed no evidence of metastases

Table 5.1.1. Location of metastases (re-staging of melanoma patients when progression was suspected clinically at time of follow-up)

Region	No. of Metastases	PET	Conventional Diagnostics[a]
Brain	02	02	02
Cervical lymph nodes	12	12	08
Lungs	23	16	20
Mediastinum/hilus (lymph nodes)	07	05	01
Liver	04	04	03
Abdomen	15	15	04
Abdominal lymph nodes	06	06	05
Peripheral lymph nodes	35	34	18
Bone	03	03	02
Skin	14	14	06
Total	121	111	69

[a] Conventional Diagnostics = CT, MRI, sonography, conventional x-ray, szintigraphy).

on the number of lesions), but on a patient-by-patient basis, all patients were correctly classified by PET as having pulmonary involvement, and the higher number of metastases found by CT did not influence further therapeutic management. For the evaluation of peripheral lymph nodes, PET is also superior to conventional diagnostics (PET 97.1 % vs. CD 51.4 %) as numerous metastases were detected at unexpected sites. In 4 patients, a successful lymph node dissection was performed on the basis of PET findings, which confirms the need for whole-body evaluation. Conventional procedures examine only single regions and thus may overlook metastases in atypical locations. A disadvantage of FDG PET is that acute inflammatory processes and abszesses show also an increased glucose metabolism which can mimick metastases and therefore reduce the general high specificity. Another limitation is the detection of brain metastases: due to high cerebral glucose uptake, small metastases can be overlooked, therefore MRI is the procedure of choice.

PET is still an expensive staging technique. However, recent studies showed (Rigo et al. 1996; Yao et al. 1994) considerable savings by replacing conventional diagnostics. For example, von Schulthess et al. (1998) realized a cost savings of 11.4 % by using whole-body PET for the staging of high-risk melanoma. Because of its diagnostic superiority (and positive cost-benefit analysis),

Table 5.1.2. Patient- and metastasis-related sensitivity (SE), specificity (SP), and diagnostic accuracy (ACC) in the follow-up of melanoma patients

	F18-FDG whole-body PET [%]			Conventional Diagnostics [%] (CT, MRI, radiography, sonography, scintigraphy)		
	SE	SP	ACC	SE	SP	ACC
In terms of patients	100	95.5	97.9	84.6	68.2	77.1
In terms of metastases	91.8	94.4	92.1	57.5	45	55.7

SE = sensitivity; SP = specificity, ACC = Diagnostic accuracy.

Table 5.1.3. Sensitivity (*SE*), specificity (*SP*) and diagnostic accuracy (*ACC*) in melanoma patients (progression suspected clinically) according to different regions (given as percentage and as absolute number of lesions)

	PET			Conventional Diagnostics		
Region	SE	SP	ACC	SE	SP	ACC
Brain	100% (2/2)	100% (13/13	100% (15/15)	100% (2/2)	100% (13/13)	100% (15/15)
Cervical lymph nodes	100% (12/12)	100% (13/13)	100% (25/25)	66,6% (8/12)	100% (13/13)	84% (21/25)
Lungs (parenchyma)	69,9% (16/23)	100% (14/14)	81,1% (30/37)	87% (20/23)	100% (14/14)	91,9% (34/37)
Mediastinum/hilus (lymph nodes)	71,4% (5/7)	100% (13/13)	90% (18/20)	20% (1/5)	86,6% (13/15)	70% (14/20)
Liver	100% (4/4)	100% (16/16)	100% (20/20)	60% (3/5)	86,6% (13/15)	80% (16/20)
Abdomen	100% (15/15)	94,4% (17/18)	97% (32/33)	26,6% (4/15)	77,7% (14/18)	54,5% (18/33)
Abdominal lymph nodes	100% (6/6)	100% (13/13)	100% (19/19)	83,3% (5/6)	100% (13/13)	94,7% (18/19)
Peripheral lymph nodes	97,1% (34/35)	100% (14/14)	97,9% (48/49)	51,4% (18/35)	92,9% (13/14)	63,3% (31/49)
Bone	100% (3/3)	100% (14/14)	100% (17/17)	66,6% (2/3)	92,9% (13/14)	88,2% (15/17)
Skin	100% (14/14)	100% (13/13)	100% (27/27)	42,9% (6/14)	100% (13/13)	70,4% (19/27)

Table 5.1.4. Recommendations of the 2nd Oncological Consensus Conference (Ulm, September 1997) for malignant melanoma

Malignant Melanoma[a]	Category
Primary tumor	3
Local recurrence	3
Lymph node staging (Breslow >1,5 mm)	1a
Distant metastases (Breslow >1,5 mm)	1a
Therapy follow up	2b

[a]Classification:
1a Appropriate and clinically usefull
1b Acceptable; peer-reviewed publications support clinical usefulness
2a Possibly helpful but benefit is not as well documented
2b No evaluation possible (to date) due to lack of data
3 Generally without benefit

FDG PET has been reimbursed by the health service in Switzerland for some time now. In the Federal Republic of Germany, FDG PET has been accorded Class Ia status for high risk melanoma (Table 5.1.4) by an oncological consensus conference (Ulm,1997), and for this indication it is reimbursed by the health insurance system upon request.

The present results indicate clearly the superiority of PET (except in brain metastases) according to a higher sensitivity, specificity and diagnostic accuracy. Therefore PET is an excellent imaging technique which can replace conventional imaging for staging high risk malignant melanoma and in the follow-up of melanoma patients with suspected recurrence.

References

Adler LP, Crowe JP, al-Kaisi NK, Sunshine JL (1993) Evaluation of breast masses and axillary lymph nodes with (F18)-2-deoxy-2-fluoro-D-Glucose PET. Radiology 187: 743–750

Armstrong BK, Kricker A (1993) How much melanoma is caused by sun exposure? Mel Res 3: 395–401

Balch CM (1988) The role of elective lymph node dissection in melanoma: rationale, results, and controversie. J Clin Oncol 6: 163–172

Blessing C, Feine U, Geiger L, Carl M, Rassner G, Fierlbeck G (1995) Positron emission tomography and ultrasonography – a comparative retrospective study assessing the diagnostic validity in lymph node metastases of malignant melanoma. Arch Dermatol 131: 1394–1398

Böni R (1996) Whole-body positron emission tomography: an accurate staging modality for metastatic melanoma. Arch Dermatol 132: 833–834

Böni R, Huch-Böni R, Steinert H, Dummer R, Burg G, von Schulthess GK (1995a) Anti-melanoma monoclonal antibody 225.28 S immunoscintigraphy in metastatic melanoma. Dermatology 191: 119–123

Böni R, Huch-Böni RA, Steinert H et al. (1995b) Staging of metastatic melanoma by whole-body positron emission tomography using 2-fluorine-18-fluoro-2-deoxy-D-glucose. Br J Dermatol 132: 556–562

Böni R, Huch-Böni RA, Steinert H, von Schulthess GK, Burg G (1996) Early detection of melanoma metastasis using fludeoxyglucose F 18 positron emission tomography. Arch Dermatol 132: 875–876

Boring CC, Squires TS, Tong T, Montgomery S (1994) Cancer statistics. CA Cancer J C 44: 7–26

Breslow A (1970) Thickness, cross-sectional areas and depth of invasion in the prognosis of cutaneous melanoma. Ann Surg 172: 902–908

Buzaid AC, Sandler AB, Mani S et al. (1993) Role of computed tomography in the staging of malignant melanoma. J Clin Oncol 11: 638–43

Chin R, Ward R, Keyes JW et al. (1995) Mediastinal staging of non-small-cell lung cancer with positron emission tomography. Am J Respir Crit Care 152: 2090–2096

Divigi CR, Larson SM (1989) Radiolabelled monoclonal antibodies in the diagnosis and treatment of malignant melanoma. Semin Nucl Med: 252–261

Fornage BD, Lorigan JG (1989) Sonographic detection and fine-needle aspiration biopsy of nonpalpable recurrent or metastatic melanoma in subcutaneous tissues. J Ultrasound Med 8: 421–424

Friedman RJ, Rigel DS, Silverman MK, Kopf AW, Vossaert KA (1991) Malignant melanoma in the 1990's. CA Cancer J Clin 41: 201–206

Godellas CV, Berman CG, Lyman G et al. (1995) The identification and mapping of melanoma regional nodal metastases: Minimally invasive surgery for the diagnosis of nodal metastases. Am Surg 61: 97–101

Gritters LS, Francis IR, Zasadny KR, Wahl RL (1993) Initial assessment of positron emission tomography using 2-fluorine-18-fluoro-2-deoxy-d-glucose in the imaging of malignant melanoma. J Nucl Med 34: 1420–7

Grünwald F, Schomburg A, Bender H et al. (1996) Fluorine-18 fluorodeoxyglucose positron emission tomography in the follow-up of differentiated thyroid cancer. Eur J Nucl Med 23: 312–319

Harris MN, Shapiro RL, Roses DF (1995) Malignant melanoma primary surgical management (excision and node dissection) based on pathology and staging. Cancer Suppl 75: 715–725

Haubold-Reuter BG, Duewell S, Schilcher BR, Marincek B, von Schulthess GK (1993) The value of bone scintigraphy and fast spin-echo magnetic resonance imaging in staging of patients with malignant solid tumors: a prospective study. Eur J Nucl Med 20: 1063–1069

Horgan K, Hughes LE (1993) Staging of melanoma. Clin Radiol 48: 297–300

Johnson N, Mant D, Newton J, Yudkin PL (1994) Role of primary care in the prevention of malignant melanoma. Br J Gen Pract 44: 523–526

Kagan R, Witt T, Bines S, Mesleh G, Economou S (1988) Gallium-67 scanning for malignant melanoma. Cancer 61: 272–274

Katsambas A, Nicolaidou E (1996) Cutaneous malignant melanoma and sun exposure – recent developments in epidemiology. Arch Dermatol 132: 444–450

Koh HK (1991) Cutaneous melanoma. N Engl J Med 325: 171–182

Kopf AW, Gross DF, Rogers GS et al. (1987) Prognostic index for malignant melanoma. Cancer 59: 1236–1241

Lyons JH, Cockerell CJ (1994) Elective lymph node dissection for melanoma. J Am Acad Dermatol 30: 467–480

MacKie RM, Hole DJ (1996) Incidence and thickness of primary tumours and survival of patients with cutaneous malignant melanoma in relation to socioeconomic status. BMJ 312: 1125–1128

Melia J, Cooper EJ, Frost T et al. (1995) Cancer Research Campaign health education programme to promote the early detection of cutaneous malignant melanoma. II Characteristics and incidence of melanoma. Br J Dermatol 132: 414–421

Reintgen, D (1998) Sentinel node biopsy: the accurate staging of the patient with melanoma. The Seventh World congress on Cancers of the Skin, Rome, 22–25 April 1998

Rigo P, Paulus P, Kaschten BJ et al. (1996) Oncological applications of positron emission tomography with fluorine-18 fluorodeoxyglucose. Eur J Nucl Med 23: 1641–1674

Rinne D, Baum RP Hör G, Kaufmann R (1998) Primary staging and follow-up of high-risk melanoma patients by whole-body F-18-FDG positron-emission-tomography (PET): results of a prospective study in 100 patients. Cancer 82: 1664–1671

Rogers GS, Kopf AW, Rigel DS et al. (1983) Effect of anatomical location on prognosis in patients with clinical stage I melanoma. Arch Dermatol 119: 644–649

Sasaki M, Ichiya Y, Kuwabara Y et al. (1996) The usefulness of FDG positron emission tomography for the detection of lymph node metastases in patients with non-small cell lung cancer: a comparative study with X-ray computed tomography. Eur J Nucl Med 23: 741–747

Schneider JS, Moore DH, Sagebiel RW (1994) Risk factors for melanoma incidence in prospective follow-up. Arch Dermatol 130: 1002–1007
Scott WJ, Gobar LS, Terry JD, Dewan NA, Sunderland JJ (1996) Mediastinal lymph node staging of non-small-cell lung cancer: a prospective comparison of computed tomography and positron emission tomography. J Thor Cardiovasc Surg 111: 642–648
Scotto J, Pitcher H, Lee JAH (1991) Indications of future decreasing trends in skin-melanoma mortality among whites in the United States. Int J Cancer 49: 490–497
Shreve PD, Grossman HB, Gross MD, Wahl RL (1996) Metastasic prostate cancer: initial findings of PET with 2-Deoxy-2-[F-18]fluoro-D-glucose. Radiology 199: 751–756
Steinert HC, Huch-Böni RA, Buck A et al. (1995) Malignant melanoma: staging with whole-body positron emission tomography and 2-(F-18)-Fluoro-2-deoxy-D-glucose. Radiology 195: 705–709
Steinert HC, Ullrich SP, Böni R, von Schulthess GK, Dummer R (1998) Kosteneffektivität beim Staging des malignen Melanoms: Vergleich Ganzkörper-PET versus Konventionelles Staging. Nuklearmedizin 37: A37 [Abstr]
Stoelben E, Sturm J, Schmoll J, Keilholz U, Saeger HD (1995) Resektion von solitären Lebermetastasen des malignen Melanoms. Chirurg 66: 40–43
Vollmer RT (1989) Malignant melanoma: a multivariate analysis of prognostic factors. Pathol Ann 24: 383–407
von Schulthess GK, Steinert HC, Dummer R, Weder W: Cost-Effectiveness of whole-body PET imaging in non-small cell lung cancer and malignant melanoma. Acad Radiol 1998; 5 (suppl 2) S300–S302
Yao WJ, Hoh JA, Glaspy F (1994) Whole-body FDG PET imaging for staging of malignant melanoma: is it cost effective? J Nucl Med 35: 8P

5.2 Head and Neck Tumors

C. Laubenbacher, R. J. Kau, C. Alexiou, W. Arnold, and M. Schwaiger

5.2.1 Introduction

Incidence, Histology, Prognosis

The incidence of ENT tumors has been increasing worldwide in recent years (Steiner 1993). The vast majority of head and neck tumors are squamous cell carcinomas that in some cases exhibit precancerous precursors. These can develop by way of non-invasive carcinomas (carcinoma in situ) into invasive carcinomas, which are classified according to their degree of differentiation as G1 (well differentiated), G2 (somewhat differentiated), G3 (poorly differentiated), or G4 (undifferentiated). Tobacco and alcohol consumption, poor oral hygiene and mechanical irritation (from dental prostheses, for example) have been described as predisposing factors for tumors of the upper GI tract (Spitz 1994). Non-squamous-cell head and neck carcinomas (salivary gland carcinoma, lymphogenous and odontogenic tumors, etc.) account for only 5 % of head and neck carcinomas and will not be considered here.

Both the prognosis and the therapy of choice are determined by site and local-regional spread of the primary tumor and any lymph node metastases. As a rule of thumb, the larger the primary tumor, the worse the prognosis. Thus, early T-1 tumors on the glottis or lips boast 5-year survival rates of up to 80 %, whereas advanced stages have a bad prognosis with survival rates between 10 % and 15 % (Baredes et al. 1993).

Recurrences appear in large numbers during the first two years, and for this reason it is essential that thorough oncological aftercare be provided during this period. It is likewise important to bear in mind that 20–30 % of patients with a head and neck tumor will develop a second carcinoma in the upper aerodigestive tract (Fitzpatrick et al. 1984; Black et al. 1983).

The most common cause of therapy failure is a local-regional recurrence or a primarily unresectable primary tumor that could not be locally controlled. Distant metastases appear fairly infrequently at the time of initial treatment, but in cases of therapeutic failure, they appear in as many as 60 % of cases, depending on localization. In particular, the highest incidence of distant metastases is associated with primary tumors of the hypopharyngeal region, followed by carcinomas at the base and tip of the tongue (Kotwall et al. 1987).

Therapy

There are few controlled prospective studies comparing differing therapy modalities in patients

Table 5.2.1. Staging of lip, oral cavity, pharynx, larynx, and maxillary sinus carcinomas (according to Hermanek and Sobin 1992). Note: malignant tumors of the salivary glands and thyroid have not been considered due to their different histology; a different staging is used for these tumor entities

Stage	T	N	M
0	is	0	0
I	1	0	0
II	2	0	0
III	1	1	0
	2	1	0
	3	0/1	0
IV	4	0/1	0
	any	2/3	0
	any	any	1

with head and neck tumors. For this reason it is difficult to provide general therapeutic recommendations for different tumor sites and stages. The best thing at the moment is to base treatment recommendations on the classification of tumors by stages (Table 5.2.1). In general, Stage I and Stage II tumors respond more or less equally well to both radiation and surgery, and given the appropriate local experience and availability that therapy should be preferred that is likely to lead to the smallest possible loss of function.

Stage III and operable Stage IV tumors are generally treated with a combination of surgery and radiation. Organ-preserving laser techniques are also being used increasingly to control tumors locally. Since only very limited survival rates can be achieved with currently available methods, these patients should be referred to a clinical therapeutic trial. With inoperable Stage IV tumors, palliative radiation is generally recommended. Because of the bad prognosis, these patients should also be referred if at all possible to clinical trials offering combined radiation and chemotherapy.

Scope of Examination

ENT physicians also debate which examinations are necessary for pre-therapeutic decision-making. According to the guidelines of the Deutsche Gesellschaft für Hals-Nasen-Ohrenheilkunde und Kopf- und Halschirurgie, the German Society for ENT Medicine and Head and Neck Surgery, necessary examinations include palpation, survey of ENT status and panendoscopy with a biopsy (see overview below).

Guidelines
for Laryngeal Carcinoma (Examinations) issued by the German Society for ENT Medicine, Head and Neck Surgery (1997)

- Necessary:
  - Palpation of soft tissue of the neck (lymph node metastases, tumor invasion)
  - ENT status
  - Indirect laryngoscopy (tumor spread, vocal cord motility)
  - Ultrasound of the soft tissue of the neck (regional metastases)
  - Chest radiography
  - Direct laryngoscopy/microlaryngoscopy (extent of tumor, infiltration)
  - Panendoscopy (ruling out a synchronous second cancer)
  - Biopsy
- Useful in certain cases:
  - Stroboscopy
  - CT/MRI: larynx, neck (extent of tumor, tumor invasion, metastases)
  - Interdisciplinary examinations: tumor staging (i.e., chest CT, abdominal sonography)

It is essential that esophagoscopy follows panendoscopy, since in 10–15 % of cases a synchronous second tumor is present, most often in the esophagus or the bronchial system (McGuirt 1982). In individual cases, morphologically oriented imaging techniques such as CT and MRI or so-called "interdisciplinary examinations" like chest CT and abdominal sonography are included (Deutsche Gesellschaft für Hals-Nasen-Ohrenheilkunde und Kopf- und Halschirurgie 1997).

5.2.2 Significance of PET

Differential Diagnosis, Detection of Primary Tumor

The initial diagnostics of ENT tumors includes both the differential diagnostic delineation of benign and malignant changes and determination of the tumor stage (especially in the case of malignancies confirmed by biopsy). Nearly all patients with head and neck tumors present with local symptoms (difficulties in speaking or swallowing). In about half the cases, the primary tumor can be found upon simple inspection. A further 45 % of primary tumors are discovered through indirect laryngoscopy or panendoscopy. Because of the superficial position of head or neck tumors, bioptic removal of tissue is usually unproblematic. Although numerous studies (Seifert et al. 1992; Benchaou et al. 1996; Braams et al. 1995; Laubenbacher et al. 1995; Rege et al. 1994; Wong et al. 1996) show that squamous cell carcinomas of the head and neck region exhibit an extraordinarily high FDG uptake and are therefore very easily imaged using PET, an elaborate examination technique like PET will not be necessary for detection or status determination of the primary tumor for the reasons noted above.

Even after careful performance of the preoperative examinations, a primary tumor cannot be found in approximately 5 % of patients; their tumor-involved cervical lymph nodes are the only manifestation of neoplastic disease. The diagnosis CUP (carcinoma of unknown primary) can only be made after a thorough examination of not only the head and neck regions, but also the esophagus, the lungs and the urogenital tract. With these patients, a methodical search for distant metastases (lungs, liver, bone) is also necessary, since the detection of metastases would dramatically alter the further course of therapy (de Braud and Al-Sarraf 1993). These patients are generally referred for radical neck dissection and/or definitive radiation, depending on local-regional involvement.

Numerous FDG PET studies have shown that head and neck tumors exhibit a very high FDG uptake. In general, these studies were not primarily directed at the visualization of unknown primary tumors. However, individual patients were included in these studies whose primary tumors were unknown before the PET scan. Rege (Rege et al. 1994) reported the successful visualization of two of four primary tumors that had eluded MRI, and Bailet (Bailet et al. 1992) also emphasizes in his work that a superficial primary tumor on the tip of the tongue eluded both MRI and CT, but was flawlessly imaged by PET. In addition to these publications, which are based on reports of individual cases, two other studies have been published that were directed specifically at the search for occult primary tumors. They were successful in detecting tumors in 9 of 19 cases (47 %) (Mukherji et al. 1996) and in 4 of 16 cases (25 %) (Schipper et al. 1996). Including the individual case reports also listed in Table 5.2.2, 45 published cases can be reviewed. The consolidated success rate of almost 50 % for a procedure performed as a diagnostic ultima ratio justifies the use of FDG PET for this indication (referred to as a 1a indication; see also Table 5.2.3).

Table 5.2.2. FDG PET studies in patients with an unknown primary tumor and histologically verified lymph node involvement in the head and neck region

Author	Primary Tumors Found	Of
Bailet et al. (1992)	1	1[a]
Jabour et al. (1993)	1	1[a]
Lindholm et al. (1993)	1	1[a]
Greven et al. (1994)	2	2[a]
Mukherji et al. (1994)	1	1[a]
Rege et al. (1994)	2	4[a]
Mukherji et al. (1996)	9	19[b]
Schipper et al. (1996)	4	16[b]
Total	21	45
	46.7 %	

[a] Study was not directed at detection of unknown primary tumors.
[b] Study was directed at detection of unknown primary tumors.

Table 5.2.3. Significance of PET, categorized by indication for head and neck tumors. Result of the PET Oncology Consensus Conference, Ulm, 1997. (After Reske, 1997)[a]

Indication	Classification
Search for unknown primary tumor, assuming otherwise negative imaging and current histology	1a
Lymph node staging (resectable primary tumor)	1b
Local recurrence (three months after radiation therapy)	2a
Lymph node staging (unresectable primary tumor)	2b
Second carcinoma	2b
Therapy monitoring	2b
Primary tumor diagnostics (Exception: see 1a)	3

[a] Classification Categories (according to a report of the American College of Cardiology 1995): *1a* Appropriate and clinically useful; *1b* Acceptable; preponderance of research supports clinical usefulness; *2a* Possibly helpful but benefit is not as well documented; *2b* No evaluation possible (to date) due to lack of data; *3* Generally without benefit.

Staging of Primary Tumor

Squamous cell carcinomas of the upper GI tract arise on the surface of the mucous membrane and spread along that surface, as well as by infiltrative growth along the deeper neck structures. T-staging of extracranial head and neck tumors is therefore based on morphological criteria (Hermanek and Sobin 1992) that determine the resectability of the tumors and consequently the primary choice of therapy. Exact T-staging is an absolute prerequisite for evaluating operability and planning the surgical approach. Superficial spreading can be adequately evaluated by (endoscopic) visual inspection. There is also the possibility of a diagnostic biopsy and histological analysis. The depth and the involvement of different cervical compartments can be evaluated by palpation and morphologically oriented imaging techniques (Wagner-Manslau et al. 1992; van den Brekel et al. 1994; and Kau et al. 1994).

Because of the primary tumor's high FDG uptake, as noted above, it is very possible to image it using FDG PET, but because of the lack of anatomical information a differentiation for purposes of T-staging is not possible with PET. Morphologically oriented imaging techniques result in correct T-staging in approximately 80–90 % of cases for CT (Steinkamp et al. 1993; Lenz et al. 1989) and for MRI (Steinkamp et al. 1993; Glazer et al. 1986). These good results were obtained with a population of patients with larger tumors. With smaller tumors (T1 and T2), these procedures are inferior to endoscopy. But endoscopy cannot satisfactorily determine the depth of large tumors. In a study of ours in which MRI, endoscopy and PET were compared, PET overestimated the size of the primary tumor in 47 % of the cases (Laubenbacher et al. 1995) and was therefore clearly inferior to endoscopy and MRI. The overestimation of tumor spread was attributable to the fact that FDG is also taken up to some degree by normal mucosa (Jabour et al. 1993).

To summarize, it can be stated as regards T-staging using PET that as a functionally orientated procedure PET cannot provide the exact anatomical information necessary for T-staging. It remains to be seen whether progress in hardware and software development can bring about an improvement through the increasing possibility of overlaying CT or MRI images and PET images to form an "anatometabolic fusion image" (Wahl et al. 1993). However, promising results have already been reported (Wong et al. 1996).

Detection of Local-Regional Lymph Node Involvement

Most clinically diagnosed tumors of the head and neck region have already undergone lymphogenic metastatic spread. This type of spread is of great prognostic significance, since the survival rate sinks by approximately one-half upon detection of lymph node involvement (Batsakis 1984). Moreover, ENT tumors are late to metastasize hematogenically, so that the detection of local-regional tumor spread and especially regional lymph node metastases has great therapeutic relevance (Dillon and Harnsberger 1991). N-staging is especially important in patients for whom neck dissection is being considered (Quetz et al. 1991).

Methods available for lymph node staging include palpation as part of the clinical examination and also morphologically oriented imaging techniques such as sonography, CT and MRI. Common to all these methods is the fact that lymph node size is included as an evaluation criterion. Depending on lymph node size, which is used to define the cut-off for malignant involvement, a decrease in specificity must be accepted in order to achieve increased sensitivity. Histopathological studies (Eichhorn et al. 1987) have shown that more than 40 % of lymph node metastases are located in lymphnodes less than 1.0 cm in diameter, and that 12 % of all tumor-positive neck dissection specimens revealed an involvement that was only microscopic in size (Feinmesser et al. 1992; Som 1992).

There is disagreement regarding the value of morphological imaging (sonography, CT, MRI) (overviews: van den Brekel et al. 1994; Dillon and Harnsberger 1991). The sensitivities and specificities reported for these diagnostic methods vary between 40 % and 90 %. Sensitivities as high as 96 % were reported for sonography (Gritzmann 1992), but specificity dropped to 53 %. If either lymph node diameter > 1.5 cm or a central inhomogeneity is used as a criterion of malignancy for CT and MRI (Dillon and Harnsberger 1991), a sensitivity of 92 % and a specificity of 73 % can be achieved (Gritzmann 1992). But it should also be noted that a central inhomogeneity can only be detected with adequate certainty when the lymph node diameter is > 1.5 cm (Quetz et al. 1991).

As a functional-morphological technique for lymph node staging of squamous cell carcinoma of the extra-cranial head and neck region, PET proves to be independent of lymph node size. The example of a patient (Fig. 5.2.1) with a carcinoma of the base of the tongue on the right side that crosses the midline shows a metastatically involved ipsilateral lymph node approximately 1.5 cm in diameter. Two more lymph nodes, lying barely caudal and dorsal to the first and measuring approximately 7 mm each in diameter, were not revealed by MRI. Because of increased FDG uptake, additional lymph node metastases had to be suspected, and these were confirmed by the histological analysis. As shown in Table 5.2.4, PET attains a sensitivity of between 72 and 91 %, and a specificity of between 88 and 99 % when applied to individual lymph nodes, and is thus clearly superior to morphologically-orientated imaging techniques such as CT and MRI (Benchaou et al 1996; Laubenbacher et al. 1995). Recently, sufficient patient numbers have been reported to attest to the fact that surgical planning for resectable primary tumors (i.e., the question of single versus double neck dissection and the type of neck dissection) can be decided or at least facilitated by PET (1b indication). By the same token, PET could be used for radiation therapy field planning for inoperable patients. However, it is still unclear whether tailoring radiation fields to individuals could be of sufficient value to justify the use of PET for a patient population with such a bad prognosis. In principle, one might envisage a dose escalation for a smaller target area, which PET could define. However, until the results of studies of this type are available, PET remains a "2b indication" in lymph node staging for unresectable primary tumors.

Detection of Distant Metastases, Synchronous and Second Tumors

Hematogenic distant metastases appear relatively infrequently with head and neck tumors at the time of the initial diagnosis. Only when local therapy has failed and neoplastic disease has advanced hematogenic metastases can be found in up to 60 % of cases, generally affecting the lungs, liver, and skeleton. At these sites they can be detected with a high degree of diagnostic accuracy using conventional diagnostic methods. Normally, however, local findings continue to determine therapy and prognosis due to local-regional complications. For this reason there is only a lim-

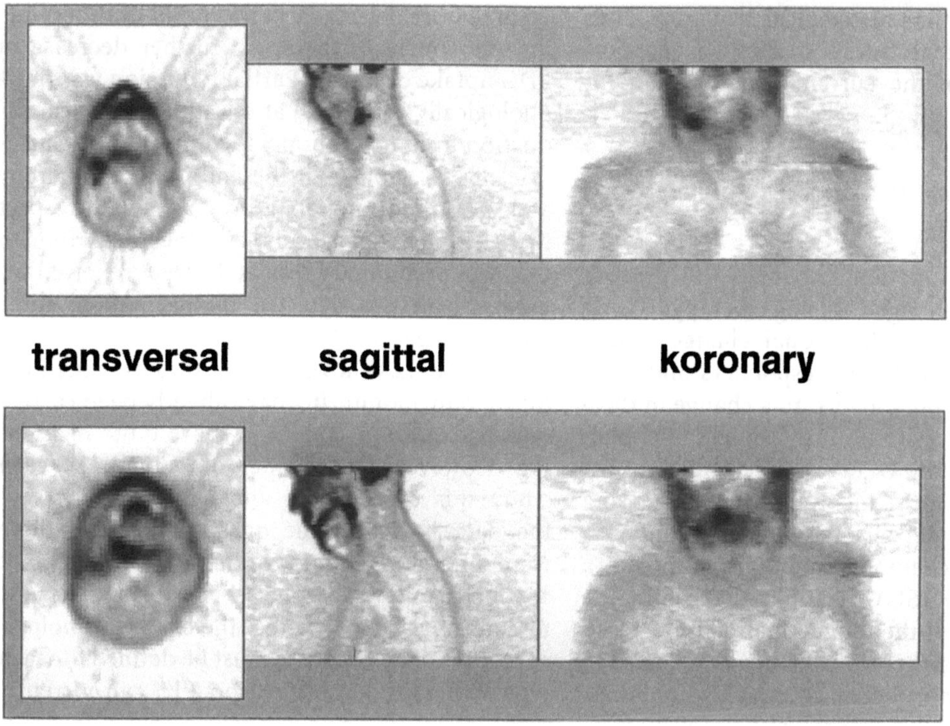

Fig. 5.2.1. FDG in a patient with a carcinoma at the base of the tongue on the right side, crossing the midline, in transverse, sagittal and coronary views, respectively. Top row: centered on the lymph node metastases. Bottom row: centered on the primary tumor. In addition to the lymph node metastasis approximately 1.5 cm in diameter that is also detectable with MRI, PET also shows two other lymph nodes with intense accumulations lying barely caudal and dorsal to the first. Metastatic involvement of these lymph nodes was also verified histologically

ited indication for using PET to search for distant metastases in patients with head and neck tumors (2b indication).

A similar situation exists in the 10–15 % of all patients with head and neck tumors who manifest a synchronous tumor of the upper aerodigestive tract at the time of first diagnosis. The majority of these synchronous tumors are localized in the esophagus (McGuirt 1982), and are detectable during the initial diagnosis by means of an esophagoscopy performed in conjunction with the requisite panendoscopy. 20–30 % of patients develop a second tumor in chronological conjunction with a local recurrence, which generally occurs within the first two years after the primary therapy (Fitzpatrick et al. 1984; Black et al. 1983). Endoscopic access can be more difficult with these previously treated patients, which would justify the use of PET. While no satisfactory studies have yet been published on the detection of distant metastases or second tumors, we can still assume that the high FDG uptake of primary tumors is applicable to second tumors, which gen-

Table 5.2.4. ^{18}F-FDG PET results from lymph node staging studies of head and neck tumors

Author	n	Sensitivity [%]	Specificity [%]
Bailet et al. (1992)	16	86	98
Jabour et al. (1993)	12	74	98
Braams et al. (1995)	12	91	88
Laubenbacher et al. (1995)	22	90	96
Benchaou et al. (1996)	48	72	99
Kau et al. (1998)	60	87	92

erally have a similar histological structure. Thus we can expect that future studies will support the upgrading of the current 2b indication for second tumors.

Therapy Monitoring, Detection of Local Recurrence, Prognosis

We expect that functional changes will precede morphological changes during therapy. Using PET to image these functional changes could help differentiate between responders and non-responders early on and lead to a change in therapeutic approach with non-responders, if applicable. Figure 5.2.2 shows an example from our own patient population of therapy monitoring using FDG PET. Only seven days after the initiation of combination chemotheraphy (cisplatin/taxol), the FDG uptake (SUV: 18.7) in the carcinoma on the left edge of the tongue that had increased massively prior to therapy had already dropped to one third. No morphological changes in tumor volume were detectable at this point in time. During the course of therapy a further decrease in FDG uptake occurred. Partial remission was morphologically confirmed at that time by a clear reduction in tumor volume. Incomplete normalization of FDG uptake at the end of chemotherapy appears to indicate a bad prognosis with respect to development of a local recurrence, according to our own preliminary results. Indeed, renewed tumor growth was detected in this patient three months later.

As table 5.2.5 shows, several studies using FDG for therapy monitoring have already been carried out. The authors' conclusions are quite heartening. However, the number of patients in each study was quite small, and a meta-analysis of the data is out of the question because there were differences in form of therapy and the point at which a follow-up exam was performed. Results to date appear to show that the exact chronological course of FDG uptake must be defined for each type of therapy. For this reason, PET can currently

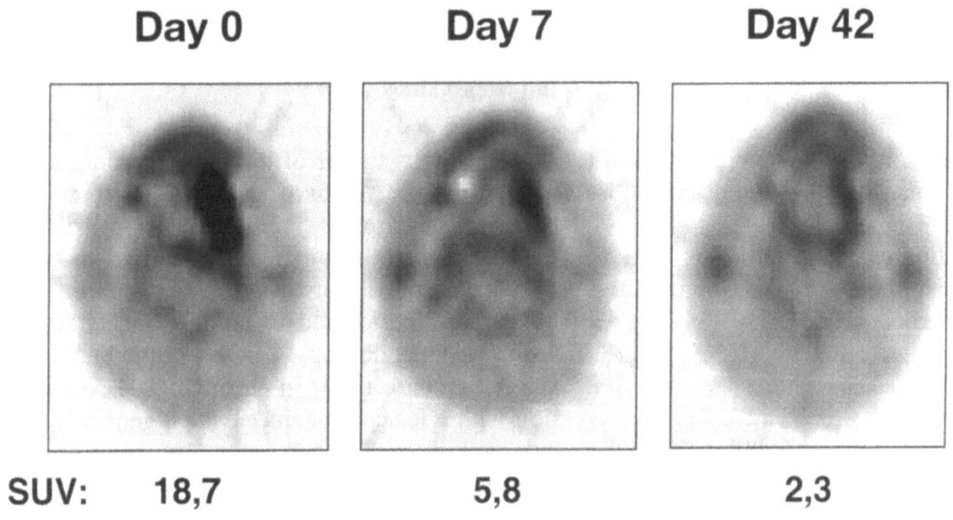

Fig. 5.2.2. Therapy monitoring during combination chemotherapy (cisplatin/taxol) using FDG PET (transverse views) of a patient with a carcinoma on the left edge of the tongue. Massively increased FDG uptake before therapy (SUV: 18.7) dropped to one-third of that level after only seven days. At that time there was no detectable morphological change in tumor volume. During the course of chemotherapy there was a further reduction in FDG uptake. Partial remission was then confirmed morphologically by a significant decrease in tumor volume. Incomplete normalization of FDG uptake at the end of chemotherapy (SUV: 2.3) appears to indicate a bad prognosis with respect to development of a local recurrence, according to our own preliminary results. Indeed, renewed tumor growth was recorded in this patient three months later

Table 5.2.5. FDG PET studies in therapy monitoring of head and neck tumors (Rtx = radiation therapy; Ctx = chemotherapy)

Author	n	Therapy	Point in Time	Result/Author's Conclusions
Minn et al. (1988)	19	Rtx	Immediately after Rtx (30 Gy)	Significant decrease in FDG uptake in responders
Seifert et al. (1992)	10	Ctx	After Ctx	Linear relationship between change in FDG uptake and growth rate of tumor
Haberkorn et al. (1993)	11	Ctx	After 1 cycle	High correlation between growth rate and FDG uptake
Rege et al. (1993)	11	Rtx	During and immediately after Rtx	Good differentiation between responders and non-responders
Berlangieri et al. (1994)	6	Ctx + Rtx	During and after 24 mos.	Suitable for recognizing early response; after two years for recurrence diagnostics
Greven et al. (1994)	25	Rtx	1 and 4 mos. after Rtx	One month: too unspecified; four months to detection of early recurrence
Reisser et al. (1995)	12	Ctx	After first cycle	Good differentiation between responders and non-responders
Chaiken et al. (1993)	15	Rtx	"During aftercare"	Suitable for evaluating local control

only be classified as a 2b indication for therapy monitoring.

Local recurrences appear in large numbers during the first two years and are difficult to detect with morphologically-orientated techniques because of the changes induced by therapy and altered anatomy. For the same reasons, it is frequently impossible to differentiate clearly between scar and recurrence. In addition, the tissue is vulnerable after therapy, which increases the rate of complications from biopsies. A non-invasive procedure is therefore desirable.

Fig. 5.2.3 shows the example of a patient with an extensive local recurrence at the base of the tongue. In addition to detecting the local recurrence, here PET also offers advantages as a whole-body examination technique. The detection of several lung metastases on the right side, which were not detected until the PET scan was made, led to a palliative approach instead of the radical local surgery that was originally planned and would have been associated with considerable loss of function. Table 5.2.6 provides an overview of studies carried out to date using FDG for local recurrence diagnosis. Half of the studies involved radiation exclusively, and half used a combined radiation/chemotherapy. The point at which the examination was performed varied from two months to several years. The results that were achieved are very encouraging. For the most part, they resolved the so-called "diagnostic problem cases," – that is, cases where morphologically-oriented techniques performed prior to PET yielded equivocal results. Yet it should be noted that a period of at least three months must elapse between radiation and PET, since inflammatory changes resulting from radiation therapy could otherwise be misinterpreted as recurrences. But a 2a indication can be derived from the good results described above and from the diagnostic uncertainties of other techniques and the increased rate of complications from biopsies.

For glioma (Di Chiro 1986), soft tissue sarcoma (Griffeth et al. 1992) and non-Hodgkins lymphoma (Okada et al. 1992), a correlation has already been described between the degree of malignancy and prognosis, on the one hand, and for the level of FDG uptake, on the other hand. Indications of a

Table 5.2.6. FDG PET studies in the detection of local recurrence of head and neck tumors. (Ctx = chemotherapy; Rtx = Radiation Therapy; "–" = not provided or calculation not useful)

Author	n	Therapy	Sensitivity [%]	Specificity [%]	Time Elapsed After Therapy
Minn et al. (1993)	1	Ctx + Rtx	–	–	4 yrs.
Greven et al. (1994)	11	Ctx + Rtx	100	100	6 mos.
Rege et al. (1994)	17	Rtx	90	100	mos.
Austin et al. (1995)[a]	10	Ctx + Rtx	67	57	mos.
Bailet et al. (1995)	10	Rtx	100	–	6 wks.
Lapela et al. (1995)	15	Rtx or OP	88	86	4–56 mos.
McGuirt et al. (1995)	13	Rtx	85	–	>3 mos.
Anzai et al. (1996)	12	Rtx	88	100	2–108 mos.

[a] Only "morphological problem cases" were studied; that is, cases where morphologically-oriented imaging techniques such as CT or MRI had yielded no clear pathological findings.

connection between proliferative activity of a tumor and the level of FDG uptake (Haberkorn et al. 1991) are also increasing for squamous cell carcinomas of the head and neck region. A univariate analysis was recently able to show an inverse correlation between prognosis and level of FDG uptake in the primary tumor (Minn et al. 1997). For example, 73 % of patients with a low FDG uptake

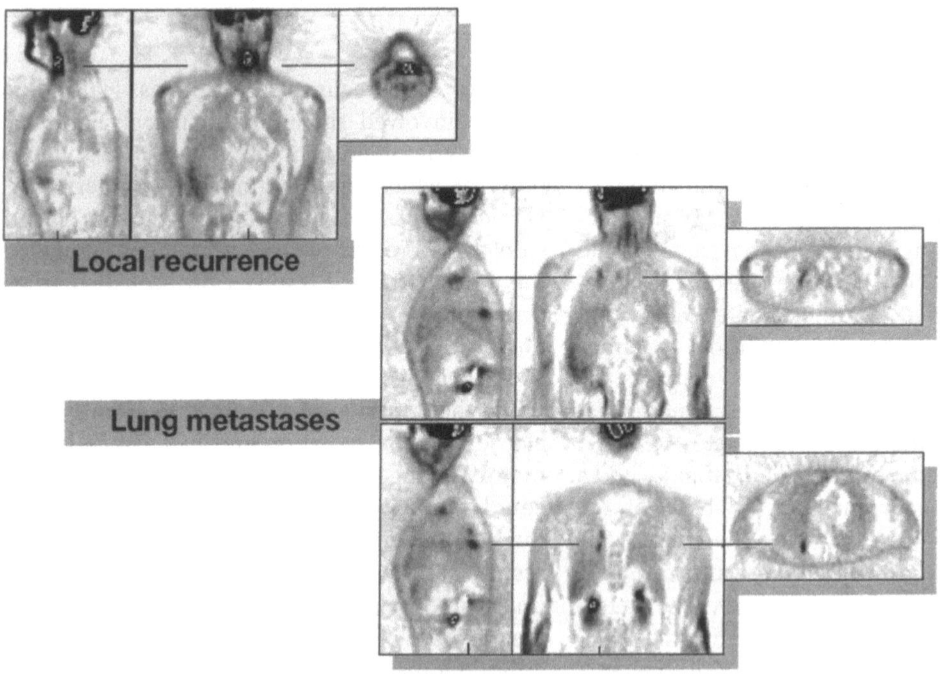

Fig. 5.2.3. Sagittal, coronal and transverse FDG PET images of a patient with an extensive local recurrence on the base of the tongue (*top left*: centered on the local recurrence; *bottom right*: centered on lung metastases). In addition to detecting the local recurrence, here PET also offers advantages as a whole-body examination technique. The detection of several lung metastases on the right side, which were not detected until the PET scan was made, led to a preference for a palliative approach over the radical local surgery that was originally planned and would have been associated with considerable loss of function

in the primary tumor (SUV $\leq$ 9) were still alive after three years compared to only 22 % of the patients with a high FDG uptake (SUV > 9). However, the small number of patients prevents us from excluding the possibility that covariant factors such as tumor size, mitotic count, etc. also influenced these results. A multivariate analysis of these data was not able to identify the extent of FDG uptake as an independent prognosis parameter, and we must therefore wait for further studies.

5.2.3 Study Protocol and Interpretation of PET

In addition to the usual preparations for FDG PET, several specifics should be noted for patients with head and neck tumors. Blood glucose testing, which should be performed on all patients before PET, is absolutely imperative with patients who have head and neck tumors, since a majority of these patients have alcohol problems and do not comply with the sobriety requirements.

The medical history taken prior to a PET examination should include medical intervention to date, since reactive changes – to biopsies, for example – can show increased FDG uptake for up to a week after surgery. Infections of the head and neck region (sinus infections, for example) should also be ruled out clinically, since they can simulate a malignant process and also mask a tumor of the paranasal sinuses. The question regarding prior therapy should be mandatory just as it is for other tumor entities. It is particularly necessary to ask about previous radiation therapy when looking for local recurrences, since prior radiation can lead to unspecific reactive inflammatory changes with increased FDG uptake.

During the 40 to 60 minute waiting period post-injection, patients should be instructed not to exert their speaking and chewing muscles; that is, they should avoid speaking if at all possible and should definitely not chew gum. The patient's position should also be comfortable so that the neck musculature is not strained. The goal of these recommendations is to minimize muscular FDG uptake and thus achieve a better tumor-muscle ratio. The area to be examined should reach from the base of the skull to the lower boundary of the liver so that any second tumors (especially esophageal carcinomas) will definitely be included. In the search for unknown primary tumors it is necessary to expand the field of view down to the symphysis, since in individual cases abdominal malignancies can cause cervical lymph node involvement. Whether attenuation correction as a prerequisite for semiquantitative evaluation justifies the necessary additional imaging time is still a point of dispute. Our own experience has shown that a purely visual evaluation with a focally increased FDG uptake in a typical location as a criterion of malignancy produces results that are identical to semiquantitative criteria (tumor/non-tumor ratio > 2.0 or SUV > 2.0) (Laubenbacher et al. 1995). When evaluating a PET image, the interpreter should note not only the usual information about size and site of the primary tumor but also any expansion across the midline and in the case of lymph nodes, the involved level. In particular, focal FDG increases at locations that cannot be reached during normal neck dissection (nuchal, lateral retroclavicular, deep retrosternal) should receive special attention. The presence of (mostly central) necroses in the primary tumor or the lymph nodes should be noted, since this can affect the surgical strategy. If there is an inhomogeneous accumulation of FDG within the tumor, then the point of maximum FDG concentration should be noted as the most suitable site for biopsy.

As regards possible pitfalls, we should mention in particular the increased muscular FDG uptake in the muscles of the neck as a consequence of an uncomfortable body position. A high uptake in the m. sternocleidomastoideus can be misinterpreted as cervical lymph node involvement, and a high uptake in the medial tract of the autochthonous spine muscles is often interpreted as an involvement of nuchal lymph nodes. It is possible to differentiate between these phenomena by noting the configuration of FDG uptake in a typical muscle track (diagonally laterocranially in m. sterno-

Table 5.2.7. Distinctive features in the execution and evaluation of FDG PET in patients with head and neck tumors

Patient preparation	
Sober	At least 6 hours (blood glucose level? C_2H_5 OH?)
Medical History	Diabetic? Biopsy, surgery, etc? previous therapy (radiation)? Existing or previous infections (sinusitis)
After Injection	No exertion of speaking and chewing muscles (not talking, no chewing gum) Comfortable body position without straining neck muscles
Examination Protocol	
Region	Base of skull to lower boundary of liver (rationale: detection of synchronous and second tumors, especially esophageal carcinomas) If primary tumor unknown: base of skull to symphysis
Lymph nodes	Size Site (level) Distant metastases? synchronous or second tumors?
Pitfalls	**Cause / Remedy**
Patient not sober (C_2H_5 OH?)	Blood glucose test required prior to injection
Biopsy prior to PET simulates tumor	Medical history
Sinusitis masks tumor, simulates tumor	Medical history
Gastritis, esophagitis simulate second tumor	Medical history
Diffuse, high level of FDG uptake in entire upper GI tract	Radiation? Wait at least three months before attempting PET
High FDG uptake in all muscles	Diabetes?
High FDG uptake in chewing and speaking muscles	Chewing gum?
Cervical lymph nodes DD: M. sternocleidomastoideus	Uncomfortable body position? Typical muscle course
Nuchal lymph nodes DD: autochthonic back	Uncomfortable body position? Lobster-mark
musculature	

cleidomastoideus; and a generally laterally symmetrical image in the small neck muscles, also known as a lobster sign). We have already discussed the possibility of a high FDG uptake in the chewing and laryngeal muscles if they are exerted during the waiting period after the injection, as well as the possible masking of a malignancy by an infection such as sinusitis. Gastric and esophageal inflammations can generally be distinguished from a second tumor (stomach carcinoma, esophageal carcinoma) by the rather diffuse distribution pattern of FDG accumulation. And the medical history can offer diagnostic support here as well. A comprehensive overview of the special problems encountered in performing and evaluating PET, including pitfalls, is provided in Table 5.2.7.

Other Radiopharmaceuticals

In addition to FDG, the PET radiopharmaceutical most frequently used as a marker for glucose utilization, other PET radiopharmaceuticals used for head and neck tumors include those for measuring protein incorporation or amino acid transport (^{11}C methionine, ^{11}C leucine and ^{11}C tyrosine), and for measuring DNA replication (^{11}C thymidine). The physiological basis for the use of labeled amino acids is the long-known fact that malignant cells exhibit an increased amino acid uptake and increased protein metabolism (Busch et al. 1959). The use of ^{11}C thymidine makes it possible to directly measure DNA replication as a measure of cell proliferation. This is an extraordinarily important prognostic factor for malignancies (Meyer et al. 1983).

Common to all these radiopharmaceuticals is the fact that a lower uptake than for FDG can theoretically be expected in inflammatory processes, and thus it is easier to differentiate between unspecific reactive changes and a malignant process when making a diagnosis. Initial results for small numbers of cases (van Eijkeren et al. 1992; Lindholm et al. 1993; and Leskinen-Kallio et al. 1994) are comparable to FDG results with respect to the imaging of primary tumors and the detection of lymph node metastases. However, only after studies are available that directly compare both procedures based on a large patient population, we will be able to make definitive statements regarding the extent to which one radiopharmaceutical is preferable to another.

5.2.4 Summary

Squamous cell carcinomas form the vast majority of the extracranial head and neck tumors and exhibit a high FDG uptake. For this reason, PET with FDG is superior to morphologically-oriented techniques such as sonography, CT and MRI in detecting malignant lymph node involvement. If neck dissection is under consideration (usually with resectable primary tumors), then PET can be classified as a 1b indication, since a negative PET result with respect to lymph node involvement could spare the patient the neck dissection. With unresectable primary tumors there is not yet sufficient data to support the use of a smaller radiation field as defined by PET. With unknown primary tumors (an otherwise negative image and current histology), FDG PET is the procedure of choice as a diagnostic ultimaratio and can detect the primary tumor in up to 50 % of cases (1a indication). PET's 2a classification for the detection of local recurrences is based on inadequate differentiation between scar tissue and local recurrence when using morphological techniques and on the increased risk of complications from biopsies of tissue that is vulnerable after therapy. It should be noted that a safety margin of at least three months should be observed after radiation in order to avoid misdiagnosis of postradiogenic inflammatory changes. Sufficient data is not yet available regarding the detection of second carcinomas and the use of PET for therapy monitoring, so that a 2b rating is given at the moment. T-staging in primary tumor diagnostics will continue to remain the realm of high-resolution morphological techniques due to the fact that PET does not provide sufficient anatomical information.

References

Anzai Y, Carroll WR, Quint DJ et al. (1996) Recurrence of head and neck cancer after surgery or irradiation: prospective comparison of 2-deoxy-2-[F-18]fluoro-D-glucose PET and MR imaging diagnoses. Radiology 200: 135–141

Austin JR, Wong FC, Kim EE (1995) Positron emission tomography in the detection of residual laryngeal carcinoma. Otolaryngol Head Neck Surg 113: 404–407

Bailet JW, Sercarz JA, Abemayor E, Anzai Y, Lufkin RB, Hoh CK (1995) The use of positron emission tomography for early detection of recurrent head and neck squamous cell carcinoma in postradiotherapy patients. Laryngoscope 105: 135–139

Bailet JW, Abemayor E, Jabour BA, Hawkins RA, Ho C, Ward P H (1992) Positron emission tomography: a new, precise imaging modality for detection of primary head and neck tumors and assessment of cervical adenopathy. Laryngoscope 102: 281–288

Baredes S, Leeman DJ, Chen TS et al. (1993) Significance of tumor thickness in soft palate carcinoma. Laryngoscope 103: 389–393

Batsakis JG (1984) Tumors of the head and neck: clinical and pathological considerations. Williams & Wilkens, Baltimore

Benchaou M, Lehmann W, Slosman DO et al. (1996) The role of FDG-PET in the preoperative assessment of N-staging in head and neck cancer. Acta Otolaryngol Stockh 116: 332–335

Berlangieri SU, Brizel DM, Scher RL et al. (1994) Pilot study of positron emission tomography in patients with advanced head and neck cancer receiving radiotherapy and chemotherapy. Head Neck 16: 340–346
Black RJ, Gluckman JL, Shumrick DA (1983) Multiple primary tumors of the upper aerodigestive tract. Clin Otolaryngol All Sci 8: 277–281
Braams JW, Pruim J, Freling NJM et al. (1995) Detection of lymph node metastases of squamous-cell cancer of the head and neck with FDG-PET and MRI. J Nucl Med 36: 211–216
de Braud F, Al-Sarraf M (1993) Diagnosis and management of squamous cell carcinoma of unknown primary tumor site of the neck. Sem Oncol 20: 273–278
van den Brekel MW, Castelijns JA, Snow GB (1994) The role of modern imaging studies in staging and therapy of head and neck neoplasms. Semin Oncol 1994; 21:340–348
Busch H, Davis JR, Honig GR, Anderson DC, Nair PV, Nyhan WL (1959) The uptake of a variety of amino-acids into nuclear proteins of tumors and other tissues. Cancer Res 19: 1030–1039
Chaiken L, Rege S, Hoh C et al. (1993) Positron emission tomography with fluorodeoxyglucose to evaluate tumor response and control after radiation therapy. Int J Radiat Oncol Biol Phys 27: 455–464
Di Chiro G (1986) Positron emission tomography using (18F)fluoro-deoxyglucose in brain tumors: a powerful diagnostic and prognostic tool. Invest Radiol 22: 360–371
Dillon WP, Harnsberger HR (1991) The impact of radiologic imaging on staging of cancer of the head and neck. Semin Oncol 18: 64–79
Deutsche Gesellschaft für Hals-Nasen-Ohrenheilkunde, Kopf- und Halschirurgie (1997) Leitlinie Kehlkopfkarzinom. HNO-Mitteilungen 47: 7–15 (auch aktuell jeweils abrufbar über Internet (AWMF-online: http://www.uni-duesseldorf. de/WWW/AWMF/II/hno)
Eichhorn T, Schroeder HG, Glanz H, Schwerk WB (1987) Histologisch kontrollierter Vergleich von Palpation und Sonographie bei der Diagnose von Halslymphknotenmetastasen. Laryngol Rhinol Otol 66: 266–274
van Eijkeren M, De Schryver A, Goethals P et al. (1992) Measurement of short-term 11C-thymidine activity in human head and neck tumours using positron emission tomography (PET). Acta Oncol 31: 539–543
Feinmesser R, Freeman JL, Feinmesser M et al. (1992) Role of modern imaging in decision-making for elective neck dissection. Head Neck 14: 173–176
Fitzpatrick PJ, Tepperman BS, Deboer G (1984) Multiple primary squamous cell carcinomas in the upper digestive tract. Int J Radiat Oncol Biol Phys 10: 2273–2279
Glazer H, Niemeyer JH, Blafes DM (1986) Neck neoplasms: MRI imaging part I. Initial evaluation. Radiology 160: 343–348
Greven KM, Williams D, Keyes JJ et al. (1994) Distinguishing tumor recurrence from irradiation sequelae with positron emission tomography in patients treated for larynx cancer. Int J Radiat Oncol Biol Phys 29: 841–845
Greven KM, Williams D, Keyes JJ et al. (1994) Positron emission tomography of patients with head and neck carcinoma before and after high dose irradiation. Cancer 74: 1355–1359
Griffeth LK, Dehdashti F, McGuire AH et al. (1992) PET evaluation of soft-tissue masses with fluorine-18 fluoro-2-deoxy-D-glucose. Radiology 182: 185–194
Gritzmann N (1992) Imaging procedures in diagnosis of laryngeal cancer with special reference to high resolution ultrasound. Wien Klin Wochenschr 104: 234–242
Haberkorn U, Strauss LG, Dimitrakopoulou A et al. (1993) Fluorodeoxyglucose imaging of advanced head and neck cancer after chemotherapy. J Nucl Med 34: 12–17
Haberkorn U, Strauss LG, Reisser C et al. (1991) Glucose uptake, perfusion, and cell proliferation in head and neck tumors: relation of positron emission tomography to flow cytometry. J Nucl Med 32: 1548–1555
Hermanek P, Sobin LH (1992) TNM classification of malignant tumors, 4th ed., 2nd Revision. Springer, Berlin Heidelberg New York
Jabour BA, Choi Y, Hoh CK et al. (1993) Extracranial head and neck: PET imaging with 2-[F-18]fluoro-2-deoxy-D-glucose and MR imaging correlation. Radiology 186: 27–35
Kau RJ, Alexiou C, Laubenbacher C, Ziegler S, Schwaiger M, Arnold W (1998) Positron-Emission-Tomography (PET) for the preoperative staging of head- and neck-tumours. Br J Cancer 77: 12
Kau RJ, Laubenbacher C, Saumweber D, Wagner-Manslau C, Schwaiger M, Arnold W (1994) Präoperatives Tumorstaging mittels Endoskopie, Magnetresonanztomographie, Somatostatinszintigraphie und Positronenemissionstomographie. Otorhinolaryngol Nova 4: 292–299
Kotwall C, Sako K, Razack MS et al. (1987) Metastatic patterns in squamous cell cancer of the head and neck. Am J Surg 154: 439–442
Lapela M, Grenman R, Kurki T et al. (1995) Head and neck cancer: detection of recurrence with PET and 2-[F-18]Fluoro-2-deoxy-D-glucose. Radiology 197: 205–211
Laubenbacher C, Saumweber D, Wagner-Manslau C, Kau RJ et al. (1995) Comparison of fluorine-18-fluorodeoxyglucose PET, MRI and endoscopy for staging head and neck squamous-cell carcinomas. J Nucl Med 36:1747–1757
Lenz M, Bongers H, Ozdoba C, Skalej M (1989) Klinische Wertigkeit der Computertomographie beim prätherapeutischen T-Staging von orofazialen Tumoren. RöFo 151: 138–144
Leskinen-Kallio S, Lindholm P, Lapela M, Joensuu H, Nordman E (1994) Imaging of head and neck tumors with positron emission tomography and (11 C)methionine. Int J Radiat Oncol Biol Phys 30: 1195–1199
Lindholm P, Leskinen KS, Minn H et al. (1993) Comparison of fluorine-18-fluorodeoxyglucose and carbon-11-methionine in head and neck cancer. J Nucl Med 34: 1711–1716
Lindholm P, Minn H, Leskinen-Kallio S, Bergman J, Ruotsalainen U, Joensuu H (1993) Influence of the blood glucose concentration on FDG uptake in cancer – a PET study. J Nucl Med 34: 1–6
McGuirt WF (1982) Panendoscopy as a screening examination for simultaneous primary tumors in head and neck cancer: a prospective sequential study and review of the literature. Laryngoscope 92: 569–576
McGuirt WF, Greven KM, Keyes JJ et al. (1995) Positron emission tomography in the evaluation of laryngeal carcinoma. Ann Otol Rhinol Laryngol 104: 274–278

Meyer JS, Friedman E, McCrate MM et al. (1983) Prediction of early course of breast carcinoma by thymidine labeling. Cancer 51: 1879–1886
Minn H, Paul R, Ahonen A (1988) Evaluation of treatment response to radiotherapy in head and neck cancer with fluorine-18 fluorodeoxyglucose. J Nucl Med 29: 1521–1525
Minn H, Aitasalo K, Happonen RP (1993) Detection of cancer recurrence in irradiated mandible using positron emission tomography. Eur Arch Otorhinolaryngol 250: 312–315
Minn H, Lapela M, Klemi PJ et al. (1997) Prediction of survival with Fluorine-18-Fluoro-deoxyglucose and PET in head and neck cancer. J Nucl Med 38: 1907–1911
Mukherji SK, Drane WE, Tart RP, Landau S, Mancuso AA (1994) Comparison of thallium-201 and F-18 FDG SPECT uptake in squamous cell carcinoma of the head and neck. Am J Neuroradiol 15: 1837–1842
Mukherji SK, Drane WE, Mancuso AA, Parsons JT, Mendenhall WM, Stringer S (1996) Occult primary tumors of the head and neck: detection with 2-[F-18] fluoro-2-deoxy-D-glucose SPECT. Radiology 199: 761–766
Okada J, Yoshikawa K, Itami M et al. (1992) Positron emission tomography using fluorine-18-fluorodeoxyglucose in malignant lymphoma: a comparison with proliferative activity. J Nucl Med 33: 325–329
Quetz JU, Rohr S, Hoffmann P, Wustrow J, Mertens J (1991) B-image sonography in lymph node staging of the head and neck area. A comparison with palpation, computerized and magnetic resonance tomography. HNO 39: 61–63
Rege S, Maass A, Chaiken L, et al. (1994) Use of positron emission tomography with fluorodeoxyglucose in patients with extracranial head and neck cancers. Cancer 73: 3047–3058
Rege SD, Chaiken L, Hoh CK et al. (1993) Change induced by radiation therapy in FDG uptake in normal and malignant structures of the head and neck: quantitation with PET. Radiology 189: 807–812
Reisser C, Haberkorn U, Dimitrakopoulou SA, Seifert E, Strauss LG (1995) Chemotherapeutic management of head and neck malignancies with positron emission tomography. Arch Otolaryngol Head Neck Surg 121: 272–276
Report of the American College of Cardiology/American Heart Association Task Force on Assessment of Diagnostic and Therapeutic Cardiovascular Procedures (Committee on Radionuclide Imaging) (1995) Task Force Report. Guidelines for Clinical Use of Cardiac Radionuclide Imaging. JACC 25: 521–527
Reske SN (1997) Konsensus-Onko-PET. Nuklearmedizin 36: 45–46
Schipper JH, Schrader M, Arweiler D, Muller S, Sciuk J (1996) Positron emission tomography for primary tumor detection in lymph node metastases with unknown primary tumor. HNO 44: 254–257
Seifert E, Schadel A, Haberkorn U, Strauss LG (1992) Evaluating the effectiveness of chemotherapy in patients with head-neck tumors using positron emission tomography (PET scan). HNO 40: 90–93
Som PM (1992) Detection of metastasis in cervical lymph nodes: CT and MR criteria and differential diagnosis. Am J Roentgenol 156: 961–969
Spitz MR (1993) Epidemiology and risk factors for head and neck cancer. Sem Oncol 21: 281–288
Steiner W (1993) Early detection of cancer in the upper aerodigestive tract, Part I. HNO 41: 360–367
Steinkamp HJ, Maurer J, Heim T, Knobber D, Felix R (1993) Magnetic resonance tomography and computerized tomography in tumor staging of mouth and oropharyngeal cancer. HNO 41: 519–525
Wagner-Manslau C, Laubenbacher C, van de Flierdt E et al. (1992) MRT bei Tumoren im Kopf-Halsbereich. Röntgenpraxis 45: 64–70
Wahl RL, Quint LE, Cieslak RD, Aisen AM, Koeppe RA, Meyer CR (1993) Anatometabolic tumor imaging: fusion of FDG PET with CT or MRI to localize foci of increased activity. J Nucl Med 34: 1190–1197
Wong WL, Hussain K, Chevretton E et al. (1996) Validation and clinical application of computer-combined computed tomography and positron emission tomography with 2-[18F]fluoro-2-deoxy-D-glucose head and neck images. Am J Surg 172: 628–632

5.3 Thyroid Carcinomas

F. Grünwald

5.3.1 Clinical Background

The most frequent forms of thyroid cancer can be divided into two main categories: tumors with follicle cell differentiation and those with C-cell differentiation. Within the category of tumors with follicle cell differentiation, a distinction is made between papillary tumors and follicular tumors. Both undifferentiated and anaplastic tumors are also included in this category, although a clear attribution to an initial cell line is not always possible for anaplastic carcinomas. Within the largest group, the papillary carcinomas, there are several types including encapsulated, minimal invasive, diffuse sclerotic and oncocytic carcinomas. Because of their generally low iodine uptake and their high mitochondrial content, Hürthle cell carcinomas have a special position, particularly in functional imaging and with respect to therapy options. Carcinomas with C-cell differentiation are partly genetically determined, either as isolated familial medullary carcinoma or in multiple endocrine neoplasia (MEN-2a/MEN-2b). The existence of mixed follicle cell/C-cell differentiated carcinomas should be mentioned, especially in the context of radioiodine therapy, since the latter can certainly offer therapeutic options. We will not discuss the rare forms of thyroid cancer or the further subcategorization of the tumor entities described above, since this information is currently not relevant to the clinical significance of PET.

The yearly incidence of malignant thyroid tumors is approximately 4/100,000 in women and 1.5/100,000 in men. Thyroid tumors comprise approximately 1.5 % of all malignant tumors in women, and approximately 0.5 % in men. Incidence increases with age: in autopsy studies occult thyroid carcinomas were found in up to 35 %. The basis for this observation is presumably the biological behavior of most of these malignancies, which frequently do not appear clinically for years. Exposure to ionizing radiation during childhood leads to a significant increase in the incidence of thyroid carcinomas, especially papillary carcinomas. An increase in the supply of adequate dietary iodine has led to a relative shift in histological findings involving an increase in papillary carcinoma and a decrease in follicular and anaplastic carcinomas. It is still unclear whether there is an absolute increase in the number of papillary tumors as a result of improved iodine supply.

In addition to age and sex, tumor stage and histopathological grading have the greatest prognostic significance. TNM classification according to the recommendations of the International Union Against Cancer/Union Internationale Contre le Cancer (UICC) (Spiessl et al. 1995) is given in Table 5.3.1. Histopathological grading is based on the evaluation of nuclear atypia, the extent of tumor necrosis, and vascular invasion (Akslen 1993). Whereas follicular carcinomas show up more frequently with distant metastases, papillary tumors tend to exhibit lymphogenic spreading that – in contrast to other tumors – is not associated with a significantly poorer prognosis. The lungs and skeletal system are affected most frequently by distant metastases. Overall, the prognosis for differentiated thyroid carcinomas is extremely good. Encapsulated papillary tumors and minimal papillary carcinomas have a long-term survival rate of over 90 %. There are different staging systems for estimating individual prognosis.

Table 5.3.1. Tumor Staging

pT[a]	
pT1	Tumor $\leq$ 1 cm, confined to the thyroid
pT2	Tumor > 1 cm, $\leq$ 4 cm, confined to the thyroid
pT3	Tumor > 4 cm, confined to the thyroid
pT4	Tumor of any size that has penetrated through the thyroid capsule
a	Unifocal tumor
b	Multifocal tumor
pN	
pN0	No lymph node metastases
pN1a	Ipsilateral lymph node metastases
pN1b	Contralateral, median or mediastinal lymph node metastases
pM	
pM0	No distant metastases
pM1	Distant metastases

[a] Largest tumor is decisive for pT classification.

Table 5.3.2 shows a clinically suitable concept in which age is the only factor considered besides primary staging for the prognosis of life expectancy. It should be emphasized especially in comparison with other tumor entities that patients under 45 years of age enjoy the relatively favorable Stage II status even when distant metastases are present. Pulmonary metastases can be treated better with high-dose radioiodine therapy than bone metastases. Radioiodine therapy is particulary

Table 5.3.2. Prognostic Staging

	$\leq$ 45 Years of Age	> 45 Years of Age
Stage I	Any T, any N, M0	T1, N0, M0
Stage II	Any T, any N, M1	T2–3, N0, M0
Stage III	–	T4, N0, M0, any T, N1, M0
Stage IV	–	Any T, Any N, M1

effective in diffuse pulmonary metastatic spread, which can be detected only by scintigraphy but not by chest radiography or CT (Menzel et al. 1996). The prognosis for anaplastic carcinomas is generally unfavorable; reported exceptions can generally be traced to the fact that a carcinoma was classified as anaplastic despite the presence of differentiated areas. A frequent limiting factor with anaplastic carcinomas is the invasive growth of the primary tumor or the local recurrence.

Carcinomas with C-cell differentiation occupy a midpoint between differentiated and anaplastic carcinomas with respect to the prognosis. In this regard, lymphogenic metastatic spread of C-cell carcinomas, which frequently also involves mediastinal lymph nodes, has a greater prognostic significance than in differentiated carcinomas, especially in papillary carcinomas.

Preoperative diagnostics of thyroid tumors will be described only briefly, since it is not related to the clinical application of PET. There is no indication for FDG PET as part of the preoperative status evaluation, as is explained in greater detail below. In addition to a physical exam, diagostics includes sonography, scintigraphy, fine needle biopsy, and both morphological imaging and the analysis of thyroid-specific laboratory parameters. Recent studies increasingly recommend checking the patient's basal serum calcitonin level when there are unclear nodular changes in the thyroid (Raue and Frank-Raue, 1997).

5.3.2 Therapy

Total thyroidectomy is the therapy of choice (Simon 1997) except in cases of highly differentiated encapsulated papillary carcinoma pT1a N0 M0 (in these cases, hemithyroidectomy is regarded as adequate by most authors). Total thyroidectomy removes tumor tissue, which is relevant especially because of its relatively frequent multifocal growth, although it has not yet been clarified whether an intrathyroidal metastatic spread is involved or the parallel development of several tumor clones. Furthermore, the radical removal of benign iodine-accumulating tissue is the precondition for effective radioiodine therapy. In the case of differentiated carcinomas, thyroidectomy includes lymph node dissection of the central compartment. If additional lymph node metastases are suspected, the lateral compartments (ipsilateral and also contralateral, if necessary) are dissected as well. C-cell carcinoma requires dissection of the lateral compartments: the ipsilateral compartment with the sporadic form of c-cell carcinoma and the contralateral compartment as well in patients suffering from the familial form. Surgical procedures for anaplastic carcinomas are largely determined by palliative factors.

An initial radioiodine therapy follows thyroidectomy. Exceptions include the constellation mentioned above (highly differentiated encapsulated papillary carcinoma pT1a N0 M0) and tumors that are not sufficiently operable. The isotope used is ^{131}I, which has a beta radiation energy (E_{max}) of .61 MeV and a gamma radiation energy of 364 keV. Beta radiation has a mean range of less than 1 mm and can be used therapeutically in order to achieve the highest possible dose – with minimal exposure to other tissues – in the follicle cells and their immediate environment, where iodine uptake ability has remained intact. Gamma radiation can be used for scintigraphy. Radioiodine therapy (RIT) should be performed at maximum TSH stimulation (> 30mU/1). A hormone withdrawal period of approximately four weeks usually results in maximum endogenous TSH secretion. Exceptions include cases with extended (usually pulmonary) metastatic spread, large amounts of remnant tissue in which a relevant hormone synthesis is still present, and pituitary insufficiency, which is rarely encountered. In such cases, recombinant TSH can be used; however, at present this substance is not yet commercially available.

The first course of RIT consists of 30–100 mCi (1.1-3.7 GBq), depending on the amount of remnant tissue. Scans are made approximately three to six days after radioiodine administration, which is usually given orally. Further RITs are carried out at intervals of approximately three months. If there is no indication that any tumor tissue remains, therapy usually consists of single doses of 100 mCi (3.7 GBq), seldom reaching 200 mCi (7.4 GBq). Besides destroying any remaining malignant cells, RIT creates optimum conditions for effective follow-up by also eliminating all benign thyroid tissue (Biersack and Hotze 1991). This affects serum thyroglobulin levels, sonography of the thyroid region, and radioiodine scintigraphy. The therapy goals are primarily a negative post-therapeutic radioiodine scan and undetectable serum thyroglobulin levels under TSH stimulation. The prognostic parameters mentioned above are the most important factor in determining to what extent one can deviate from these goals in patients in whom no remaining malignant tissue is suspected. In many cases Huerthle cell carcinomas take up radioiodine in small amounts or not at all, so that these tumors frequently evade effective therapy. But an attempt at therapy should be made in any case, especially when no other curative therapy options exist.

Suspected or detected metastatic spread or recurrence is treated with single doses of up to 300 mCi (11.1 GBq) (Grünwald et al. 1988). Pulmonary metastases respond better than bone and other metastases, especially if the spread is disseminated (Menzel et al. 1996; Reiners 1993; Georgi et al. 1993). High doses should be administered as early as possible, since radioiodine uptake generally decreases during the course of the disease.

In general, C-cell carcinomas do not take up radioiodine, but in the follicular type the use of radioiodine should be tried. The thyroglobulin immunohistochemistry of the primary tumor and of metastases, where applicable, can provide clinically useful information. Anaplastic carcinomas seldom take up radioiodine, and RIT rarely results in an appreciable effect on tumor growth even when tumors are radioiodine-positive.

Surgical intervention is a curative option for single metastases and can be used in multiple metastases for the purpose of reducing tumor size (to optimize the radioiodine effect before RIT). Percutaneous radiation is used less often in therapy for thyroid carcinoma than it was in the past. It is indicated for inoperable tumors, local tumor compression, and skeletal metastases, particularly in cases with risk of a fracture. There is still disagreement concerning the prophylactic radiation therapy of the lymph vessels with respect to the prognosis for all pT4 tumors.

Chemotherapeutic agents can be used in certain circumstances for undifferentiated carcinomas and the progression of multiple metastases of differentiated carcinomas. Initial studies with 13-cis retinoic acid – a substance that has already been used widely in the field of hematooncology – show that its use can induce radioiodine uptake in -negative tumor localizations in some patients (Grünwald et al. 1998; Simon et al. 1996). This is particularly interesting with respect to FDG PET, since PET can be used here to test whether radioiodine uptake was induced in all tumor sites.

5.3.3 Use of FDG PET

There are no preoperative indications (evaluation of unclear lesions) for FDG PET in thyroid tumors, in contrast to other tumor entities. Increased FDG uptake in malignant thyroid tumors has often been observed incidentally, and some authors also describe a differentiation between malignant and benign tumors based on semiquantitative data. But the specificity of FDG PET is too low to insist on its use for malignant thyroid tumors, since even benign adenomas frequently show an increased tracer uptake and some carcinomas (particularly those with papillary growth patterns) take up no FDG at all (Feine et al. 1996; Joensuu and Ahonen 1987; Sisson et al. 1993; Adler and Bloom 1993).

The sensitivity and specificity of FDG PET increase if the scan is performed postoperatively when no large amounts of thyroid remnant tissue remain. Therefore, the scan should generally not be done earlier than approximately two months after the first RIT. At that time the rate of false positive findings due to unspecific postoperative changes is also significantly lower.

Studies on the value of FDG PET for differentiated thyroid carcinoma have often focused in part on the situation involving a negative radioiodine scan with the suspicion of metastatic spread (based on an increase in the serum thyroglobulin value or unclear morphological findings) (Feine et al. 1996; Baqai et al. 1994; Messa et al. 1996; Easton et al. 1995; Grünwald et al. 1996, 1997; Tatsch et al. 1996; Conti et al. 1996; Platz et al. 1995). Morphological imaging methods (sonography, CT, MRI) can be used to detect radioiodine-negative tissue. But they have the disadvantage that only limited areas can be studied and that their specificity is extremely limited in patients with altered anatomical conditions (for example, after neck dissection) (Schober et al. 1986). The value of CT is also reduced by the fact that with respect to further RIT, no iodine-containing contrast medium may be used. The specificity of CT in particular is comparatively low in these cases.

This necessitates the use of tumor-seeking tracers. Thallium-201 (T1), technetium-99m methoxyisobutylisonitrile (^{99m}Tc-MIBI), and technetium ^{99m}1,2-bis [bis(2-ethoxyethyl)phosphino]ethane (tetrofosmin) have emerged as suitable, single-photon-emitting tracers (Dadparvar et al. 1995; Briele et al. 1991; Gallowitsch et al. 1996: Nemec et al. 1996). MIBI exhibits a sensitivity of approximately 80-90 % and is especially well suited for imaging tumor tissue in Huerthle cell carcinoma. Whereas most authors describe a high sensitivity in local recurrence, Nemec et al. (1996) report that MIBI is especially sensitive in distant metastases, particularly in bone metastases.

Many studies dealing with groups of approximately 50 patients each have shown that FDG PET has a sensitivity of over 90 % in cases with a negative radioiodine scintiscan (Feine et al. 1996; Grünwald et al. 1997; Dietlein et al. 1997). It has been found that tumor localisations very often take up either only radioiodine or only FDG (Fig. 5.3.1-5.3.5). This holds true for both the interindividual comparison of patients with a single tumor site and for cases with several localizations, some of which are radioiodine-positive and some FDG-positive. The reason for this alternating uptake behavior is presumably a varying degree of differentiation in the tumor clone. Like other tumor entities (especially neuroendocrine tumors), poorly differentiated tumors take up FDG to a great extent, while well differentiated tumors prefer the organ-specific tracer radioiodine, which indicates that the Na/I symporter is still present. A significant correlation has been demonstrated between primary tumor grading and differences in sensitivity for radioiodine and FDG PET (Grünwald et al. 1996).

At this point we will present a detailed comparison of FDG PET and scintigraphy using tumor-seeking radiopharmaceuticals (specifically MIBI) with respect to an optimal diagnostic process. The following aspects should be considered.

Spatial Resolution

Spatial resolution is approximately 5 mm for PET under clinical conditions, while SPECT with a dual head camera achieves a maximum resolution of approximately 10 mm. Thus PET should be preferred for any problem requiring tomographic examination. In regions where planar imaging usually suffices (for example, superficially located cervical lymph node metastases), the difference between PET and SPECT due to varying tomographic resolution is not so significant. In contrast, there are definite advantages in using PET for mediastinal and pulmonary processes.

Tumor Tracer Uptake Mechanisms

FDG uptake correlates frequently with proliferative activity and is determined by glucose metabolism in both the tumor cells and the macrophages associated with tumors, among others. (Kubota et al. 1995; Kubota et al. 1994). Quickly growing tumors therefore usually exhibit a higher sensitivity with FDG PET. Yoshioka et al. (1994) demonstrated that FDG uptake in various gastrointestinal tumors increases with the loss of differentiation. Most differentiated thyroid carcinomas, espe-

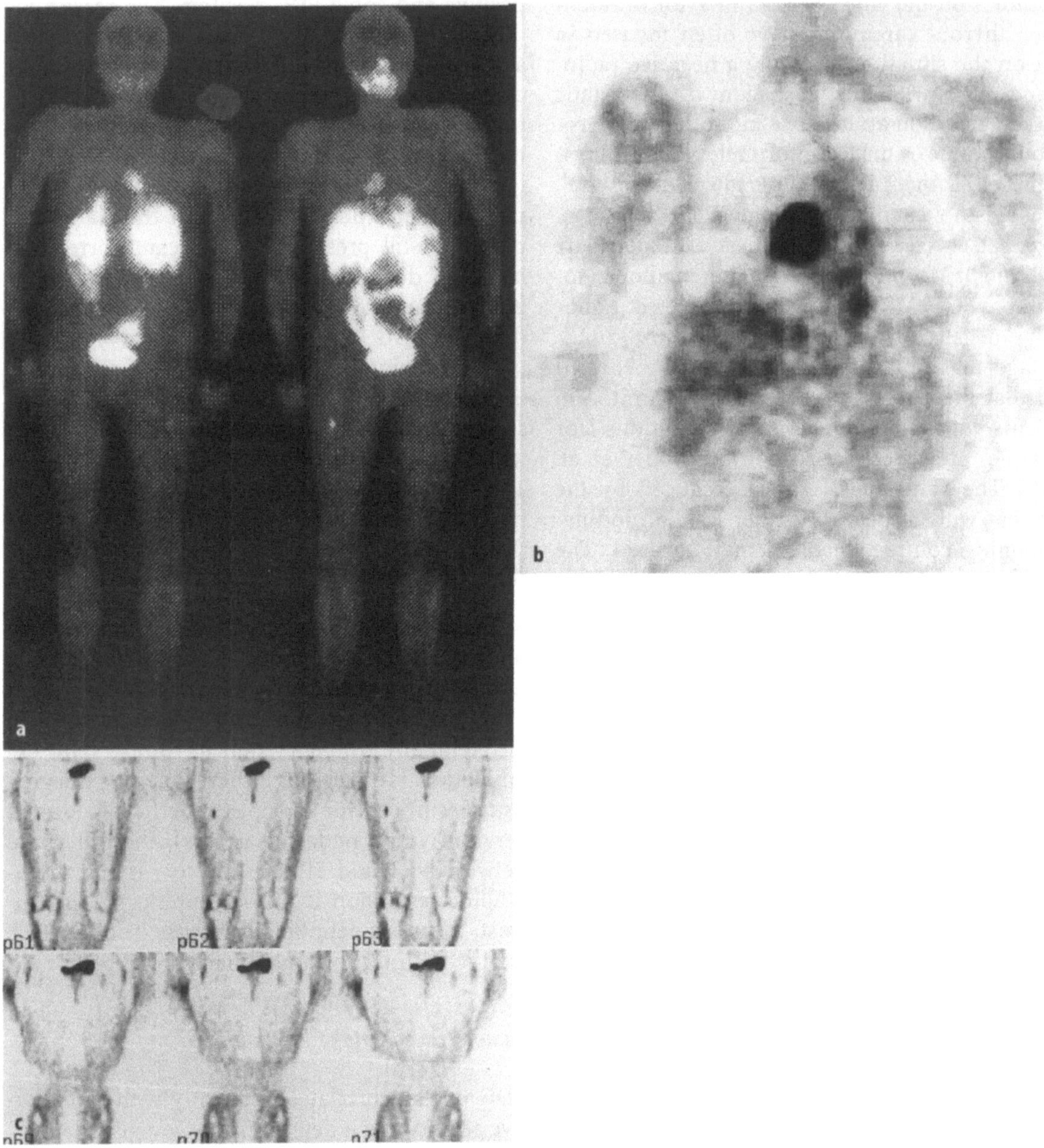

Fig. 5.3.1a-c. Huerthle cell follicular thyroid carcinoma (pT4NxM1) with pulmonary and bone metastases; serum thyroglobulin: > 10,000 μg/l. MIBI scintigraphy (**a**: dorsal projection on the left, ventral projection on the right) showed pathological accumulations in the mediastinum (right paramedian) and in the right femur. FDG PET shows a clearly positive finding in the mediastinum (right paramedian), a small nodule left paramedian, a suspicious finding in the right lung (**b**), which was confirmed as positive during subsequent follow-up, and a metastasis in the right femur (**c**). In the radioiodine scan, the localizations were partly positive and partly negative

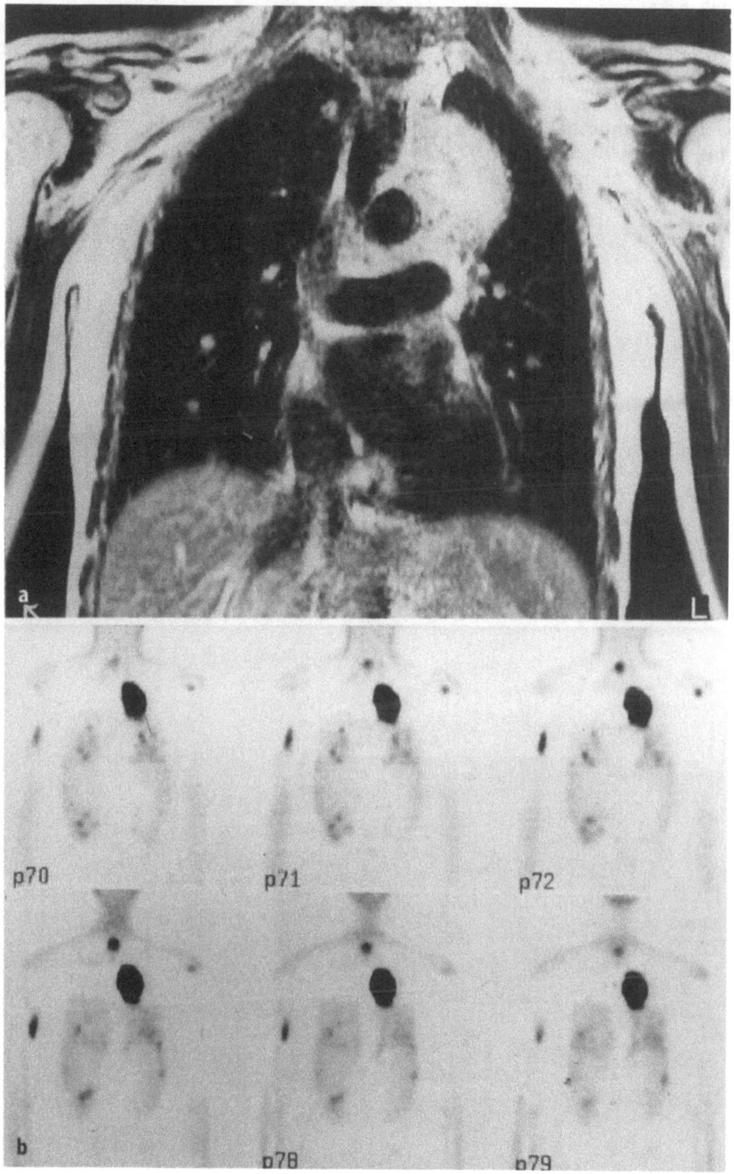

Fig. 5.3.2a, b.
Papillary thyroid carcinoma (pTxN1M1) with metastases in the lymph nodes, lung, bone, liver, spleen, and kidneys. Serum thyroglobulin: $134\,\mu g/l$. **a** MRI shows a large mediastinal metastasis as well as multiple pulmonary metastases. **b** with FDG PET, metastases can be detected in the jugulum, mediastinum, lung, right humerus, left shoulder joint, liver, spleen and kidneys. Only a small percentage of the tumor localizations showed any radioiodine uptake

cially G1 tumors, are relatively slow-growing and are therefore frequently FDG-negative, whereas they can be detected in a radioiodine scan because of their intact Na/I symporters (Dai et al. 1996). MIBI uptake is, above all, a function of mitochondrial potential. More than 90 % of the tracer is taken up in the inner mitochondrial matrix (Piwnica-Worms et al. 1990). Therefore mitochondrial content and metabolic requirements, which determine potential, have a significant influence on the sensitivity of MIBI scintigraphy. This would lead to the expectation that Huerthle cell carcinomas in particular (which are frequently radioiodine-negative) would show a pronounced MIBI uptake (Ba-

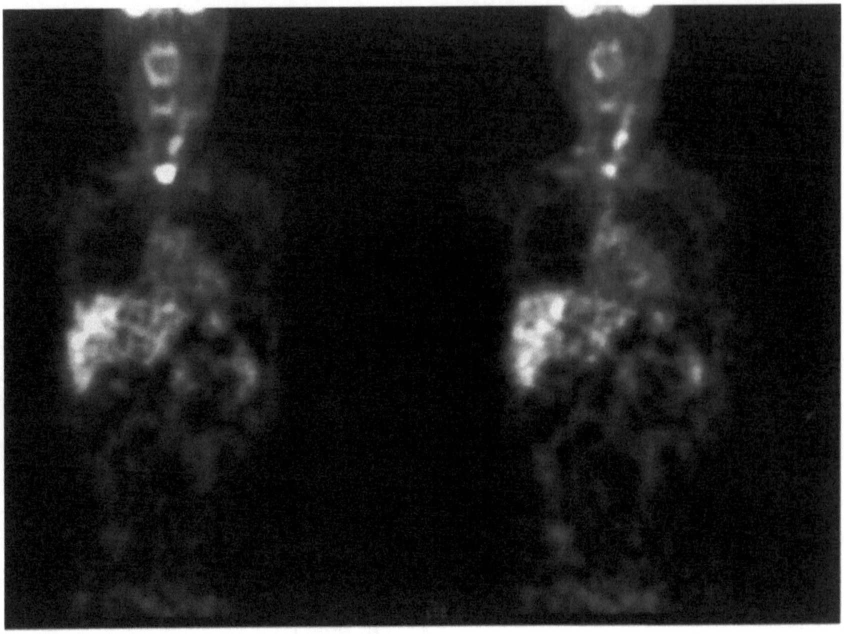

Fig. 5.3.3.
Follicular thyroid carcinoma (pT4N1Mx). Serum thyroglobulin: 850 μg/l. Local recurrence (median) and cervical lymph node metastases on both sides were detectable using FDG PET

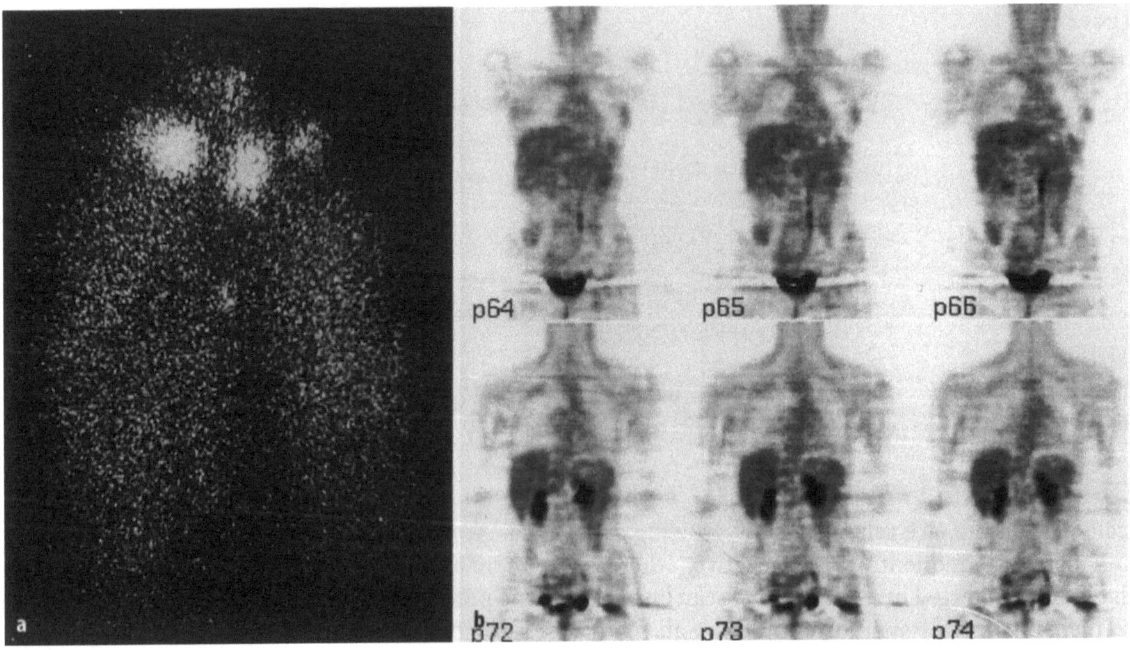

Fig. 5.3.4a, b. Papillary thyroid carcinoma (pT4N1M1). Serum thyroglobulin: 334 μg/l. Radioactive iodine-positive disseminated pulmonary and regional lymph node metastases (**a**). No increase in glucose metabolism was detectable with FDG PET (**b**)

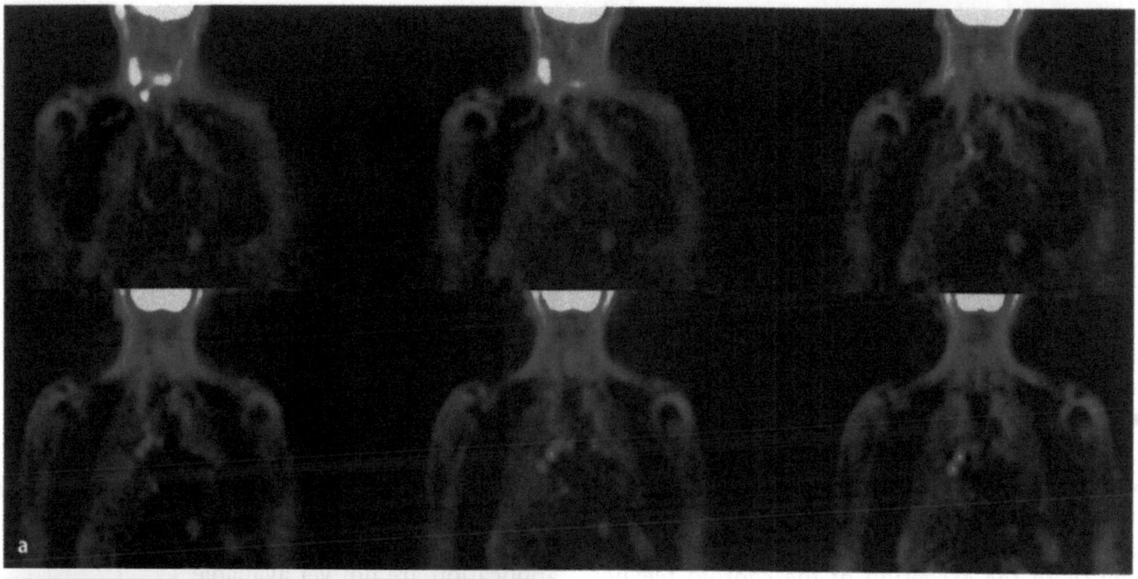

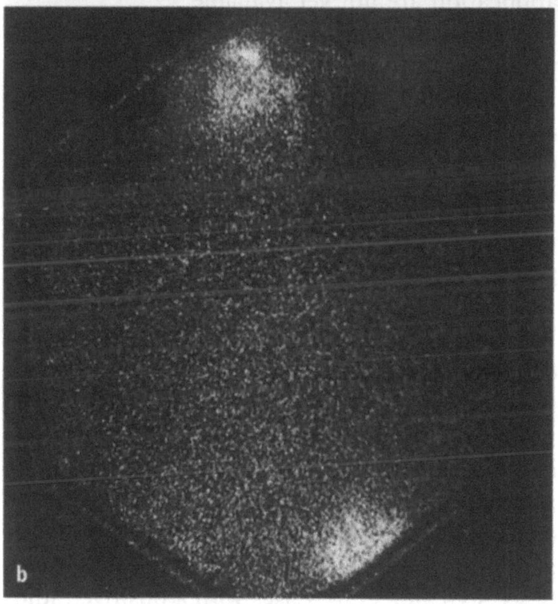

Fig. 5.3.5a, b. Papillary thyroid carcinoma (pT4N1M1). Serum thyroglobulin: . 10,000 μg/l. Using FDG PET (**a**) pulmonary and bilateral cervical lymph node metastases were detected; radioiodine scintigraphy showed no pathological findings (**b**)

lone et al. 1992). However, MIBI scintigraphy has not been proven to be clinically superior to FDG PET in Huerthle cell carcinomas.

Tracer Uptake in Other Organs

Physiological accumulation of both FDG and MIBI is very low in the neck and upper mediastinum, so that clinical evaluation of local recurrences and regional lymph node metastases is not significantly affected by high levels of background activity (with the exception of the problems described below). In other organs where FDG PET and MIBI scintigraphy can be used for detecting distant metastases, physiological tracer uptake is extremely variable. MIBI uptake in the myocardium is high, with the result that pericardial pulmonary metastases can be detected with an inferior sensitivity. In this situation it is especially important that FDG is administered in a fasted state, so that predominantly free fatty acids will be metabolized in the myocardium and FDG uptake will be minimized. In contrast, FDG uptake is always very high in the brain, so that sensitivity (with respect to hot lesions) is very low for distant metastases, whereas MIBI accumulation in the brain is low (with the exception of the choroid plexus), making scintigraphy with tumor-seeking single-photon-emitters clearly superior for detecting cerebral metastases. The detection of distant metastases in the kidneys and lower urinary tract is made difficult by renal excretion of FDG, but this plays a smaller role with thyroid carcinomas than with other tumors since metastases of differentiated thyroid carcinomas seldom appear at this particular localization. MIBI uptake is extremely high in the liver. FDG uptake, on the other hand, is relatively low (especially with late acquisition of emission images), so that FDG PET is superior for this localization (Briele et al. 1991; Dietlein et al. 1997; and Pirro et al. 1994).

Radioiodine uptake has a significant prognostic relevance, with the result that a prognostic statement can be made on the basis of the detection of radioiodine-negative and FDG-positive tumor localizations. Even though a current radioiodine scan is essential for therapy planning, information about FDG-positive and radioiodine-negative tumor cells is extremely important, since we must consider a selection pressure on the different clones that favors the poorly differentiated FDG-positive cells, while the well differentiated are exposed to a higher radiation effect.

Serum calcitonin and CEA levels are the most important parameters in the follow-up of carcinomas with C-cell differentiation (Becker et al. 1986). It has been shown that for these tumors FDG PET can detect tumor tissue with approximately the same sensitivity as MRI (Köster et al. 1996). FDG PET findings and the "tissue-specific" methods – somatostatin receptor scintigraphy and scintigraphy with pentavalent DMSA (Adams et al. 1998) – provide an indication of the current degree of differentiation in C-cell carcinomas just as they do in carcinomas with follicle cell differentiation. It has been demonstrated through correlation with Ki-67 antigens associated with cell cycles that tumors with a high proliferation tendency tend to be FDG-positive. In addition, MIBI scintigraphy offers an alternative scintigraphic method for these tumors as well. However, studies comparing scintigraphy with FDG PET for this application are not yet available.

Nothing has been published yet regarding experiences with FDG PET for anaplastic carcinoma. However, this method does not yet seem to have any appreciable significance for either prognosis or changes in procedure.

5.3.4 Indications

Indications for clinical use were evaluated at the consensus conference in Ulm at the end of 1997 (Consensus-Onco-PET 1997, Table 5.3.3). Of note is the highest classification – 1a – for differentiated thyroid carcinomas when radioiodine scintigraphy is negative and there is an indication of recurrence due to an increase in serum thyroglobulin and/or unclear morphological findings (Figs. 5.3.5 and 5.3.6). Cases with a positive radioiodine scintiscan are also an indication for FDG PET – in spite of the 1b rating (Fig. 5.3.1 and 5.3.2) – since it is crucial to the further course of treatment to know whether there are poorly differentiated tumor cell clones, which are frequently only detectable with FDG, in addition to well differentiated cells. Carcinomas with C-cell differentiation are not shown in this evaluation because there is not enough data. The indications for C-cell carcinoma are both preoperative and post-

Table 5.3.3. Indications for FDG PET in differentiated thyroid carcinomas

Suspicion of recurrence / metastases when a radioiodine scan shows no pathological findings (but serum thyroglobulin is elevated and/or morphological imaging reveal suspicous findings)	1a
Detection of further tumor manifestations when recurrence and / or metastases are detected by radioiodine scan	1b
Primary lymph node staging	2b
Therapy monitoring	2b
Primary tumor staging	3
Primary tumor detection	3

1a: appropriate;
1b: acceptable;
2b: no evaluation possible to date;
3: without benefit

operative in connection with staging or when recurrence or metastases are suspected during follow-up. In particular, changes in the calcitonin level (basal and after pentagastrin stimulation) and serum CEA level are decisive. FDG PET is especially sensitive in cases with a rapidly rising CEA level, which indicates a high proliferation tendency (Adams et al. 1998).

5.3.5 Results and Interpretation

The results of clinical studies are described in detail above. The information shown in Table 5.3.4 is important for interpreting FDG PET findings in carcinoma with follicle cell differentiation and should therefore be available. Evaluation of PET findings in the thyroid region and lymph node compartments requires a great deal of experience, particularly in view of the limitations mentioned

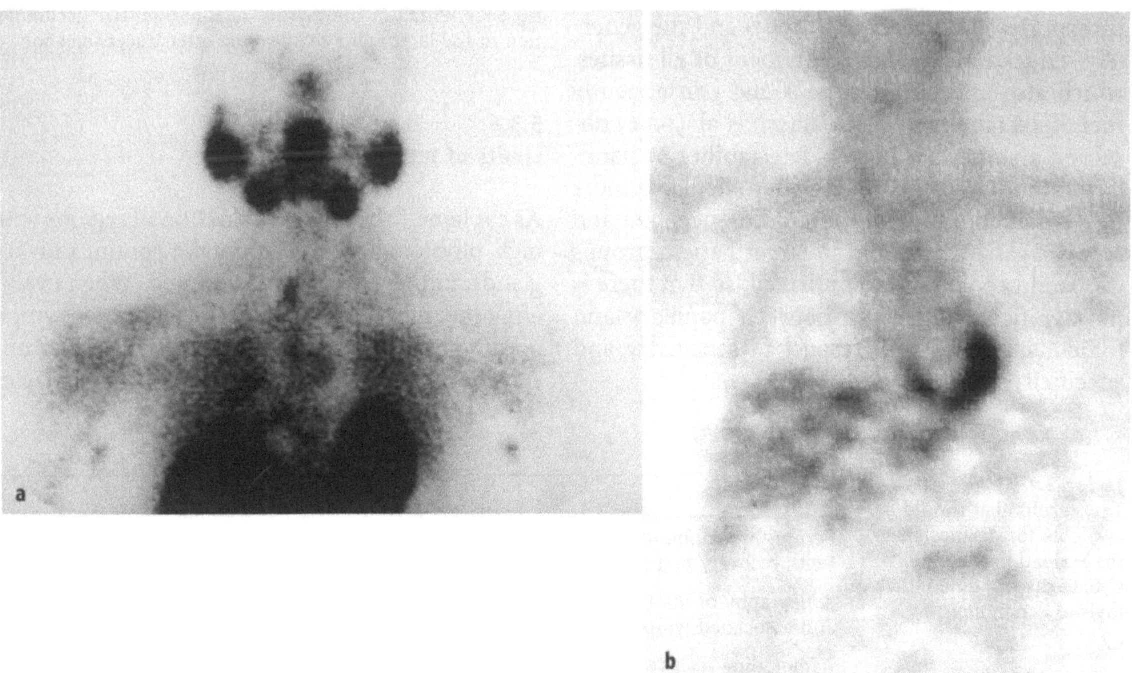

Fig. 5.3.6a, b. Suspected local recurrence after thyroidectomy and multiple radioiodine therapy for papillary thyroid carcinoma (pT2N1M0) and known tubercular lymph node changes right cervical; serum thyroglobulin: 2 µg/l. **a** A positive finding is visible right paratracheal in MIBI scintigraphy. **b** FDG PET shows negative findings (confirmed as correct in subsequent follow-up)

below. For this reason, PET results should in principle only be evaluated by a practiced well trained physician.

While TSH stimulation is essential for radioiodine scintigraphy, FDG PET (and also MIBI scintigraphy or thallium scintigraphy) can be performed while the patient is being medicated with thyroid hormones. It appears that PET has a higher sensitivity even with low TSH levels, in direct comparison with radioiodine scintigraphy under TSH stimulation (Grünwald et al. 1997). In contrast, Sisson et al. (1993) report on a case involving several sequential FDG PET scans in which there was a higher FDG PET sensitivity for individual tumor localizations under TSH stimulation. If we assume that metabolism is TSH-dependent even in malignant follicle cells and that the functional activity of glucose transport is increased in hypothyroidism (Matthaei et al. 1995), then we would expect a higher sensitivity during TSH stimulation. But what is more decisive with hypothyroidism is the absolute decrease in glucose transporters (Matthaei et al. 1995) and the generally reduced metabolic requirement of all tissues, which also affects tumor cells and consequently their detectability by FDG. Tatsch et al. (1996) observed a somewhat higher detectability of papillary tumors in comparison with follicular tumors in a small collective of radioiodine-negative and MIBI-negative cases. But in larger patient groups this trend could not be confirmed, so that there is no significant difference between papillary and follicular tumors with respect to sensitivity and specificity.

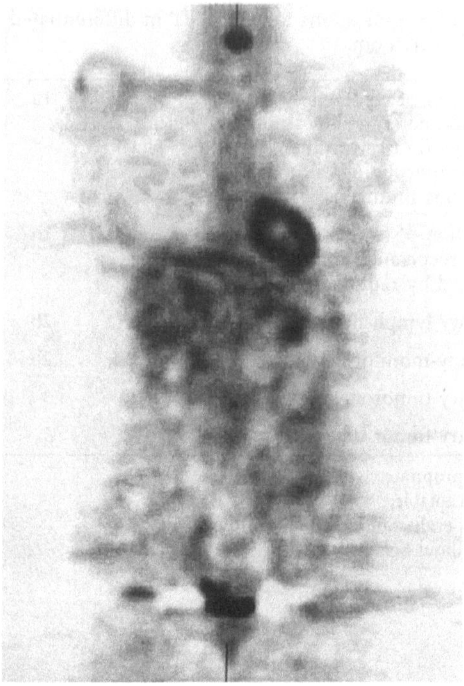

Fig. 5.3.7. Pitfall in the thyroid region: intensive accumulation in the larynx due to speaking after tracer injection

5.3.6 Limits of Interpretation

As explained above, the evaluation of regions with high physiological tracer uptake (brain, salivary glands, kidneys, bladder) is limited. When evaluating the thyroid region and the associated lymph node compartments, we should also consider unspecific uptake in the larynx, the neck muscles

Table 5.3.4. Test results that should be available for diagnosis and the evaluation of an FDG PET scan in cases of differentiated thyroid carcinoma

Obligate	Facultative
Serum thyroglobulin level (with recovery and recovery testing)	Neck/chest CT (without contrast medium!)
Sonography of the thyroid bed and associated lymph node compartments	MRI of the neck
Radioiodine scan (with therapeutic doses if possible)	MIBI-/tetrofosmin-/thallium scintigraphy, including SPECT of the neck and chest
Chest X-ray	Bone scintigraphy Morphological imaging of other organ systems if metastases e.g. are suspected

and occasionally the thymus. It is therefore important during the examination that the patient does not talk after the tracer injection has been given in order to avoid activating the musculature of the larynx (Fig. 5.3.7) and that the patient is as relaxed as possible to minimize glucose utilization by the neck muscles. Beyond this, the general guidelines for whole-body FDG PET should of course be followed.

References

Adams S, Baum R, Rink T, Schumm-Dräger PM, Usadel KH, Hör G (1998) Limited value of fluorine-18 fluorodeoxyglucose positron emission tomography for the imaging of neuroendocrine tumours. Eur J Nucl Med 25: 79–83

Adler LP, Bloom AD (1993) Positron emission tomography of thyroid masses. Thyroid 3: 195–200

Akslen LA (1993) Prognostic importance of histological grading in papillary carcinoma. Cancer 72: 2680–2685

Balone HR, Fing-Bennett D, Stoffer SS (1992) ^{99m}Tc-sestamibi uptake by recurrent Hürthle cell carcinoma of the thyroid. J Nucl Med 33: 1393–1395

Baqai FH, Conti PS, Singer PA, Spencer CA, Wang CC, Nicoloff JT (1994) ^{18}F-FDG-PET scanning – a diagnostic tool for detection of recurrent and metastatic differentiated thyroid cancers. Abstract, 68th annual meeting of the American Thyroid Association, Chicago, p 9

Becker W, Spiegel W, Reiners C, Börner W (1986) Besonderheiten bei der Nachsorge des C-Zell-Karzinoms. Nuklearmediziner 9: 167–181

Biersack HJ, Hotze A (1991) The clinician and the thyroid. Eur J Nucl Med 18: 761–778

Briele B, Hotze AL, Kropp J et al. (1991) A comparison of ^{201}Tl and ^{99m}Tc-MIBI in the follow-up of differentiated thyroid carcinoma. Nucl Med 30: 115–124

Conti PS, Durski JM, Grafton ST, Singer PA (1996) PET imaging of locally recurrent and metastatic thyroid cancer. J Nucl Med 37: 135P

Dadparvar S, Chevres A, Tulchinsky M, Krishna-Badrinath L, Khan AS, Slizofski WJ (1995) Clinical utility of technetium-99 m methoxisobutylisonitrile imaging in differentiated thyroid carcinoma: comparison with thallium-201 and iodine-131 Na scintigraphy, and serum thyroglobulin quantitation. Eur J Nucl Med 22: 1330–1338

Dai G, Levy O, Carrasco N (1996) Cloning and characterization of the thyroid iodide transporter. Nature 379: 458–460

Dietlein M, Scheidhauer K, Voth E, Theissen P, Schicha H (1997) Fluorine-18 fluorodeoxyglucose positron emission tomography and iodine-131 whole-body scintigraphy in the follow-up of differentiated thyroid cancer. Eur J Nucl Med 24: 1342–1348

Easton E, Coates D, McKusick A, Borchert R, Zuger J (1995) Concurrent FDG F-18 thyroid PET imaging in I-131 therapy patients. J Nucl Med 36: 197

Feine U, Lietzenmayer R, Hanke JP, Held J, Wöhrle H, Müller-Schauenburg W (1996) Fluorine-18-FDG and iodine-131-iodide uptake in thyroid cancer. J Nucl Med 37: 1468–1472

Gallowitsch HJ, Kresnik E, Mikosch P, Pipam W, Gomez I, Lind P. (1996) Tc-99 m tetrofosmin scintigraphy: an alternative scintigraphic method for following up differentiated thyroid carcinoma – preliminary results. Nucl Med 35: 230–235

Georgi P, Emrich D, Heidenreich P, Moser E, Reiners C, Schicha H (1992) Radiojodtherapie des differenzierten Schilddrüsenkarzinoms. Empfehlungen der Arbeitsgemeinschaft Therapie der Deutschen Gesellschaft für Nuklearmedizin. Nuklearmedizin 31: 151–153

Grünwald F, Menzel C, Bender H et al. (1998) Redifferentiation induced radioiodine uptake in thyroid cancer. J Nucl Med, im Druck

Grünwald F, Menzel C, Bender H et al. (1997) Comparison of ^{18}FDG-PET with ^{131}Iodine and ^{99m}Tc-sestamibi scintigraphy in differentiated thyroid cancer. Thyroid 7: 327–335

Grünwald F, Ruhlmann J, Ammari B, Knopp R, Hotze A, Biersack HJ (1988) Experience with a high-dose concept of differentiated metastatic thyroid cancer therapy. Nucl Med 27: 266–271

Grünwald F, Schomburg A, Bender H et al. (1996) Fluorine-18 fluorodeoxyglucose positron emission tomography in the follow-up of differentiated thyroid cancer. Eur J Nucl Med 23: 312–319

Joensuu H, Ahonen A (1987) Imaging of metastases of thyroid carcinoma with fluorine-18 fluorodeoxyglucose. J Nucl Med 28: 910–914

Konsensus – Onko-PET (1997) Ergebnisse der 2. interdisziplinären Konsensuskonferenz im Ulm, 12.9.97. Nuklearmedizin 36: 45–46

Köster C, Ehrenheim C, Burchert W, Oetting G, Hundeshagen H (1996) F-18-FDG-PET, MRT und CT in der Nachsorge des medullären Schilddrüsenkarzinoms. Nuklearmedizin 35: A60

Kubota R, Kubota K, Yamada S, Tada M, Ido T, Tamahashi N (1994) Microautoradiographic study for the differentiation of intratumoral macrophages, granulation tissues and cancer cells by the dynamics of fluorine-18-fluorodeoxyglucose uptake. J Nucl Med 35: 104–112

Kubota R, Kubota K, Yamada S, Tada M, Takahashi T, Iwata R, Tamahashi N (1995) Methionine uptake by tumor tissue: a microautoradiographic comparison with FDG. J Nucl Med 36: 484–492

Matthaei S, Trost B, Hamann A et al. (1995) Effect of in vivo thyroid hormone status on insuline signalling and GLUT1 and GLUT4 glucose transport systems in rat adipocytes. J Endocrinol 144: 347–357

Menzel C, Grünwald F, Schomburg A, Palmedo H, Bender H, Späth G, Biersack HJ (1996) „High-dose" radioiodine therapy in advanced differentiated thyroid carcinoma. J Nucl Med 37: 1496–1503

Messa C, Landoni C, Fridrich L, Lucignani G, Striano G, Riccabona G, Fazio F (1996) [F-18]FDG uptake in metastatic thyroid carcinoma prior and after I-131 therapy. Eur J Nucl Med 23: 1097

Nemec J, Nyvltova O, Blazek Tb et al. (1996) Positive thyroid cancer scintigraphy using technetium-99 m methoxyisobutylisonitrile. Eur J Nucl Med 23: 69–71
Pirro JP, Di Rocco RJ, Narra RK, Nunn AD (1994) Relationship between in vitro transendothelial permeability and in vivo single-pass brain extraction. J Nucl Med 35: 1514–1519
Piwinica-Worms D, Kronauge JF, Chiu ML (1990) Uptake and retention of hexakis (2-methoxyisobutyl isonitrile) technetium (I) in cultured chick myocardial cells, mitochondrial and plasma membrane potential dependence. Circulation 82: 1826–1838
Platz D, Lübeck M, Beyer W, Grimm C, Beuthin-Baumann B, Gratz KF, Hotze LA (1995) Einsatz der [^{18}F]-deoxyglucose-PET (FDG-PET) in der Nachsorge von Patienten mit differenziertem und medullärem Schilddrüsencarcinom. Nucl Med 34: 152
Raue F (1997) Chemotherapie bei Schilddrüsenkarzinomen: Indikation und Ergebnisse. Onkologe 3: 55–58
Raue F, Frank-Raue K (1997) Gehört die Calcitoninbestimmung zur Abklärung der Struma nodosa? Dtsch Ärztebl 94: 855–856
Reiners C (1993) Radiojodtherapie – Indikation, Durchführung und Risiken. Dtsch Ärztebl 90: 2217–2221
Schober O, Heintz P, Schwarzrock R, Dralle H, Gratz KF, Döhring W, Hundeshagen H (1986) Schilddrüsen-Carcinom: Rezidiv- und Metastasensuche; Sonographie, Röntgen und CT. Nuklearmediziner 9: 139–148
Simon D (1997) Von limitierter bis erweiterter Radikalität der Operation beim Schilddrüsenkarzinom. In: Roth et al. (eds) Klinische Onkologie. Huber, Bern: 347–357
Simon D, Köhrle J, Schmutzler C, Mainz K, Reiners C, Röher HD (1996) Redifferentiation therapy of differentiated thyroid carcinoma with retinoic acid: basics and first clinical results. Exp Clin Endocrinol Diabetes 104 [Suppl 4]: 13–15
Sisson JC, Ackermann RJ, Meyer MA (1993) Uptake of 18-fluoro-2-deoxy-D-glucose by thyroid cancer: implications for diagnosis and therapy. J Clin Endocrin Metabol 77: 1090–1094
Spiessl B, Beahrs OH, Hermanek P, Hutter RVP, Scheibe O, Sobin LH, Wagner G (1993) TNM-Atlas. Illustrierter Leitfaden zur TNM/pTNM-Klassifikation maligner Tumoren/International Union Against Cancer/Union Internationale Contre le Cancer (UICC). Springer, Berlin Heidelberg New York, p 58
Tatsch K, Weber W, Rossmüller B, Langhammer H, Ziegler S, Hahn K, Schwaiger M (1996) F-18 FDG-PET in der Nachsorge von Schilddrüsencarcinom-Patienten mit hTg-Anstieg aber fehlender Iod- und Sestamibi-Speicherung. Nuklearmedizin 35: A34
Yoshioka T, Takahashi H, Oikawa H et al. (1994) Accumulation of 2-deoxy-2[^{18}F]fluoro-D-glucose in human cancer heterotransplanted in nude mice: comparison between histology and glycolytic status. J Nucl Med 35: 97–103

5.4 Pulmonary Nodules and Non-Small-Cell Bronchial Carcinoma

R. P. Baum, N. Presselt, and R. Bonnet

Diagnostic imaging of lung cancer has been the province of morphologically oriented techniques almost exclusively, especially high-resolution CT, which today is increasingly performed using the spiral technique.

Nuclear medical modalities have played a role in the surgical planning phase (quantification of perfusion or ventilation deficiency) and have also been used for the detection of bone metastases (skeletal scintigraphy), for isolated instances of status determination of focal lung changes (^{201}Tl-SPECT, gallium scintigraphy, immunoscintigraphy), and for recurrence diagnosis. But scintigraphic methods have not yet been widely accepted for the general diagnosis of bronchial carcinoma.

With the introduction of PET, an imaging technique is available for the first time that is based on biochemical changes and can detect primary tumors and metastases on the basis of metabolic changes with relatively high resolution in whole-body mode.

5.4.1 Epidemiology and Etiology of Lung Cancer

Lung cancer is one of the most common cancers: around the world, over a million deaths per year are attributable to it.

In Germany lung cancer continues to be the most frequent cause of death from cancer in men over 45 years of age (approximately 26,000 lung cancer deaths annually, although recently a plateau or slight decrease is noticeable due to changes in smoking habits); in women the frequency of lung carcinoma has strongly increased in tandem with cigarette consumption and has overtaken breast cancer as a cause of cancer mortality in many western countries. In England more than 30,000 people die every year of lung cancer, in the U.S. more than 150,000 (with more than 170,000 new cases annually).

In Germany the incidence exceeds 50 per 100,000. Lung cancer is (still) four to five times more common in men than in women. The peak of frequency occurs in the 60 to 70-year age group (median age: about 61). More than 36,000 people die annually from this disease in the former West Germany.

Etiologically, the inhalation of exogenous chemical carcinogens – primarily inhalational tobacco smoking – plays the biggest role: 85 % of all deaths from lung cancer are traceable to smoking. Genetic factors also play a role: discussion focuses on familial predisposition, among other factors.

5.4.2 Prognosis, Histology and Staging

The mean survival time for untreated lung cancer is a mere 6 months. The 5-year survival rate is about 17 % for men and 9 % for women; for both sexes (all lung carcinoma), it is only 13 %.

Decisive prognostic parameters include the histological tumor type (Table 5.4.1), tumor spread (by stage; see Table 5.4.2), and the patient's performance status (Karnofsky score, ECOG scale). Other factors are the degree of malignity (grading), tumor doubling time, and the presence of clinical symptoms, among others.

Table 5.4.1. Histological classification of bronchial carcinoma. (After WHO)

Histological Classification	ICD Number
Squamous cell carcinoma Variant: spindle cell carcinoma	ICD No. 8070/3
Adenocarcinoma Acinar adenocarcinoma Papillary adenocarcinoma Solid carcinoma with myxopoiesis	ICD No. 8140/3
Large-cell carcinoma Giant cell carcinoma Clear cell carcinoma	ICD No. 8012/3
Adenosquamous carcinoma	ICD No. 8560/3
Bronchoalveolar adenocarcinoma	ICD No. 8250/3
Adenocystic carcinoma	ICD No. 8200/3
Mucoepidermoid carcinoma	ICD No. 8320/3

Table 5.4.2. Clinical Staging of Bronchial Carcinoma. (After UICC/AJCC/ISSLC 1997)

Stage		Grouping of Stages	
Occult carcinoma	TX	N0	M0
No primary tumor	T0	–	M0
Stage 0 Carcinoma in situ	Tis	N0	M0
Stage I A	T1	N0	M0
Stage I B	T2	N0	M0
Stage II A	T1	N1	M0
Stage II B	T2	N1	M0
Stage III A	T1 T2 T3	N2 N2 N1, N2	M0 M0 M0
Stage III B	any T T4	N3 any N	M0 M0
Stage IV	any T	any N	M1

The 5-year survival rate for lung carcinoma treated by chemotherapy is only 5–10 % (Whitehouse 1994; Cullen 1995), which is largely traceable to early metastatic spread. Even after apparently complete surgical tumor resection, the 5-year survival rate does not exceed 40 % (Lee and Hong 1992). In Stage I survival rates of 70 % are reported, and in Stage II survival rates of 40 %. In Stage IIIa (when mediastinoscopy is negative), a 5-year survival rate of 30 % has been reported (Morgan 1995).

5.4.3 Diagnosis of Lung Cancer

Screening

There is general agreement that early detection programs do little to increase the survival rate for persons with lung cancer. However, a study at the Mayo Clinic showed that the mortality rate for patients who underwent surgical therapy at an early stage (because a lung carcinoma was discovered during screening) was approximately

18 % lower than it was for a comparison group (Flehinger and Melamed 1994).

Clinical Symptoms and Examination

There are hardly any characteristic early symptoms. A dry cough, bronchial hemorrhage, fever, and excessive sweating at night are the most frequent symptoms, followed by weight loss, weakness, chest pain, dyspnea, dysphagia, hoarseness, superior vena cava syndrome, and Horner's or Pancoast's syndrome.

The medical history should be taken and the physical exam performed according to applicable oncological guidelines, with questioning and investigation focusing particularly on the above-listed symptoms. In addition, there should be careful palpation of the accessible lymph node groups.

Instrument-Based Diagnostics

The diagnosis and staging of bronchial carcinoma involves numerous examinations. The possible therapeutic consequences of these tests and the patient's individual tolerance for them should always be the primary focus. A breakdown of these examinations into basic diagnostics (see overview), continuing diagnostics (see overview) and functional diagnostics (lung function, body plethysmography, lung perfusion scintigraphy, ventilation scintigraphy, and EKG) has been standard clinical practice (Drings 1988).

5.4.4 Therapy for Non-Small-Cell Bronchial Carcinoma

Surgical Treatment

Nonsmall cell bronchial carcinoma predominates among lung cancers with 75 % of cases. The recommended treatment is an anatomically appropriate radical surgical resection of the tumor-bearing lobe or lobes of the lung, with an oncological objective of R_0. This applies to all tumor

Basic Diagnosis for Bronchial Carcinoma

- Medical history (risk factors: inhalational smoking, familial disposition, noxious substances in the workplace)
- Clinical examination (pulmonary, thoracic, paraneoplastic, unspecific symptoms)
- Laboratory tests
- Chest radiography on two planes
- CT of the chest and upper abdomen (with contrast medium)
- Bronchoscopy (with extraction of material for cytological and histological examination and staging biopsy for central tumors)
- Skeletal scintigraphy
- Cardiac functional diagnosis (spirometry or body plethysmography), arterial blood gas analysis, EKG
  - Stress EKG (facultative)
  - Spiroergometry (facultative)
  - Echocardiography (facultative)
  - Heart catheter (facultative)

Instrument-Based and Imaging Diagnosis for Bronchial Carcinoma

- Whole-body PET
- CT of the chest and upper abdomen (with contrast medium)
- Bronchoscopy
- Sonography of the upper abdomen
- Possible head CT (depending on symptoms and/or for adenocarcinoma)
- Skeletal scintigraphy
- Quantitative lung perfusion scintigraphy (facultative)
- Mediastinoscopy (facultative)
- Thoracoscopy (facultative)
- Pulmonary angiography, upper cavography (facultative)
- MRI (facultative)

Surgical Therapy for Nonsmall Cell Bronchial Carcinoma (According to the Guidelines of the Gesellschaft für Thoraxchirurgie)

- Surgical Indication
  - Non-small-cell bronchial carcinoma in tumor Stage I and II and for T3No and T3N1 tumors in Stage IIIA (especially if T3 is located above the main carina)
  - If N2 is suspected (i.e., CT reveals lymph nodes with diameter > 1 cm), mediastinoscopy should be performed. A positive result requires multimodal treatment. Mediastinal bulky disease should primarily not be surgically treated.

A precondition for a surgical indication is functional operability.

- Surgical Principle
  - Resection of the involved lobe or lobes of the lung: for example, lobectomy, bilobectomy, bronchial sleeve resection, pneumonectomy
  - Only if lung function is very limited: segment resection, wedge resection

A systematic lymphadenectomy is a component of surgery.
There must be an opportunity for rapid section diagnosis during surgery.

stages in which contralateral lymph node involvement of the N_3 type was ruled out preoperatively. Systematic lymphadenectomy of the mediastinum (see overview) is a regular surgical component of anatomically appropriate radical resection in any case. However, only 10–20 % of all patients are primarily operable in the strictest sense (Morgan 1995). In order to achieve the stated goal of an R_0 resection (no histological evidence of tumor cells at the periphery of the resection and successful radical lymph node dissection), the surgeon must be experienced in bronchoplastic and angioplastic techniques including expanded resection techniques for neighbor organs to the lung, especially the mediastinum and/or chest wall.

Some centers follow a more aggressive surgical approach even in advanced stages such as IIIB and T4 (Ginsberg 1991), i.e., extended T3/T4 and N2/N3 stages and extrathoracic metastases (especially isolated brain metastases). Cures have been achieved in some cases.

Chemotherapy

Chemotherapy offers a palliative and sometimes life-prolonging option, given the great frequency of metastatic spread. However, standard chemotherapeutic agents have only limited effectiveness with non-small-cell bronchial carcinoma: substances such as ifosfamide, mitomycin, cisplatin, etoposide, vinblastine and vindesine show a major response in only 15–20 % of patients when used singly (Cullen 1995). Newer chemotherapeutic agents such as paclitaxel, vinorelbine and gemcitabine are more promising (response rates of over 30 %). Response rates to combined chemotherapy (with cisplatin) are in the range of 25–50 % (with complete remission occurring in 10 % or less of patients), but in this regard there is scarcely a statistically verified significant survival advantage (Crino 1995; Thatcher et al. 1995).

There are randomized studies (and meta-analyses) of adjuvant chemotherapy after a "curative" resection, of neoadjuvant therapy before the extirpation of enlarged carcinomas, of chemotherapy for inoperable (but localized) carcinomas, and of combined radiotherapy and chemotherapy.

Radiotherapy

Primary radiation therapy is the (potentially curative) treatment for medically inoperable patients (or those who do not agree to surgery). Five-year survival rates of 5–40 % are achievable with tumor doses of 60 Gy and more. Radiotherapy is performed as a supplementary measure on patients with mediastinal lymph node metastases or incomplete tumor resection; it can reduce the rate of local recurrence by approximately 10 %.

Tumor doses of 40 – 50 Gy are sufficient for palliative therapy and can temporarily have a favorable affect on secondary tumor symptoms in a majority of patients.

Combined radiation therapy and chemotherapy is being studied intently, in particular for Stage III patients.

5.4.5 Positron Emission Tomography

Metabolic Tracers

2-F-18-fluoro-2-deoxy-D-glucose (^{18}F-FDG) is widely accepted in clinical practice. Because of its high uptake in tumors (SUV, Table 5.4.3) and associated high sensitivity – resulting in a detection rate of nearly 100 % for primary tumors – this glucose analogue has been used successfully in many types of examinations including the differential diagnosis of pulmonary nodules, the detection of primary bronchial carcinoma, the detection of lymph nodes and distant metastases, recurrence diagnosis, and the evaluation of response to therapy.

However, an increased glucose metabolism is detectable in acute inflammatory reactions (e.g., florid lymph node tuberculosis) as well as in malignant tumors. Some groups have therefore recommended S-methyl-C-11 – methionine (MET) because of its supposedly lower uptake in inflammatory lesions; moreover, it exhibits faster blood clearance than FDG. But recent studies by Weber et al. (1998) examining 19 patients with lung carcinoma using FDG PET, MET PET (and CT) intraindividually in direct comparison showed that the lower MET tumor uptake (SUV 4.3) does not lead to a higher image contrast compared with FDG (SUV 7.9), despite its faster clearance, and that FDG is even superior in the detection of mediastinal lymph node metastases. Additionally, MET is even concentrated in florid inflamed lymph nodes, just like FDG.

Other PET tracers – such as positron-marked antibodies (Immune-PET) or receptor ligands (Receptor-PET), for example – and labeled amino acids or chemotherapeutic agents have only been used preclinically in isolated instances to date and do not yet play a role in routine diagnostics.

PET Scanning Technique

The accurate technical execution of whole-body PET is of great significance in achieving a high diagnostic sensitivity (and specificity). Optimal patient preparation must be strictly observed (fasting, hydration, administration of diuretics, physical immobility), as should a sufficient waiting period (Lowe et al. 1995) before image acquisition (FDG blood clearance, especially in the mediastinum and lung) and the optimal imaging time for the emission and transmission scans (see overview for details).

Our experience suggests that is it critical to obtain an attenuation-corrected image of the chest area at a minimum and of the whole body if possible, since small mediastinal lymph node metastases, in particular, can occasionally only be detected in attenuation-corrected images. If there is very intensive uptake in primary bronchial car-

Table 5.4.3. FDG PET in patients with malignant and benign pulmonary nodules: standardized uptake values (SUV)

Author	Number	Malignant	Benign	SUV
Gupta (1992)	20	5,62,38	0,560,27	<0,001
Gupta (1993)	32	5,52,38	1,20,9	<0,001
Patz (1993)	51	6,52,9	1,71,2	
Hübner (1993)	52	6,43,0	2,82,2	<0,001
Minn (1995)	10	8,33,8	no data provided	no data provided

Procedure for FDG Whole-Body PET Scanning

- Patient Preparation
  - Fasting period of 12 hours (at least 4–6 hours), check blood glucose level *before* FDG administration (blood glucose if possible 90 mg/dl)
  - Noncaloric beverages (mineral water) are permitted
  - Injection of 300–500 MBq ^{18}F-FDG (2D technique, full ring scanner)
  - Rest period (physical immobility) of at least 45–60 minutes (optimal: 90–120 minutes) before emission scan
  - Hydration (0.75–1 liter of mineral water, beginning approximately 15 minutes before the FDG injection)
  - I.v. administration of a diuretic (furosemide [Lasix]: 20–40 mg) approximately 20 minutes after FDG injection)
- Imaging Technique
  - Transmission scan (5–10 minutes, approximately 50 % of the time required for the emission scan) in the form of a "hot transmission scan," if necessary also after the emission scan.
  - Emission scan: 8–15 minutes per bed position (calculated by elapsed time post-injection) from mid-thigh to base of skull
- Options
  - Transmission scan before the FDG injection ("cold transmission scan"), possibly with subsequent repositioning of the patient
  - Separate image of the brain (beginning approximately 30–45 minutes post-injection)
  - Reduced ^{18}F activity for 3D scanning or coincidence cameras

cinomas, massive reconstruction artifacts (distortion, particularly in non-iterative reconstruction) occasionally appear in a lone emission image, making it difficult to correctly evaluate surrounding regions or localized lymph node metastases near the primary tumor.

Evaluation and Documentation of Whole-Body FDG PET

- *Always:* evaluation by the *physician* at the *monitor*
- Viewing of *all* transverse and coronal (and sagittal) slices from the base of the skull to the femurs
- Correlation with morphological tomographic methods (spiral CT), if possible as co-registered images on the same display screen or as image fusion, especially when evaluating lymph node metastases
- Documentation of all pathological findings in the form of al color printout (zoomed slices); also as PET-CT fusion image, if available.
- Visual evaluation is sufficient for routine; additional quantitative evaluations (standardized uptake value [SUV] or Patlak plot) are necessary for specific scientific problems. A semi-quantitative evaluation of characteristic tumor nodules (> 1.5–2 cm in diameter, if possible) using an SUV curve is very helpful for purposes of therapy monitoring.

Of equally great importance is a painstaking evaluation of the scan (see overview), which can be quite time-consuming when detecting metastases (especially for image overlays with CT). It is advisable to evaluate transmission-corrected and non-transmission-corrected scans separately since the contrast is sometimes higher in superficially located metastases in images that are not attenuation-corrected (Bengel et al. 1997).

As to whether a quantitative or semiquantitative evaluation is superior to a purely visual image evaluation, it can be stated that a visual image evaluation generally has the same sensitivity (or even a higher sensitivity) (Lowe et al. 1994). An improvement of approximately 10 % in specificity can be produced through Patlak analyses (expensive), but at the sacrifice of sensitivity (Hübner et al. 1996).

5.4.6 Clinical Indications for Positron Emission Tomography

Solitary Pulmonary Nodules and Primary Tumor Detection (*Fig. 5.4.1*)

Nearly 75 % of pulmonary nodules are found incidentally. They are frequently discovered during routine chest radiography occasioned by disease that is not pulmonary. Signs and symptoms indicating a lung problem are found in only approximately 20–25 % of patients with solitary pulmonary nodules (coughing, hemoptysis or thoracic pain appearing as uncharacteristic symptoms). According to earlier examinations of over 1,000 patients with peripheral nodules, an average time period of seven months elapsed until a definitive diagnosis was reached, whereby the younger the patient and the smaller the nodule, the longer the delay until diagnosis. Since in central Europe approximately 50 % of patients have a malignant genesis of a pulmonary lung nodule, valuable time is being lost.

In terms of differential diagnosis, approximately 80 diseases in varying degrees of frequency are cited in the literature as sources of a pulmonary nodule. Age, medical history, and even patient nationality can provide clues (echinococcus cysts in the orient, for example, or fungal infections in various parts of the American continent).

In an analysis of 950 solitary pulmonary nodules (Toomes et al. 1981), half of the pulmonary nodules revealed a malignant tumor and the other half revealed benign findings (Tables 5.4.4 and 5.4.5). According to estimates (Dewan et al. 1993), approximately 130,000 solitary pulmonary nodules (SPN) are discovered annually in the U.S. (incidence: approximately 52 per 100,000 inhabitants), of which approximately 30–50 % are malignant. Before the era of CT, approximately 60 % of all surgically removed SPN were benign. This high rate was reduced by 20–40 % through the use of high-resolution CT, but even today invasive diagnosis is routine in many places.

Bronchoscopy achieves a sensitivity of only 65 % in the detection of malignant nodules, and even transbronchoscopic biopsy increases the sensitivity to only 79 % (Salathe et al. 1992).

Transthoracic fine needle biopsy (TTFB) achieves a sensitivity of 94–98 % and a specificity

Table 5.4.4. Benign histological findings in 955 surgically treated pulmonary nodules (Toomes et al. 1981)

Benign Diseases	n = 486
Benign Tumors	n = 132
Chondromas	74
Neurogenic tumors	22
Bronchial adenomas	11
Benign mesotheliomas	5
Other	20
Tuberculosis	n = 225
Other	n = 129
Chronic pneumonias (abscess)	23
Echinococcus cysts	22
Bronchial cysts	21
Aspergillomas	13
Diaphragmatic hernias	11
Other	39

Table 5.4.5. Malignant histological findings in 955 surgically treated pulmonary nodules (Toomes et al. 1981)

Malignant Diseases	n = 469
Bronchial carcinomas	n = 364
Squamous cell carcinomas	74
Adenocarcinomas	127
Alveolar cell carcinomas	22
Other	44
Other	20
Metastases	n = 89
Adenocarcinomas	40
Squamous cell carcinomas	32
Sarcomas	12
Other	5
Other	n = 16
Primary lung sarcomas	6
Solitary myelomas	2
Hodgkin's disease	2
Teratomas	2
Other	4

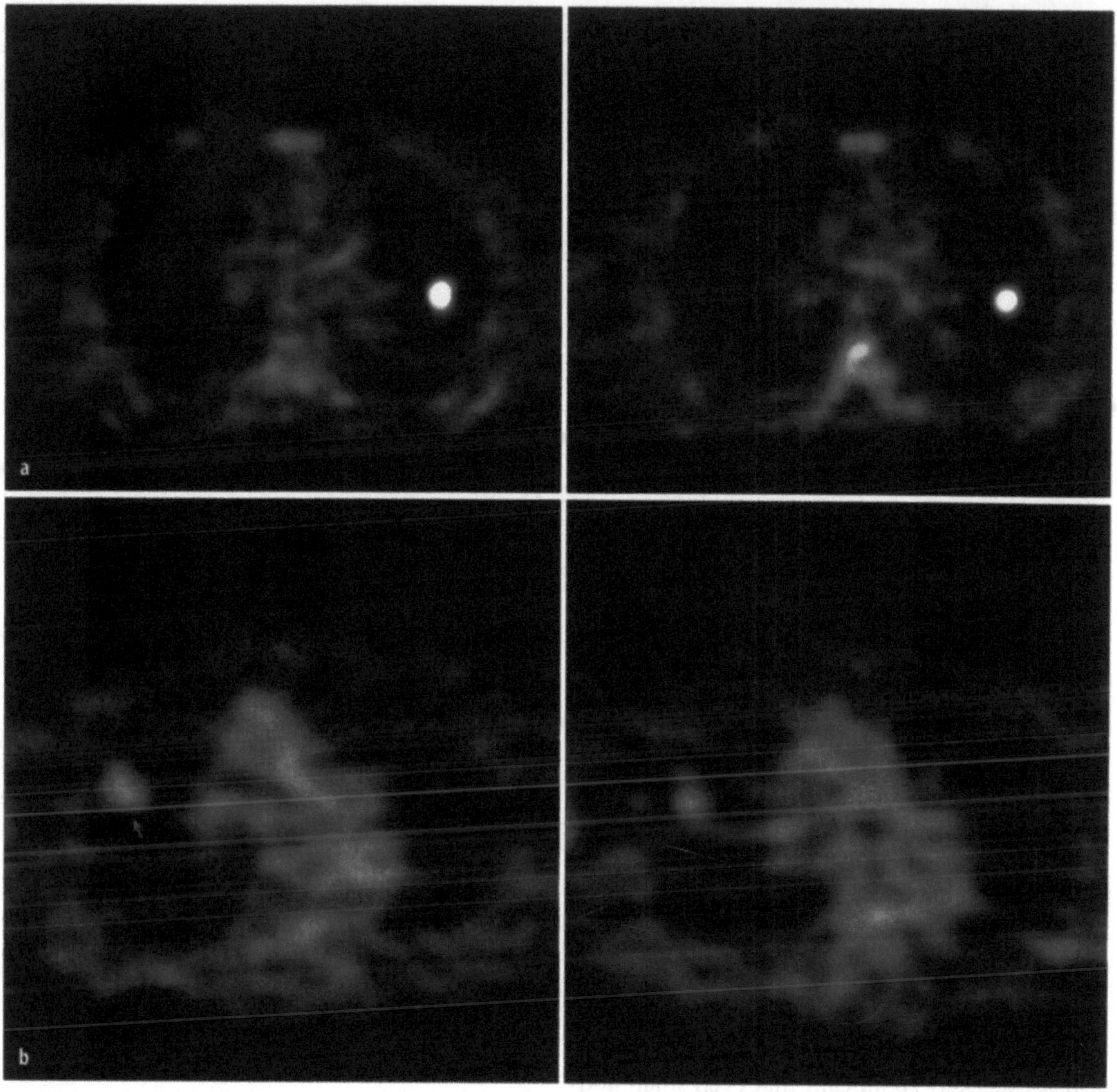

Fig. 5.4.1. a Solitary nodule of unclear etiology localized left pulmonary (indeterminate SPN in chest CT). Highly hypermetabolic focal findings typical of a tumor (SUV: 7.8) in transmission-corrected transverse FDG PET. Histological diagnosis: moderately differentiated adenosquamous carcinoma (diameter 1.6 cm). **b** Solitary pulmonary nodule right pulmonary; CT findings ambiguous as regards genesis; transthoracic aspiration was unsuccessful. The attentuation-corrected FDG PET (transverse slice sequence) shows focal findings with low glucose consumption (SUV: 2.3). Definitive diagnosis: active tuberculoma

of 91–96 % (Wang et al. 1988) but harbors a 19–26 % risk of pneumothorax. 10–15 % of patients with this problem require pleural drainage, which means a hospital stay and therefore considerable extra expense. In a study of 181 patients with discrete pulmonary lesions that were diagnosed using TTFB, TTFB could not definitively rule out a tumor in 40 % of those biopsies, and malignant findings appeared later histologically in 40 % of the nodules (Winning et al. 1986).

The basic possibility of differentiating between benign and malignant pulmonary nodules using

Table 5.4.6.
Lung carcinoma: solitary pulmonary nodules and detection of primary lung carcinoma using FDG PET

Patients (n)	Sensitivity [%]	Specificity [%]	Author
20	100	100	Gupta (1992)
30	95	80	Dewan (1993)
51	89	100	Patz (1993)
33	100	78	Dewan (1995)
87	97	82	Duhaylongsod (1995)
23	100	67	Hübner (1995)
61	93	88	Gupta (1996)
48	100	63	Knight (1996)
82	100	52	Sazon (1996)
46	94	86	Guhlmann (1997)
109	98	89	Rigo (1997)
98	92	90	Lowe (1998)
$\Sigma = 682$	97	81	Average

FDG PET (Table 5.4.6) was demonstrated some years ago (Kubota et al. 1990; Gupta et al. 1992, 1993; Patz et al. 1993; and Dewan et al. 1993). A multi-institutional prospective study at nine university centers in the U.S. was published in March 1998 in the *Journal of Clinical Oncology*, one of the most highly regarded oncological journals (Lowe et al. 1998). Visual evaluation of PET scans of 89 patients with solitary pulmonary nodules of unresolved etiology (despite previously completed lung survey radiography and CT examinations) yielded a sensitivity for PET of 98 % for tumor detection. Semiquantitative SUV analyses resulted in a sensitivity of 92 % and a specificity of 90 %.

It is especially significant that even small nodules (< 1.5 cm) can be detected with very high sensitivity (100 % in visual evaluation).

This multi-institutional prospective study came to the conclusion that FDG PET is able to differentiate between individual pulmonary nodules as regards etiology (benign/malignant) with a high degree of diagnostic accuracy and that by this means unnecessary invasive surgery can be avoided. According to estimates of the Institute for Clinical PET (ICP), approximately 10,126 unnecessary surgeries (for benign pulmonary nodules) could be avoided and 30–236 million U.S. dollars could be saved (Fig. 5.4.2). Among other things, the abovementioned prospective study resulted in Medicare reimbursement of PET examinations for SPN (and for primary staging of lung carcinoma as well) effective January 1998. Switzerland's health care system also reimburses the costs of FDG PET for this indication. Only in Germany (in spite of a clear position taken by the consensus conference: see Table 5.4.10) is it still necessary for patients covered by the statutory health insurance system to file a separate application.

Lymph Node Staging

In addition to differential diagnosis of solitary pulmonary nodules and associated primary tumor detection, preoperative lymph node staging is another indication for FDG PET that is clinically extremely significant.

There are a number of reasons for this:

- Decisions about the operability or inoperability of a patient based on which lymph nodes are involved with tumor (especially the distinction between ipsilateral and contralateral involvement, i.e., between Stage N1, N2, and N3).

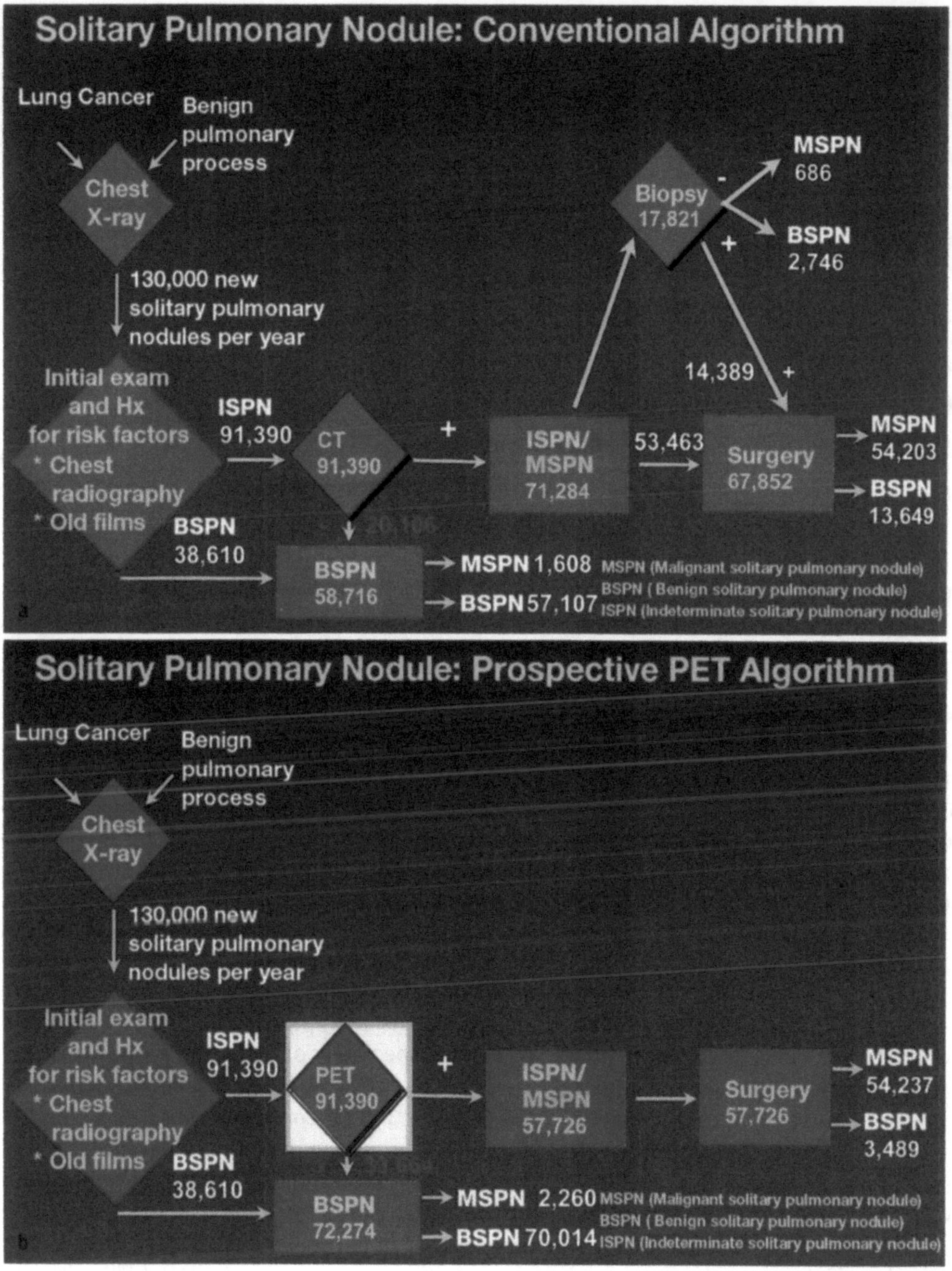

Fig. 5.4.2a, b. Diagnostic algorithm and cost savings using FDG PET for nonsmall cell lung carcinoma (ICP 1994)

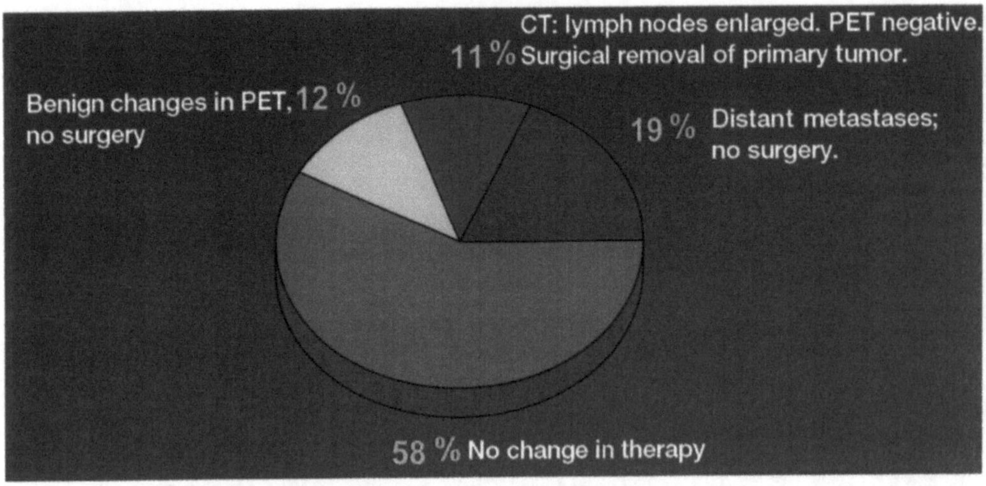

Fig. 5.4.3. Staging of non-small-cell bronchial carcinoma using FDG PET. Therapeutic procedure was changed for 11 of 26 patients (42 %)

- Whereas ipsilateral involvement (Stage N1 or limited N2) is regarded as an indication for surgery, contralateral involvement (or cervical lymph node metastases) is seen as a contraindication, since these patients do not profit prognostically from the operation. In 1978 the incidence of lymph node metastases in surgically treated lung carcinoma was still 31–71 % and reached 75–94 % at postmortem examinations (Naruke et al. 1978).
- Lymph node status is a significant prognostic parameter.

It is recognized that the established imaging techniques (especially CT) have insufficient sensitivity and specificity for detecting lymph node metastases since lymph node size correlates poorly with tumor involvement. A prospective RDOC study carried out with the support of the NIH (Webb et al. 1991) showed a low sensitivity for CT and MRI in the detection of mediastinal lymph node metastases (approximately 50 %) with an equally insufficient specificity (65 %). On the other hand, approximately 30 % of all enlarged lymph nodes (diameter 2–4 cm) exhibit no tumor cells (Schiepers 1997) histopathologically.

Initial studies by the Heidelberg group (Knopp et al. 1992) have already noted PET's high diagnostic accuracy for mediastinal staging of bronchial carcinoma. This group reported a sensitivity of 98 % and a specificity of 94 % (histologically verified) in 49 patients, for example. In 33 % of cases, a change was made in the patient's CT classification after the PET examination. The Frankfurt group (Fig. 5.4.3) reported a change in therapeutic procedure for 30 % of all patients studied (Baum et al. 1996b) and for 42 % when distant metastases were included (Baum et al. 1996a).

Prospective studies by Wahl et al. (1994) have already shown that the metabolic characterization of mediastinal lymph node involvement as revealed by FDG metabolism was more accurate than CT scans: in 23 patients PET had a sensitivity of 82 %, a specificity of 81 %, and a diagnostic accuracy of 81 % (CT: 64/44/52 %). Subsequent studies (Table 5.4.7) all confirmed FDG PET's higher diagnostic accuracy when compared with CT (even in spiral technique). The recent publication by the Zürich group (Steinert et al. 1997) should be emphasized in particular since it includes a direct preoperative comparison of FDG PET with CT (newest generation), including image overlay and definitive histological verification (classified by lymph node stations: lymph node sampling of 599 lymph nodes from 199 lymph node stations). This prospective study found a PET sensi-

Table 5.4.7. Lung carcinoma: mediastinal/hilar lymph node staging using FDG PET; comparison with CT

	PET		CT		
Patients (n)	SE [%]	SP [%]	SE [%]	SP [%]	Author
23	82	81	64	44	Wahl (1994)
30	78	81	56	86	Chin (1995)
29	76	98	65	87	Sasaki (1996)
16	100	100	81	56	Sazon (1996)
47	89	99	57	94	Steinert (1997)
46	80	100	50	75	Guhlmann (1997)
75	88	88	73	68	Rigo (1997)
50	93	97	67	59	Vansteenkiste (1997)
$\Sigma = 316$	86	93	64	71	Average

tivity of 89 % in the detection of mediastinal N2 or N3 lymph node metastases (CT 57 %), while specificity for PET was as high as 99 % (CT 94 %). The use of PET resulted in a 96 % rate of correct lymph node status determination in patients with bronchial carcinoma, whereas the rate for CT was only 79 %.

Detection of Distant Metastases (Fig. 5.4.4)

A major advantage of PET over other imaging techniques is that PET is a basically whole-body scanning method and can detect distant metastases in addition to the primary tumor and lymph node metastases. It is especially significant that metastases of bronchial carcinoma are imaged with very good contrast (high FDG uptake) and for the most part independent of localization („all organ imaging"). For example, adrenal gland metastases can be detected with a high sensitivity (and specificity), as can liver and bone metastases and parenchymatous lung metastases (Bury et al. 1997), but also abdominal and cervical lymph node metastases and brain metastases, as our own experience has shown.

This permits better selection of patients before a planned primary tumor surgery. Although the literature on distant metastases is not as extensive as that on SPN problems or lymph node staging, available data show unilaterally a very high diagnostic accuracy for PET when used to detect distant metastases (Valk et al. 1996) and a change in therapeutic procedure in 10–18 % of patients resulting from PET detection of previously unknown distant metastases (Table 5.4.8).

Table 5.4.8. Lung carcinoma: detection of distant metastases in primary staging using FDG PET

Patients (n)	Result	Author
34	10 patients (23 %) with additional lesions, change in therapeutic procedure with 14 patients (41 %), of whom 6 patients (18 %) had no surgical therapy because of PET findings.	Lewis (1994)
61	Compared with conventional diagnosis: change of N-stage in 13 patients (21 %) and of M-stage in 6 patients (10 %)	Bury (1996)
39	59 lesions (liver, bone, lung, adrenal gland, lymph nodes, various). Sensitivity 100 %, specificity 94 %. PET resulted in change of M-Stage in 14 % of patients.	Rigo (1997)
99	Detection of previously unknown distant metastases in 11 of 99 (11 %) of patients. Confirmation of uncertain metastases in 7 patients. Histologically benign findings in 16 of 17 patients with suspected metastases in CT but no increased FDG uptake.	Valk (1996)

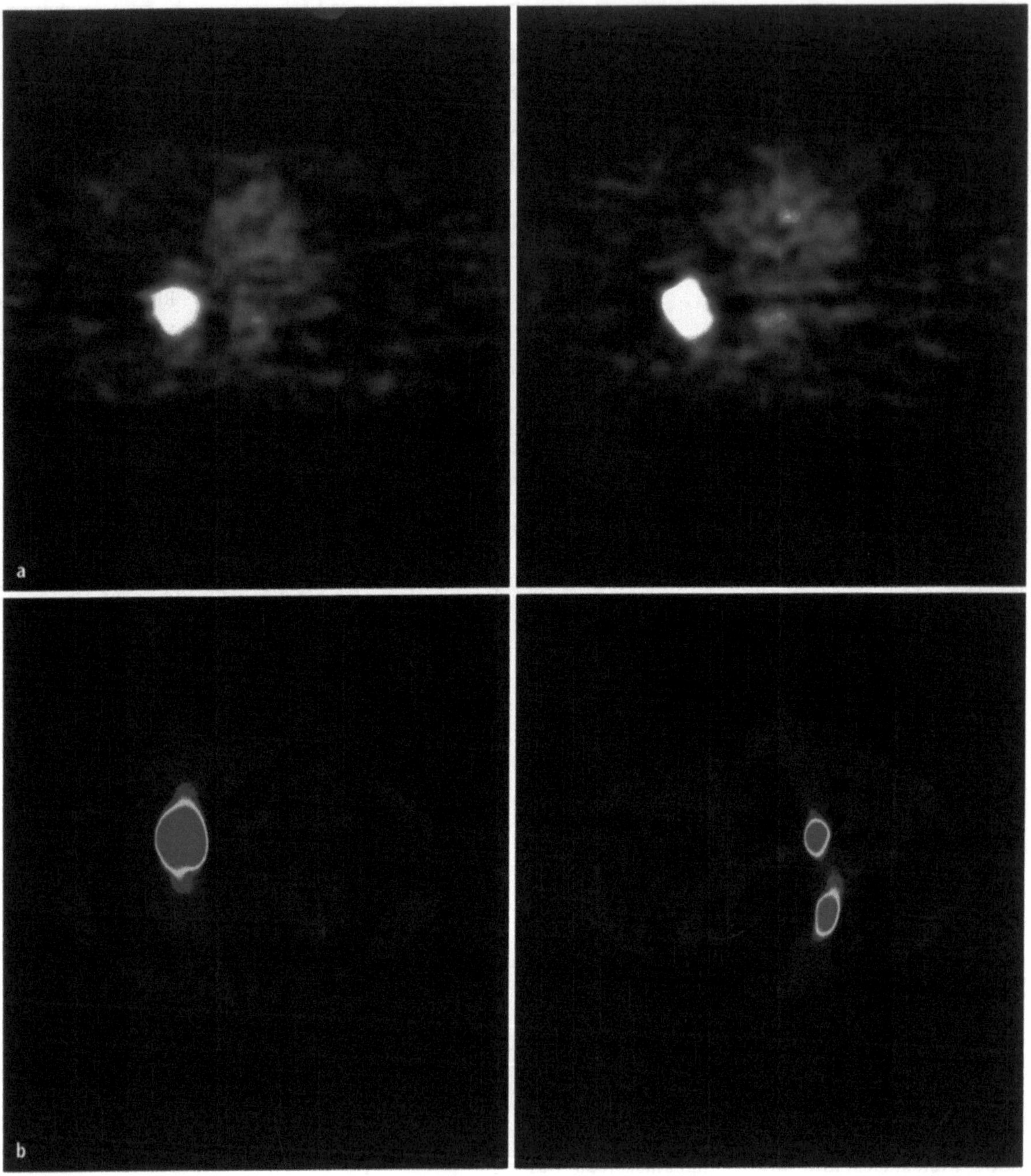

Fig. 5.4.4. a Squamous cell carcinoma in right inferior lobe of the lung, verified using transbronchoscopic biopsy. Chest CT reveals contralaterally enlarged hilar lymph nodes (Stage N3). Transmission-corrected PET shows the primary tumor with its greatly increased FDG uptake (SUV: 6.4) but no lymph node metastases. The subsequent surgery initiated on the basis of the PET scan confirmed a Stage N0 tumor. The primary tumor (diameter: 4.3 cm) was resected completely. To date the patient has been free of recurrence (period of observation: 32 months). **b** Highly FDG-consumptive squamous cell carcinoma in the right inferior lobe of the lung (pT2) and synchronous large cell adenocarcinoma of the left lung with mediastinal lymph node metastases (with CT, only the tumor in the right lung was detected initially)

Recurrence Diagnostics

The detection of a local recurrence of a previously surgically treated lung carcinoma is possible with a sensitivity of 83–100 % (average 95 %) and a specificity of 62–100 % (average 81 %), according to statements in the published literature (Table 5.4.9).

Of great interest clinically is the possibility of using whole-body scanning to detect distant metastases in addition to the local recurrence, which can be of great significance for subsequent therapy decisions (radiation therapy/chemotherapy or further surgical resection).

Therapy Monitoring

Changes in metabolism fundamentally precede changes in morphology. The fact that amino acid metabolism, tumor perfusion, and glucose metabolism can be ascertained using PET means that we are able in principle to determine accurately a tumor's response to therapy (Strauss 1996).

In 21 patients with lung carcinoma (43 scans), Kubota et al. (1993) showed that a group of patients with early recurrence can be distinguished from a group with late recurrence if ^{11}C-methionine PET is used after chemotherapy or radiation therapy. Using FDG PET, Hebert et al. (1996) determined tumor volume before radiotherapy in 20 patients with much greater accuracy than is possible using CT. There was also a decrease in FDG metabolism that correlated with therapeutic success.

Table 5.4.9. Lung carcinoma: detection of a local recurrence or residual tumor using FDG PET

Patients (n)	SE [%]	SP [%]	Author
43	97	100	Patz (1994)
16	100	82	Duhaylongsod (1995)
38	100	62	Inoue (1995)
13	83	80	Hübner (1995)
Σ = 110	95	81	Average

Inflammatory changes in the first few weeks after radiation therapy ("radiation pneumonitis") pose a problem since they can also lead to increased glucose metabolism. It is therefore advisable not to repeat PET examinations until 4–6 weeks after chemotherapy and 3 months after radiation therapy. An EORTC group (PET Study Group) is devoting itself specifically to this problem.

5.4.7 Positron Emission Tomography: Limitations and Pitfalls

Even though FDG PET has the potential to revolutionize the diagnosis and therapy monitoring of lung cancer, a careful diagnosis must be made – primarily, at the moment, for reasons of capacity. According to the recommendations of the consensus conference (Ulm 1997; Table 5.4.10), FDG PET is suitable for the diagnosis of unclear pulmonary nodules and for primary (above all, lymph node) staging, and – as newer studies show – for the detection of distant metastases and recurrences. Future studies incorporating larger numbers of patients must determine whether FDG PET is capable of evaluating therapeutic success wth higher sensitivity and with greater accuracy than has been possible with CT.

Because PET images contain limited anatomical information, a supplementary CT chest exam-

Table 5.4.10. Lung carcinoma: recommendations of the consensus conference (Ulm 1997)[a]

Primary Tumor	Classification
Peripheral nodule	1a
Local recurrence	1a
Staging	
N	1a
M	2b
Therapeutic monitoring	2a

[a] Classification:
1a. Appropriate and clinically useful
1b. Acceptable; preponderance of research supports clinical usefulness
2a. Possibly helpful but benefit is not as well documented
2b. No evaluation possible (do date) due to lack of data
3. Generally without benefit

ination should always be performed. Optimal information is obtained from an image overlay of PET (metabolism) and CT (morphology), with the result that image fusion will be incorporated in the future as a routine method, above all preoperatively (Fig. 5.4.5).

In spite of the relatively simple interpretability of PET scans (attested to by a low interobserver variance of less than 5 %), considerable experience in interpreting FDG scans is necessary due to the generally high tumor contrast, and there are a number of pitfalls that must be noted (see overiew). Nor should the time requirements of PET scanning be underestimated – up to two hours, including preparation time (particularly with whole-body examinations).

FDG PET in Lung Cancer. Pitfalls: Increased Glucose Metabolism in Benign Diseases

- Active tuberculosis (especially lymph node tuberculosis)
- Active sarcoidosis or nocardiosis
- Inflammatory anthrosilicosis
- Putrid bronchiectasis, florid pneumonia
- Other nodules with increased glucose metabolism (abscesses, inflammatory hematomas, radiogenic pneumonitis)

Whether coincidence technology using dual head cameras will be able to achieve a high sensitivity similar to that of ring tomographs is still

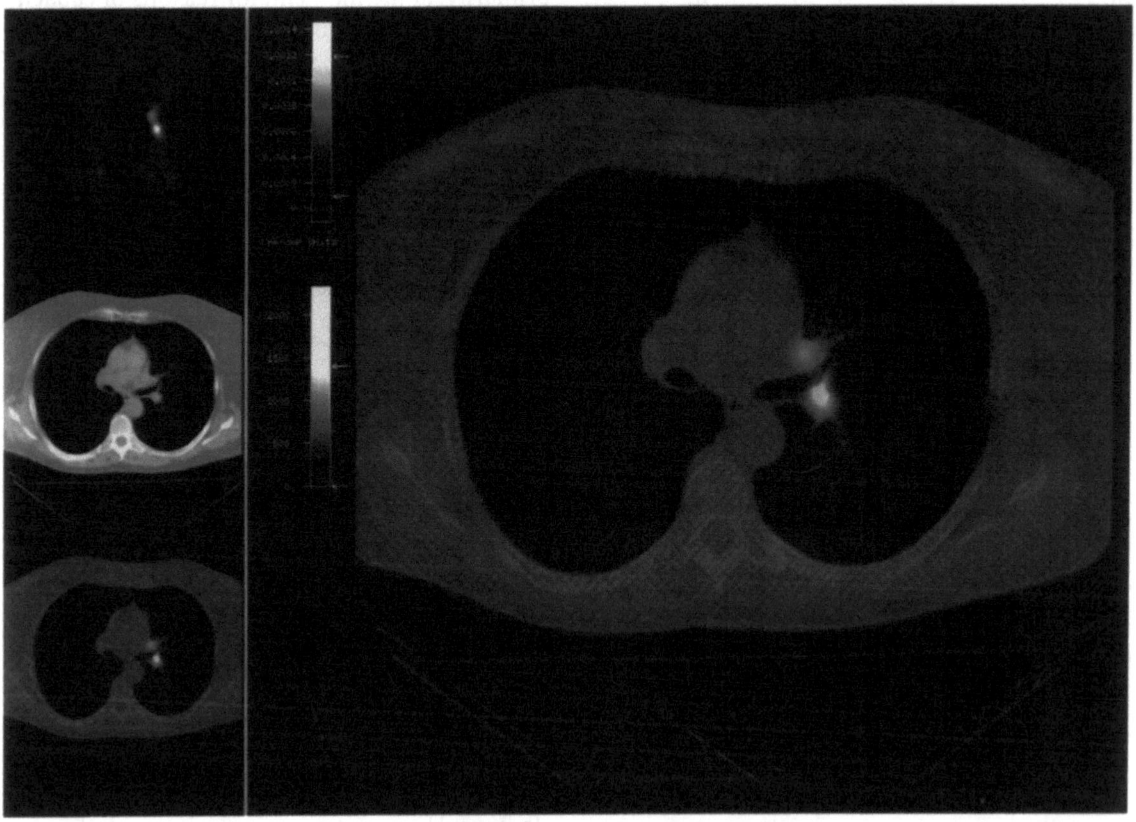

Fig. 5.4.5. Central bronchial carcinoma left bronchohilar (approximately 15 mm in diameter). Initial detection by FDG whole-body PET for initial existing UPT syndrome (neck lymph node metastases of unknown primary tumor). Further detection of an isolated lymph node metastasis left paraaortal (diameter 13 mm). Only the PET/CT image fusion allows the exact anatomical classification of the tumor focus

an open question. Early results (Shreve et al. 1998) show a markedly lower sensitivity for coincidence cameras (55 % that of „dedicated" PET). Pulmonary tumor lesions were detected most successfully (13 of 14 = 93 %), but only 20 of 31 (65 %) mediastinal lymph node metastases were detected.

Technological advancements such as attenuation correction (Karp et al. 1995) will also be able to bring about further improvements in this area in the future.

References

Abe Y, Matzuzawa T, Fujiwara T (1990) Clinical assessment of therapeutic effects on cancer using FDG and PET: preliminary study of lung cancer. Int J Radiat Oncol Bio Phys 19: 1005–1010

Abdel-Dayem HM, Scott A, Macapinlac H, Larson S (1995) Tracer imaging in lung cancer. Eur J Nucl Med 22: 1355

Baum RP, Rust M, Adams S et al. (1996a) Wertigkeit der Fluor-18-Fluor-Deoxy-Glukose (FDG) Ganzkörper-PET zum präoperativen Staging von Bronchialkarzinomen und Einfluß auf das therapeutische Procedere. Nucl Med 35: A19

Baum RP, Rust M, Adams S et al. (1996b) Influence on patients' management by whole-body F-18 FDG PET for preoperative staging of non small cell lung cancer. J Nucl Med 37: 121P

Bengel FM, Ziegler SI, Avril N, Weber W, Laubenbacher C, Schwaiger M (1997) Whole-body positron emission tomography in clinical oncology: comparison between attenuation-corrected and uncorrected images. Eur J Nucl Med 24: 1091–1098

Bleehan NM (1992) Current radiotherapy for non-small-cell lung cancer. Lung Cancer Ther 1: 1–3

Bury T, Dowlati A, Paulus P, Hustinx R, Radermecker M, Rigo P (1996) Staging of non-small-cell lung cancer by whole-body fluorine-18 deoxyglucose positron emission tomography. Eur J Nucl Med 23: 204–106

Castella J, Buj J, Puzo C, Antón PA, Burgués C (1995) Diagnosis and staging of bronchogenic carcinoma by transtracheal and transbronchial needle aspiration. Ann Oncol 6 [Suppl 3]: S21–S24

Chin R, Ward R, Keyes JW et al. (1995) Mediastinal staging of non-small-cell lung cancer with positron emission tomography. Am J Respir Crit Care Med 152: 2090–2096

Clorius HH, Lührs H (1990) Das Bronchialkarzinom – Nuklearmedizinische Diagnostik. Radiologe 30: 164–168

Crino L (1995) Chemotherapy on advanced non-small cell lung cancer. The experience of Italian Cooperative Groups. Ann Oncol 6 [Suppl 3]: S45–S47

Cullen MH (1995) Adjuvant and neo-adjuvant chemotherapy of non-small cell carcinoma. Ann Oncol 6 [Suppl 1]: S43–S48

Dewan NA, Gupta NC, Redepenning LS, Phalen JJ, Frick MP (1993) Diagnostic efficacy of PET-FDG imaging in solitary pulmonary nodules. Potential role in evaluation and management. Chest 104/4: 997–1002

Dewan NA, Reeb SD, Gupta NC, Gobar LS, Scott WJ: (1995) PET-FDG imaging and transthoracic needle lung aspiration biopsy in evaluation of pulmonary lesions. Chest 108: 441–446

Duhaylongsod FG, Lowe VL, Patz EF, Vaugh AL, Coleman RE, Wolfe WG (1995) Detection of primary and recurrent lung cancer by means of F-18 fluorodeoxyglucose positron emission tomography (FDG PET). J Thorax Cardiovasc Surg 110: 130–140

Drings P, Voigt-Moykopf I (1988) Das nicht kleinzellige Bronchialkarzinom. Dtsch Ärztebl 85: B-1469–B-1473

Flehinger BJ, Melamed MR (1994) Current status of screening for lung cancer. Chest Surg Clin North Am 4: 1–15

Frank A, Lefkowitz D, Jaeger S (1995) Decision logic for retreatment of asymptomatic lung cancer recurrence based on positron emission tomography findings. Int J Radiat Oncol Biol Phys 32: 1495–1512

Gambhir SS, Hoh CK, Phelps ME, Madar I, Maddahi J (1996) Decision tree sensitivity analysis for cost – effectiveness of FDG-PET in the staging and management of non-small-cell lung carcinoma. J Nucl Med 37: 1428–1436

Ginsberg RJ (1991) Surgery of higher stage lung cancer. Chest Surg Clin North Am 1: 61–69

Graham EA, Singer JJ (1933) Successfull removal of an entire lung for carcinoma of the bronchus. JAMA 101: 1371

Guhlmann A, Storck M, Kotzerke J, Moog F, Sunder-Plassmann L, Reske SN (1997) Lymph node staging in non-small-cell lung cancer: evaluation by F-18 FDG positron emission tomography (PET). Thorax 52: 438–441

Gupta NC, Frank AR, Dewan NA et al. (1992) Solitary pulmonary nodules: detection of malignancy with PET with 2-(F-18)-Fluoro-2-deoxy-D-glucose. Radiology 184: 441–444

Gupta NC, Dewan NA, Frank A (1993) Diagnostic evaluation of suspected solitary nodules (SPN) using PET FDG imaging. Chest 104: 119 S

Gupta NC, Maloof J, Gunel E (1996) Probability of malignancy in solitary pulmonary nodules using fluorine-18-FDG and PET. J Nucl Med 37: 943–948

Hebert ME, Lowe VJ, Hoffmann JM, Patz EF, Anscher MS (1996) Positron emission tomography in the pretreatment evaluation and follow-up of non-small-cell lung cancer patients treated with radiotherapy: preliminary findings. Am J Clin Oncol 19: 416–421

Hoh CK, Hawkins RA, Glaspy JA at al. (1993) Cancer detection with whole-body PET using 2-(F-18)-fluoro-2-deoxy-D-glucose. J Comput Assist Tomogr 17: 582–589

Hoh CK, Schiepers C, Seltzer MA et al. (1997) PET in oncology. Will it replace the other modalities? Sem Nucl Med 27: 94–106

Hör G (1993) Positronen-Emissions-Tomographie (PET) – Von der Forschung zur Klinik. Dtsch Ärztebl 90: 1883–1892

Hör G, Adams S, Baum RP, Hertel A, Adamietz IA, Böttcher HD, Kollath J (1994) Impact of single-photon-emission computed tomography and positron emission tomography on diagnostic oncology. Diagn Oncol 4: 297–321

Hübner KF, Buonocore E, Singh SK, Gould HR, Cotten DW (1995) Characterization of chest masses by FDG positron emission tomography. Clin Nucl Med 20: 293–298

Hübner KF, Buonocore E, Gould HR, Thie J, Smith GT, Stephens S, Dickey J (1996) Differentiating benign from malignant lung lesions using "quantitative" parameters of FDG PET images. Clin Nucl Med 21/12: 941–949

Hughes JMB (1996) F-18-fluorodeoxyglucose PET scans in lung cancer. Thorax 51: S16–S22

Ichiya Y, Kuwabara Y, Otsuka M et al. (1991) Assessment of response to cancer therapy using fluorine-18-fluorodeoxyglucose and positron emission tomography. J Nucl Med 32: 1655–1660

Inoue T, Kim EE, Komaki R et al. (1995) Detection of recurrent or residual lung cancer with FDG-PET. J Nucl Med 36: 788–793

Karp JS, Muehllehner G, Qu H, Yan XH (1995) Singles transmission in volume-imaging PET with ^{137}Cs source. Phys Med Biol 40: 929–944

Knight SB, Delbeke D, Stewart JR, Sandler MP (1996) Evaluation of pulmonary lesions with FDG-PET. Chest 109: 982–988

Knopp MV, Strauss LG, Haberkorn U (1990) PET of the thorax: assessment of its clinical application in tumor staging. Radiology 177: 174

Knopp MV, Bischoff H, Ostertag H et al. (1992) Mediastinal lymph node mapping using F-18 deoxyglucose PET. J Nucl Med 33: 828

Knopp MV, Bischoff H, Oberdorfer F, van Kaick G (1992) Positronen Emissions Tomographie des Thorax. Derzeitiger klinischer Stellenwert. Radiologe 32: 290–295

Kubota K, Matsuzawa T, Fujiwara T et al. (1990) Differential diagnosis of lung tumors with positron emission tomography: a prospective study. J Nucl Med 31/12: 1927–32

Kubota K, Yamada S, Ishiwata K, Ito M, Ido T (1992) Positron emission tomography for treatment evaluation and recurrence detection compared with CT in long-term follow-up cases of lung cancer. Clin Nucl Med 17: 877–881

Kubota K, Yamada S, Ishiwata K et al. (1993) Evaluation of the treatment response of lung cancer with positron emission tomography and L-(methyl-C-11) methionine: a preliminary study. Eur J Nucl Med 20: 495–501

Lee JS, Hong WK (1992) Prognostic factors in lung cancer. N Engl J Med 327: 47–48

Lewis P, Griffin S, Marsden P, Gee T, Nunan T, Malsey M, Dussek J (1994) Whole-body F-18 fluorodeoxyglucose positron emission tomography in preoperative evaluation of lung cancer. Lancet 344: 1265–1266

Lowe VJ, Hoffman JM, De Long DM, Patz EF, Coleman RE (1994) Semiquantitative and visual analysis of FDG-PET images in pulmonary abnormalities. J Nucl Med 35/11: 1771–1776

Lowe VJ, De Long DM, Hoffman JM, Coleman RE (1995) Optimum scanning protocol for FDG-PET evaluation of pulmonary malignancy. J Nucl Med 36/5: 883–887

Lowe VJ, Duhaylongsod FG, Patz EF, Delong DM, Hoffmann JM, Wolfe WG, Coleman RE (1997) Pulmonary abnormalities and PET data analysis: A retrospective study. Radiology 202: 435–439

Lowe VJ, Fletcher JW, Gobar L et al. (1998) Prospective investigation of positron emission tomography in lung nodules. J Clin Oncol 16: 1075–1084

Maul FD, Müller D, Lorenz W, Hör G (1980) Erste Erfahrungen mit Tl-201 in der szintigraphischen Diagnostik von Bronchialtumoren. Nuklearmediziner 4: 335–339

Morgan WE (1995) The surgery of lung cancer. Ann Oncol 6 [Suppl 1]: S33–S36

Mountain CF (1986) A new international staging system for lung cancer. Chest 89 [Suppl 4]: 225 S–233 S

Mountain CF (1997) Revisions in the international system for staging lung cancer. Chest 111: 1710–1717

Naruke T, Suemasu K, Ishikawa S (1978) Lymph node mapping and curability at various levels of metastasis in resected lung cancer. J Thor Cardiovasc Surg 76: 832–839

Nolop KB, Rhodes CG, Brudin LH, Peaney RP, Krausz T, Jones T, Hughes JMB (1987) Glucose utilization in vivo by human pulmonary neoplasms. Cancer 60: 2682–2689

Patz EF Jr, Lowe VJ, Hoffman JM, Paine SS, Burrowes P, Coleman RE, Goodman PC (1993) Focal pulmonary abnormalities: evaluation with F-18 fluorodeoxyglucose PET scanning. Radiology 188/2: 487–490

Patz EF, Lowe VJ, Hoffmann JM, Paine SS, Harries LK, Goodman PC (1994) Persistent or recurrent bronchogenic carcinoma: detection with PET and 2-(F-18)-2-deoxy-D-glucose. Radiology 191: 379–382

Quint LE, Francis IR, Wahl RL, Gross BH, Glazer GM (1995) Preoperative staging of non-small-cell carcinoma of the lung: imaging methods. AJR 164: 1349–1359

Ramanna L (1986) Interest growing in new aerosol imaging methods. Diagn Imag Int 3/4: 3437

Rege SD, Hoh CK, Glaspy JA et al. (1993) Imaging of pulmonary mass lesions with whole-body positron emission tomography and fluorodeoxyglucose. Cancer 72: 82–90

Salathe M, Soler M, Bolliger CT et al. (1992) Transbronchial needle aspiration in routine fiberoptic bronchoscopy. Respiration 59: 5–8

Sasaki M, Ichiya Y, Kuwabara Y et al. (1996) The usefulness of FDG positron emission tomography for the detec- tion of mediastinal lymph node metastases in patients with non-small-cell lung cancer: a comparative study with x-ray computed tomography. Eur J Nucl Med 23: 741–747

Sazon DA, Santiago SM, Soo Hoo GW (1996) FDG-PET in the detection and staging of lung cancer. Am J Respir Crit Care Med 153: 417–421

Schiepers C (1997) Role of positron emission tomography in the staging of lung cancer. Lung Cancer 17 [Suppl 1]: S29–S35

Scott WJ, Schwabe JL, Gupta NC, Dewan NA, Reeb SD, Sugimoto JT (1994) Positron emission tomography of lung tumors and mediastinal lymph nodes using F-18 fluorodeoxyglucose. Ann Thorac Surg 58: 698–703

Scott WJ, Gobar LS, Hauser LG, Sunderland JJ, Dewan NA, Sugimoto JT (1995) Detection of scalene lymph node metastases from lung cancer. Chest 107: 1174–1176

Shreve PD, Steventon RS, Deters EC, Kison PV, Gross MD, Wahl RL (1998) Oncologic diagnosis with 2-[fluorine-18]fluoro-2-deoxy-D-glucose imaging: dual-head coincidence gamma camera versus positron emission tomographic scanner. Radiology 207: 431–437

Siegelman SS, Khouri NF, Leo FP, Fishman EK, Braverman RM, Zerhouni EA (1986) Solitary pulmonary nodules : CT assessment. Radiology 160: 307–312

Steinert HC, Hauser M, Allemann F, Engel H, Berthold T, von Schulthess GK, Weder W (1997) Non-small cell lung cancer: nodal staging with FDG PET versus CT with correlative lymph node mapping and sampling. Radiology 202: 441–446
Steinert HC, von Schulthess GK, Wedder W (1998) Effektivität der Ganzkörper-PET mit FDG beim Staging des nicht-kleinzelligen Bronchuskarzinoms bei 100 Patienten. Nuklearmedizin 37: A37
Strauss LG (1996): Die Positronen-Emissions-Tomographie in der onkologischen Therapie- kontrolle. Nuklearmediziner 19: 281–285
Thatcher N, Ranson M, Lee SM, Niven R, Anderson H (1995) Chemotherapy in non-small cell lung cancer. Ann Oncol 6 [Suppl 1]: S83–S95
Toomes H, Delphendal A, Manke HG, Vogt-Moykopf I (1981) Der solitäre Lungenrundherd. Dtsch Ärztebl 37: 1717–1722
Valk PE, Pounds TR, Tesar RD, Hopkins DM, White RI, Orringer MB (1994) Staging of mediastinal non-small-cell lung cancer with FDG-PET, CT, and fusion images: preliminary prospective evaluation. Radiology 191: 371–377
Valk PE, Pounds TR, Tesar RD, Hopkins DM, Haseman MK (1996) Cost-effectiveness of PET imaging in clinical oncology. Nucl Med Biol 23: 737–743
Vansteenkiste JF, Stroobants SG, De Leyn PR, Dupont PJ, Verschakelen JA, Nackaerts KL, Mortelmans LA and the Leuven Lung Cancer Study Group (1997) Mediastinal lymph node staging with FDG-PET scan in patient with potentially operable non-small-cell lung cancer. A prospective analysis of 50 cases. Chest 112: 1480–1486
Wahl RL, Quint LE, Greenough RL, Meyer CR, White RI, Orringer MB (1994) Staging of mediastinal non-small cell lung cancer with FDG-PET, CT, and fusion images: preliminary prospective evaluation. Radiology 191: 371–377
Wang, KP, Kelly SJ, Britt JE (1988) Percutaneous needle aspiration biopsy of chest lesions. New instrument and new technique. Chest 93: 993–997
Wang H, Maurea S, Mainolfi C et al. (1997) Tc-99m-MIBI scintigraphy in patients with lung cancer, comparison with CT and fluorine-18 FDG PET imaging. Clin Nucl Med 22: 243–249
Webb WR, Gatsonis C, Zeerhouni EA (1991) CT and MR imaging in staging of non-small cell bronchogenic carcinoma: report of the Radiological Diagnostic Oncology Group. Radiology 178: 705–713
Weber W, Voll B, Treumann T, Watzlowik P, Präuer H, Schwaiger M (1998) Positronen-Emissions-Tomographie mit C-11-Methionin und F-18-Fluordeoxyglukose in der Diagnostik des Bronchialkarzinoms. Nuklearmedizin 37: A37
Whitehouse JMA (1994) Management of lung cancer. Standing Medical Advisory Comittee
Winnig AJ, McIvor J Seed WA et al. (1986) Interpretation of negative results in fine needle aspiration of discrete pulmonary lesions. Thorax 41: 875–879
Zasadny KR, Kison PV, Quint LE, Wahl RL (1996) Untreated lung cancer: quantification of systematic distortion of tumor size and shape on non-attenuation-corrected 2-(fluorine-18) fluoro-2-deoxy-D-glucose PET scans. Radiology 201: 873–876

5.5 Breast Cancer

P. Willkomm, H. Palmedo, M. Bangard, P. Oehr, and H.-J. Biersack

5.5.1 Introduction, Clinical Background, Prognosis

Breast cancer is the most common malignant tumor in women in the western world. The incidence of breast cancer has increased over the last decades. It is curable if it is discovered very early. But the diagnosis of primary breast cancer can be difficult in young women with dense breasts, since the mammary gland can obscure a tumor from view during a mammogram. On the other hand, the specificity of mammography is relatively low because there are many false positive findings, some of which are benign lesions (fibroadenomas, for example). Many unnecessary biopsies are performed as a result (Herman 1987). Neither MRI (Gilles et al. 1994) nor sonography (Jackson 1990) can solve this problem.

Breast carcinoma is frequently multicentric (30%) or bilateral (7%). The size of the primary tumor is recognized as a clinical predictor of outcome. Tumors less than 2 cm in size are associated with the most favorable outcome. The presence and extent of axillary metastases is the most important prognostic factor (Henderson et al. 1989). Lymph node involvement is found in 38% of primary tumors < 1.5 cm, usually as micrometastases, but in 70% when the primary is greater than 5.5 cm (Avril et al. 1996). The five-year survival rate drops from 80% to 35% if regional lymph nodes are involved with tumor and even to 10% if distant metastases are present. In many cases of breast cancer, systemic disease is already present at the time of diagnosis (Table 5.5.1).

Table 5.5.1. Disease-free survival related to lymph node involvement

Axillary node status	Percentage of patients surviving disease-free	
	5 years	10 years
Negative	82	76
Positive	35	24
1–3 nodes	50	35
≥ 4 nodes	21	11

Therapy

The classic principle of breast cancer treatment is mastectomy including axillary dissection. Today small lesions are often treated by breast lumpectomy and axillary node dissection. But it is particularly difficult to identify tumor tissue in soft tissues using conventional methods. Early identification of a recurrent tumor and the presence of lymph node metastases indisputably have a significant influence on therapy: local recurrence and limited axillary lymph node involvement are treated with surgical resection and frequently radiation therapy or neoadjuvant therapy, whereas clavicular or mediastinal metastases or other distant metastases (lung, liver, bone) are treated with chemotherapy or local radiation (Henderson et al. 1989; Bastert and Costa 1995).

The classic tumor screening usually consists of palpation of the breast, the axilla and mammography and in addition sonography tumor markers. Every pathological mass should be assessed with aspiration cytology. If a tumor is detected, primary evaluation of the stage of disease and follow-up examinations are performed; these include physical exams, axillary lymph node sonography, mammography, CT, MRI, skeletal scintigraphy and tumor markers (Henderson et al. 1989; Moore and Kinne 1996; Mintun et al. 1988; Kallinowski et al. 1989).

The appropriate therapy depends mainly upon early tumor detection and correct tumor staging und re-staging after therapy (Baum 1998).

FDG PET is a new and promising imaging technology that offers the possibility of discovering primary breast cancer, regional metastases, distant metastases and local recurrences. Moreover, FDG PET offers the possibility of differentiating between a scar and viable tumor tissue. It is very important to make early predictions regarding therapeutic response, and to monitor therapeutic success.

5.5.2
Technical Aspects

Patients must fast for at least 12 hours since elevated blood glucose levels can lead to reduced FDG uptake in existing tumors. Thus, a blood sugar test is recommended for each patient. Sufficient FDG uptake in tumors occurs only when fasting has induced relatively low blood sugar levels. Moreover, patients should lie quietly during incubation to prevent increased FDG uptake in the muscles.

The usual dose of FDG for adults undergoing PET varies between 6–20 mCi (222–740 MBq). FDG is administered intravenously, if possible in the contralateral arm using a butterfly. After the injection, patients remain in a supine position for approximately 45–60 minutes and are asked to drink one liter of water to prevent artifacts from the kidneys as FDG is excreted by the urinary tract. The bladder must be emptied immediately before scanning

If a diagnosis of primary breast cancer is being considered, then patients are studied in the prone position with the breasts suspended in a special cup and the arms extended above the head. Images are taken in two bed positions and include the axillary region and the breasts.

If distant metastatic spread is suspected, patients are scanned in a supine position with the arms next to the torso. The scan is performed in „move-out“ mode to minimize artifacts resulting from bladder activity, i.e., the bladder region is scanned first and the neck area last.

A transmission scan is required so that quantification is possible. In our clinic all patients undergo a transmission scan of the torso (5–6 bed positions) at 10 minutes per bed position.

The emission scan begins 45–60 minutes after the FDG injection and lasts ten minutes per bed position. Our scans are performed using an ECAT EXACT 927/47 scanner (Siemens-CTI, Knoxville, TN, USA) which has a field of view of 16.2 cm with a slice thickness of 3.2 mm in transaxial projection. The current resolution averages 7–8 mm. Emission data are usually reconstructed without scatter correction using filtered back-projection with a Hanning filter and a cut-off frequency of 0.4. Attenuation correction is performed using the transmission data. The physician evaluates the images at the monitor in the "volume viewer" mode, which consists of three views (transaxial, coronal, sagittal) and permits interactive selection of slices. All images are documented in transaxial, coronal and sagittal views. The standard uptake value (SUV) was specified as the parameter of regional radioactivity distribution for quantitative evaluation.

SUV definition:

$$\frac{\text{tissue activity}}{\text{Volume}} \times \frac{\text{Body weight}}{\text{Injected activity}}$$

5.5.3 Indications

Primary Breast Cancer

An example of primary breast cancer is shown in Figure 5.5.1. Multiple PET studies have evaluated data from breast cancer patients (Palmedo et al. 1997; Leskinen Kallio et al. 1991; Holle et al. 1996; Kubota et al. 1989; Wahl et al. 1991a,b, 1993, 1994; Adler et al. 1993; Nieweg et al. 1993; Dedashti et al. 1995; Scheidhauer et al. 1996; Bassa et al. 1996; Utech et al. 1996; Hoh et al. 1993; Bruce et al. 1995; Crowe et al. 1994; Avril et al. 1996; Chaiken et al. 1993, Bender 1997). These data are summarized in Table 5.5.2. Tumors with a size > 3 cm were detected with a high sensitivity (67–100%) and specificity (70–100%) (Minn et al. 1989; Wahl et al. 1991a,b; Kubota et al. 1989). A resolution threshold of approximately 1–1.2 cm has been reported (Avril et al. 1996; Adler et al. 1993; Utech et al. 1996; Wahl 1998). Lesions smaller than 1 cm were frequently false negative (Avril et al. 1996; Nieweg et al. 1993).

FDG-PET is assumed to be a sensitive and accurate functional imaging method for detecting primary breast cancer, although its use in screening is limited by its low sensitivity to lesions under 1 cm in size.

Table 5.5.2. Clinical studies evaluating FDG PET in diagnosis of primary breast cancer

Author/Year/Reference	Patients/ Lesions	Sensitivity [%]	Specificity [%]
Kubota et al., 1989	1/1	n.a.[a]	n.a.
Wahl et al., 1991	10/12	100	100
Tse et al., 1992	14/14	86	100
Hoh et al., 1993	15/17	88	–
Nieweg et al., 1993	11/11	91	–
Chaiken et al., 1993	4/4	100	100
Crowe et al., 1994	28/37	96	100
Dedashti et al., 1995	32/24	88	87–100
Bruce et al., 1995	14/15	93	–
Holle et al., 1996	50/–	67	82
Bassa et al., 1996	16	75	100
Scheidhauer et al., 1996	30/23	91	86
Avril et al., 1996	71/95	74	98
Utech et al., 1996	124/n.a.	100	n.a.
Adler et al., 1997	50/	95	66
Palmedo et al., 1997	20/22	92	86

[a] n.a. = not available

Benign Changes in the Breast

One important diagnostic problem consists of differentiating between cancer and benign changes (fibroadenomas, adenomas, fibrocystic changes). Several groups described correct negative findings in fibroadenomas (Palmedo et al. 1997; Holle et al. 1996; Adler et al. 1993; Dedashti et al. 1995). Adler et al. (1993) described 5 benign cysts that were

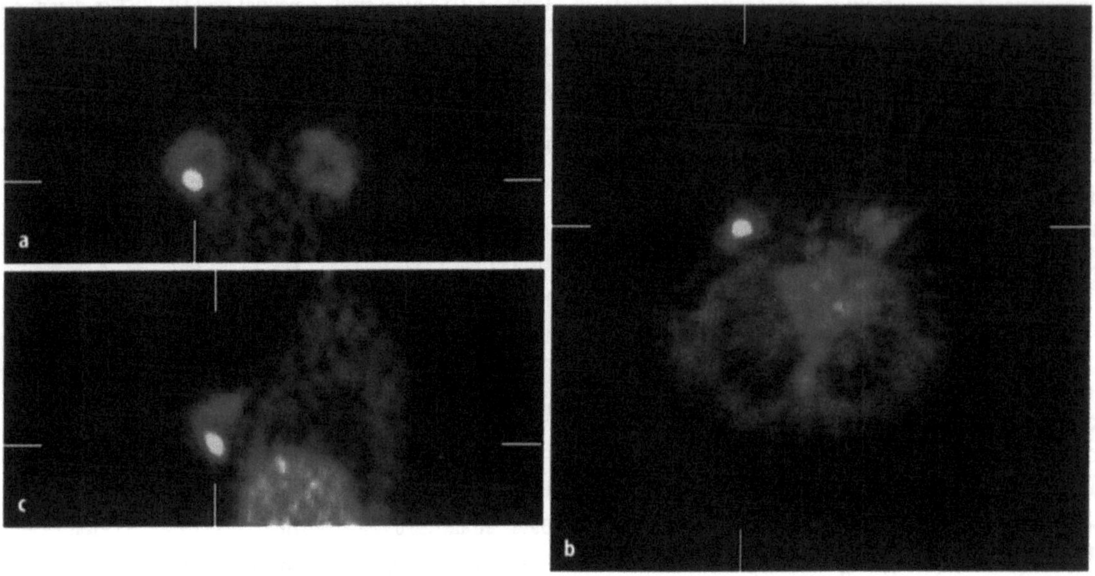

Fig. 5.5.1. Increase in glucose utilization in a primary tumor in the right breast. Transmission-corrected images in coronal (**a**), transverse (**b**), and sagittal (**c**) views of the tumor

photopenic areas. Silicone implants complicate detection of breast cancer because of their radiodensity.

Local Recurrence

An example of local recurrence is shown in Fig. 5.5.2. Suspected tumor recurrence can also be another clinical indication for FDG-PET (Moon 1998; Bender 1997; Avril 1997). To date, only a few patients with suspected local recurrence have been examined under clinical study conditions. Thus, clinical and therapeutic relevance still need to be substantiated by further studies.

Axillary Lymph Nodes

FDG-PET is a sensitive method for detecting lymph node metastases (Fig. 5.5.3) and offers an excellent possibility for lymph node staging, especially in combination with CT/MRI. Moreover, the evaluation of parasternal and mediastinal lymph nodes is of great significance for cancers of the mesial quadrants, in particular. Recent studies have shown considerable promise in detecting the presence or absence of axillary adenopathy in patients with breast cancer. To date investigators have reported sensitivities of 57–100% and specificities of 91–100% (Table 5.5.3) (Avril et al. 1996; Holle et al. 1996; Palmedo et al. 1997;

Table 5.5.3. Evaluation of FDG PET as regards detection of axillary lymph node involvement

Author/Year	Patients/ Lesions	Sensitivity [%]	Specificity [%]
Wahl et al., 1991	1/3	n.a.	n.a.
Wahl et al., 1991	4/n.a.	100	100
Tse et al., 1992	14/7	57	100
Avril et al., 1996	51	94	100
Palmedo et al., 1996	3/3	100	100
Utech et al., 1996	124	100	n.a.
Romer et al., 1997	n.a.	79	96
Bender et al., 1997	75/51	97	91
Crippa et al., 1998	68	85	91
Smith et al., 1998	50/n.a.	90	97

n.a. = not available; LN = lymph nodes; F+ = false positive; F− = false negative; MIBI* = scintimammography with ^{99m}TcMIBI)

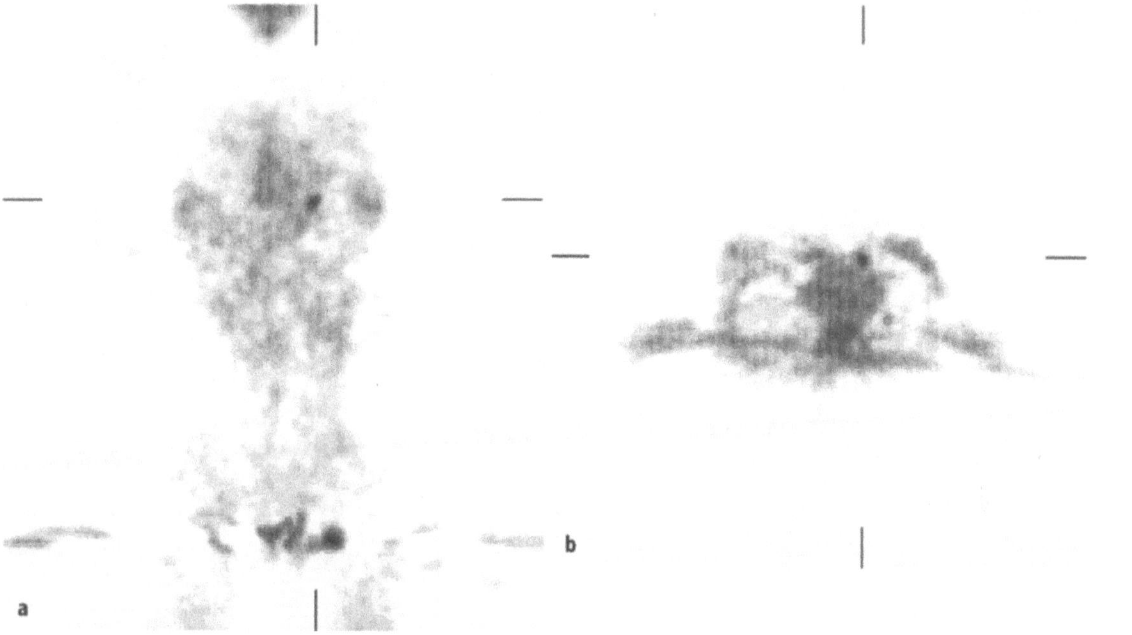

Fig. 5.5.2. Scar recurrence in the chest wall/left breast. Transmission-corrected images in coronal (**a**) and transverse (**b**) views

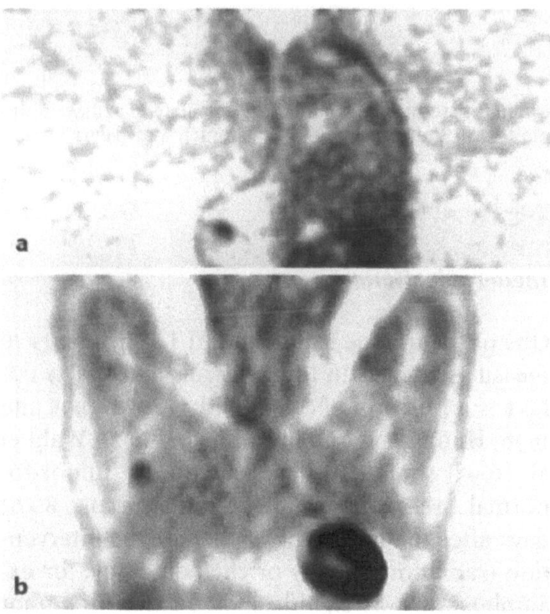

Fig. 5.5.3 a, b. An 85 year-old woman with cancer in the right breast, detected by palpation and confirmed by mammography. FDG-PET shows a hypermetabolic focus in the lateral right upper quadrant (**a**). Additionally, PET demonstrates an increased uptake in the right axilla (**b**). Histology confirmed right breast cancer with one invaded axillary lymph node

Wahl et al. 1991a,b, 1993; Scheidhauer et al. 1996; Utech et al. 1996; Adler et al. 1993; Nieweg et al. 1993; Crowe et al. 1994; Bender et al. 1997; Crippa et al. 1998; Smith et al. 1998).

However, sensitivity for small tumors (< 1 cm) was found to be low. Some authors have noted that sensitivity in detecting lymph node metastases is a function of the size of the primary tumor. Avril et al. (1996) observed a high sensitivity and specitivity in detecting axillary lymph node involvement in breast cancer. However, in small breast cancer (stage pT1) axillary lymph node metastases could not be diagnosed with sufficient accuracy using PET (sensitivity 33%). Crippa et al. 1998 confirmed these results. Thus, detection of micrometastases and small tumor-infiltrated lymph nodes is limited due to the spatial resolution of PET-imaging.

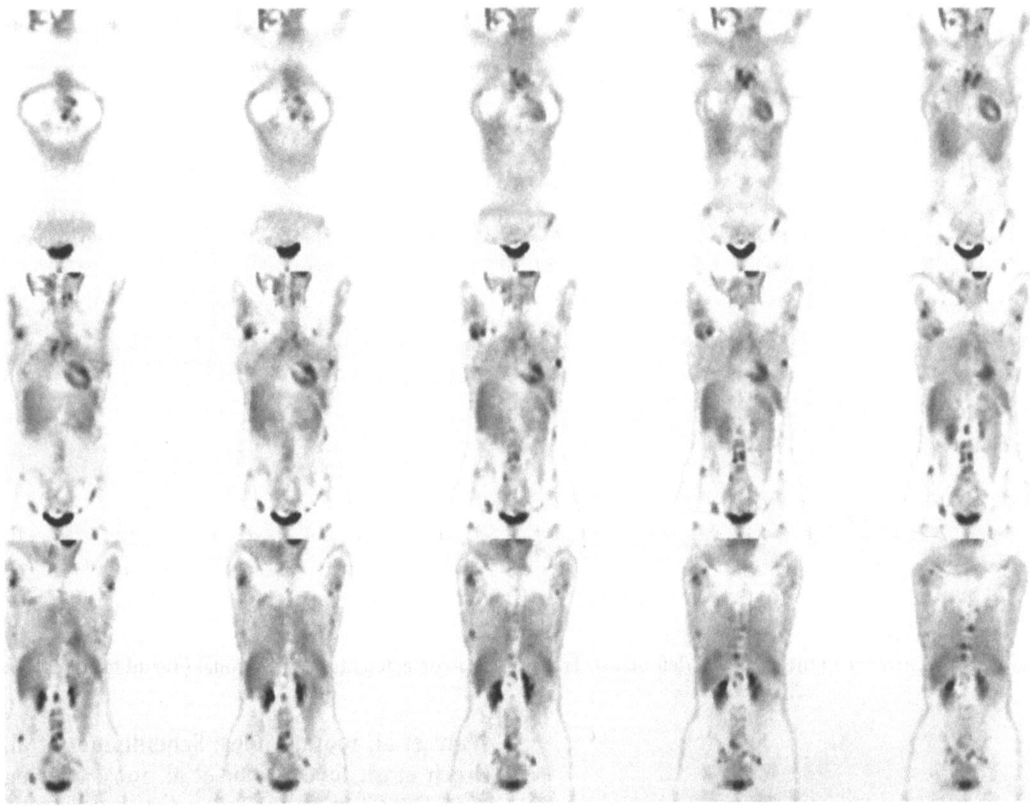

Fig. 5.5.4. Multiple metastasized breast cancer. Emission scans of the torso. Coronal slices from ventral to dorsal: increased glucose utilization typical of malignancy left cervical, in the sternum, the mediastinum, bilateral axillae, multiple foci in the spinal column, abdomen and pelvis

Distant Metastases

An example of distant metastases is shown in Figure 5.5.4. FDG PET has the potential to detect distant metastases, for example in the lung, the skeleton, the liver and distant lymph node metastases. This results in the detection of many lesions that elude conventional imaging procedures (Bender et al. 1997; Wahl et al. 1991a,b; Dedashti et al. 1995; Jansson et al. 1995) (Table 5.5.4).

Therapy Monitoring

One of the unique features of PET is its ability to measure changes in tumor tissue, since FDG uptake is a function of cell vitality (Brown 1995 and 1996; Huovinen et al. 1993; Zincke 1997). Wahl et al. (1993) showed that a reduction of tumor-to-normal breast tissue uptake ratios occurs 8–63 days after the beginning of therapeutic intervention (radiation therapy or chemotherapy, for example), whereas significant reduction of tumor size requires time (Minn and Soini 1989; Nieweg et al. 1993).

Several studies have shown that FDG uptake declines in patients responsive to treatment, while no significant decline was seen in the non-re-

Table 5.5.4. FDG PET in the diagnosis of distant metastases – clinical studies (n. a. = not available)

Author/Year	Patients/ Lesions	Sensitivity	Specificity	Notes
Minn et al. (1989)	17/n. a.	88	n. a.	(Planar images) lymph nodes, lung, liver, bone
Wahl et al. (1991a)	1/3	n. a.	n. a.	Bone
Wahl et al. (1991b)	3/n. a.	100	100	Bone, pleura
Dedashti et al. (1995)	19/45	89	100	Metastases n=13, recurrences n=4
Jansson et al. (1995)	16/n. a.	n. a.	n. a.	Lymph nodes, liver, pleura
Bender et al. (1997)	75/21	80	97	Lymph nodes, bone, lung, liver

sponding patients (Wahl 1998; Wahl et al. 1993; Bassa et al. 1996; Jansson et al. 1995; Chaiken et al. 1993; Bruce et al. 1995) (Table 5.5.5). These data indicate that PET is of clinical value in predicting response to chemotherapy. Additional studies with larger populations are needed to verify the clinical relevance of FDG-PET in monitoring early tumor response to chemotherapy.

Estrogen Receptors

Scans performed using ^{18}F-labeled progesterone have yielded discouraging results with a sensitivity of 50 % (Dedashti et al. 1991). The estrogen analog 16 alpha (^{18}F) fluoroestradiol (FES) has already proven to be an effective imaging agent for estrogen receptor positive tumors. Some studies have focused on the development of estrogen and progestin radiopharmaceuticals for imaging breast cancer (Mintun et al. 1988; Nieweg et al. 1993).

Table 5.5.5. FDG PET for therapy monitoring (Met^{a}= ^{11}C-methionine, n. a. = not available)

Author/Year	Patients/ Lesions	Sensitivity	Specificity	Notes
Wahl et al. (1993)	11/n. a.	n. a.	n. a.	FDG uptake decreases in lesions that are sensitive to therapy
Chaiken et al. (1993)	4/4	n. a.	n. a.	FDG uptake in recurrences only
Huovinen et al. (1993)	8/n. a.	n. a.	n. a.	Met. uptake decreases in metastases that are sensitive to therapy
Bruce et al. (1995)	14/15	93	n. a.	Reduced quotient of tumor to normal tissue
Jansson et al. (1995)	16/n. a.	n. a.	n. a.	FDG uptakte decreases in lesions that are sensitive to therapy
Jansson et al. (1995)	16/n. a.	n. a.	n. a.	Met uptake decreases in lesions that are sensitive to therapy
Bassa et al. (1996)	16/n. a.	75	100	FDG uptake decreases in lesions that are sensitive to therapy

[a] ^{11}C-Methionin.

There was a good correlation between FES-uptake and in-vitro receptor status (Mintun et al. 1998; Dedashti et al. 1995; Chaiken et al. 1993). Katzenellenbogen et al. described an interesting relationship between tumor metabolic response (assessed with FDG) and tumor estrogen receptor levels (assessed with FES). Finally, some studies have focused successfully on ^{18}F-labeled tamoxifen, which has also been used in animal studies (Yang et al. 1994). However, further studies are needed to substantiate its clinical and therapeutic relevance.

5.5.4 Summary

Primary Breast Cancer: As part of preoperative staging, FDG-PET is an excellent method of detecting primary breast cancer over 1 cm in diameter in addition to conventional imaging techniques.

Benign Lesions: FDG-PET offers the possibility of differentiating indeterminate mammographic findings (dense breasts, fibrocystic changes).

Axillary Lymph Nodes: FDG-PET improves preoperative staging. A considerable number of lymph node dissections can probably be avoided.

Distant Metastases: PET is useful for complete tumor staging. The whole-body technique can prevent unnecessary examinations and consequently has a major impact on therapeutic management.

Tumor Recurrence: The use of PET for recurrent disease is highly advisable for detecting lymph node metastases and confirming or ruling out distant metastases (bone, lung, liver) that might alter therapeutic regimen options.

Tumor Response: Current evaluation of therapeutic response relies on evaluation of tumor size. PET offers the possibility of monitoring early tumor response to chemotherapeutic agents, since response to therapy is accompanied by a decrease in FDG uptake but resistance to therapy is accompanied by unchanged or increasing glucose utilization.

References

Adler LP, Crowe JP, al Kaisi NK, Sunshine JL (1993) Evaluation of breast masses and axillary lymph nodes with [F-18] 2-deoxy-2-fluoro-D-glucose PET. Radiology 187: 743–750

Avril N, Dose J, Janicke F et al. (1996a) Assessment of axillary lymph node involvement in breast cancer patients with positron emission tomography using radiolabeled 2-(fluorine-18)-fluoro2-deoxy-D-glucose. J Natl Cancer Inst 88: 1204–1209

Avril N, Dose J, Janicke F et al. (1996b) Metabolic characterization of breast tumors with positron emission tomography using F-18 fluorodeoxyglucose. J Clin Oncol 14: 1848–1857

Bassa P, Kim EE, Inoue T et al. (1996) Evaluation of preoperative chemotherapy using PET with fluorine-18-fluorodeoxyglucose in breast cancer. J Nucl Med 37: 931–938

Bastert G, Costa SD (1995) Therapie des Mammakarzinoms. In: Zeller WJ, zur Hausen H (Hrsg) Onkologie. Grundlagen, Diagnostik, Therapie, Entwicklungen. Ecomed, Landsberg

Beaney RP, Lammertsma AA, Jones T, McKenzie CG, Halnan KE (1984) Positron emission tomography for in-vivo measurement of regional blood flow, oxygen utilisation, and blood volume in patients with breast carcinoma. Lancet 1: 131–134

Bender H, Kirst J, Palmedo H, Schomurg A, Wagner U, Ruhlmann J, Biersack HJ (1997) Value of 18F-fluorodeoxyglucose positron emission tomography in the staging of recurrent breast carcinoma. Anticancer Res 17: 1687–1692

Brown RS, Leung JY, Fisher SJ, Frey KA, Ethier SP, Wahl RL (1951) Intratumoral distribution of tritiated fluoro-deoxyglucosein breast carcinoma: 1. are inflammatory cells important. J Nucl Med 36: 1854–1861

Brown RS, Leung Y, Fisher SJ, Frey KA, Ethier SP, Wahl RL (1996) Intratumoral distribution of tritiated-FDG in breast carcinomae-correlation between Glut-1 expression and FDG uptake. J Nucl Med 37: 1042–1047

Bruce DM, Evans NT, Heys SD et al. (1995) Positron emission tomography: 2-deoxy-2 F18-fluoro-D-Glucose uptake in locally advnaced breast cancers. Eur J Surg Oncol 21: 280–283

Chaiken L, Rege S, Hoh C et al. (1993) Positron emission tomography with fluorodeoxyglucose to evaluate tumor response and control after radiation therapy. Int J Radiat Oncol Biol Phys 27: 455–464

Cherry SR, Carnochan P, Babich JW, Serafini F, Rowell NP, Watson IA (1990) Quantitative in vivo measurements of tumor perfusion using rubidium-81 and positron emission tomography. J Nucl Med 31: 1307–1315

Crowe JP Jr, Adler LP, Shenk RR, Sunshine J (1994) Positron emission tomography and breast masses: comparison with clinical, mammographic, and pathological findings. Ann Surg Oncol 1: 132–140

Dedashti F, McGuire AH, Van Brocklin HF et al. (1991) Assessment of 21-[18F] fluoro-16 alphaethyl-19-norprogesterone as a positron-emitting radiopharmaceutical for the detection of progestin receptors in human breast carcinomas. J Nucl Med 32: 1532–1537

Dedashti F, Mort-Imer JE, Siegel BA et al. (1995) Positron tomographic assessment of estrogen receptors in breast cancer: comparison with FDG-PET and in vitro receptor assays. J Nucl Med 36: 1766–1774

Gallagher BM, Fowler JS, Gutterson NI, MacGregor RR, Wan CN, Wolf AP (1978) Metabolic trapping as a principle of radiopharmaceutical design: some factors responsible for the biodistribution of 2-Deoxy-2-(18F) fluoro-D-glucose. J Nucl Med 19: 1154–1161

Gilles R, Guinebretiere JM, Lucidarme O et al. (1994) Nonpalpable breast tumors: diagnosis with contrastenhanced substraction dynamic MR imaging. Radiology 191: 625–631

Henderson IC, Harris JR, Kinne DW, Hellman S (1989) Cancer of the breast. In: DeVita VT, Hellman S, Rosenberg SA (eds) Cancer. Principles and practice of oncology. Lippincott, Philadelphia, p 925X

Herman G, Janus CL, Schwarz IS, Kriviski S, Bier J, Rabinowitz G (1987) Non-palpable breast lesions – accuracy of prebiopsy mammographic diagnosis. Radiology 65: 323–326

Hoh CK, Hawkins RA, Glaspy JA et al. (1993) Cancer detection with whole-body PET using 2-(18F) fluor-2-deoxy-D-glucose. J. Comput Assist Tomogr 17: 582–589

Holle LH, Trampert L, Lung Kurt S, Villena Heinsen CE, Puschel W, Schmidt S, Oberhausen E (1996) Investigations of breast tumors with fluorine-18-fluorodeoxyglucose and SPECT. J Nucl Med 37: 615–622

Huovinen R, Leskinen Kallio S, Nagren K, Lehikoinen P, Ruotsalainen U, Teras M (1993) Carbon-11-methionine and PET in evaluation of treatment response of breast cancer. Br J Cancer 67: 787–791

Inoue T, Kim EE, Wong FC et al. (1996) Comparison of fluorine-18-fluorodeoxyglucose and carbon-11-methionine PET in detection of malignant tumors. J Nucl Med 37: 1472–1476

Jacobs M, Mantil J, Peterson C et al. (1995) FDG-PET in breast cancer. J Nucl Med 35: 142P

Jackson VP (1990) The role of ultrasound in breast imaging. Radiology 177: 305–311

Jansson T, Westlin JE, Ahlstrom H, Lilja A, Langstrom B, Bergh J (1995) Positron emission tomography studies in patients with locally advanced and/or metastatic breast cancer – a method for early therapy evaluation? J Clin Oncol 13: 1470–1477

Kallinowski F, Schlenger KH, Runkel S, Kloes M; Stohrer M; Okunieff P; Vaupel P (1989a) Blood flow, metabolism, cellular microenvironment, and growth rate of human tumor xenografts. Cancer Res 49: 3759–3764

Kallinowski F, Schlenger KH, Kloes M, Stohrer M,Vaupel P (1989b) Tmor blood flow: the principle modulator of oxidative and glycolytic metabolism, and of the metabolic milieu of human tumor xenografts in vivo. Int J Cancer 44: 266–272

Kubota K, Matsuzawa T, Amemiya A et al. (1989) Imaging of breast cancer with [18F]fluorodeoxyglucose and positron emission tomography. J Comput Assist Tomogr 13: 1097–1098

Leskinen Kallio S, Nagren K, Lehikoinen P, Ruotsalainen U, Joensuu H (1991) Uptake of 11C-methionine in breast cancer studied by PET. An assaciation with the size of S-phase fraction. Br J Cancer 64: 1121–1124

Lindholm P, Min E, Leskinen Kallio S, Bergmann J, Ruotsalainen, Joensuu H (1993) Influence of the blood glucose concentration on FDG uptake in cancer – a PET study. J Nucl Med 34: 1–6

McGuire AH, Dedashti F, Siegel BA et al. (1991) Positron tomographic assessment of 16 alpha [18F] fluoro-17 beta-estradiol uptake in metastatic breast-carcinoma. J Nucl Med 32: 1526–1531

Minn H, Soini I (1989) [18F] fluorodeoxyglucose scintigraphy in diagnosis and follow up of treatment in advanced breast cancer. Eur J Nucl Med 15: 61–66

Minn H, Leskinen Kallio S, Lindholm P, Bergmann J, Ruotsalainen U, Teras M, Haaparanta M (1993) (18F) fluorodeoxyglucose uptake in tumors: kinetic vs. steady-state methods with reference to plasma insulin. J Compu Assist Tomogr 17: 115–123

Mintun MA, Welch MJ, Siegel BA, Mathias CJ, Brodack JW, McGuire AH, Katzenellenbogen JA (1988) Breast cancer: PET imaging of estrogen receptors. Radiology 169: 45–48

Moore MP, Kinne DW (1996) Is axillary lymph node dissection necessary in the routine management of breast cancer? Yes. Important Adv Oncol 19: 245–250

Nieweg OE, Kim EE, Wong WH, Broussard WF, Singletary SE, Hortobagyi GN, Tilbury RS (1993) Positron emission tomography with fluorine-18-deoxyglucose in the detection and staging of breast cancer. Cancer 71: 3920–3925

Palmedo H, Bender H, Grünwald F, Mallmann P, Zamora PO, Krebs D, Biersack HJ (1997) Comparison of fluorine-18 fluorodeoxyglucose positron emission tomography and technetium-99 m methoxyisobutylisonitrile scintimammography in the detection of breast tumors. J Nucl Med, in press

Phelps ME, Mazziotta JC, Schelbert HR (eds) (1986) Positron emission tomography and autoradiography. In: Principles and applications for the brain and heart. Raven, New York

Scheidhauer K, Scharl A, Pietrzyk U, Wagner R, Gohring UJ, Schomacker K, Schicha H (1996) Qualitative [18F] FDG positron emission tomography in primary breast cancer: clinical relevance and practicability. Eur J Nucl Med 23: 618–623

Schelstraete K, Simons M, Deman J et al. (1982) Uptake of 13N-ammonia by human tumors as studied by positron emission tomography. Br J Radiol 55: 797–804

Thomas DG, Duthie NL (1968) Use of 2-deoxy-D-glucose to test for the completeness of surgical vagotomy. Gut 9: 125–128

Utech Cl, Young CS, Winter PF (1996) Prospective evaluation of fluorine-18 fluorodeoxyglucose positron emission tomography in breast cancer for staging of the axilla related to surgery and immunocytochemistry. Eur J Nucl Med 23: 1588–1593

Wahl RL, Kaminski MS, Ethier SP, Hutchins GD (1990) The potential of 2-deoxy-2-[18F]fluoro-D-glucose (FDG) for

the detection of tumor involvement in lymph nodes. J Nucl Med 3/l: 1831–1835
Wahl RL, Cody R, Hutchins G, Mudgett E (1991a) Positron emission tomographic scanning of primary and metastatic breast carcinoma with the radiolabeled glucose analogue 2-deoxy-2-[18F] fluoro-D-glucose [letter]. N Engl J Med 324: 200
Wahl RL, Cody RL, Hutchins GD, Mudgett E (1991b) Primary and metastatic breast carcinoma: initial clinical evaluation with PET with the radiolabeled glucose analogue 2-[F-18]-fluoro-2-deoxy-D-glucose. Radiology 179: 765–770
Wahl RL, Henry CA, Ethier SP (1992) Serum glucose: effect on tumor and normal tissue accumulation of 2F -[18] fluoro-2-deoxy-D-glucose in rodents with mammary carcinoma. Radiology 183: 643–647
Wahl RL, Zasadny K, Helvie M, Hutchins GD, Weber B, Cody R (1993) Metabolic monitoring of breast cancer chemohormonotherapy using positron emission tomography: initial evaluation. J Clin Oncol 11: 2101–2111
Wahl RL, Helvie MA, Chang AE, Andersson I (1994) Detection of breast cancer in women after augmentation mammoplasty using fluorine-18-fluorodeoxyglucose-PET. J Nucl Med 35: 372–875
Warburg o (1930) The metabolism of tumours. Constabel, London
Warburg o (1956) On the origin of cancer cells. Science 123: 309–314
Wilson CB, Lammertsma AA, McKenzie CG, Sikora K, Jones T (1992) Measurements of blood flow and exchanging water space in breast tumors using positron emission, tomography: a rapid and noninvasive dynamic method. Cancer Res 52: 1592–1597
Yang D, Kuang LR, Cherif A et al. (z) Synthesis of 18F-fluoroalanine and 18F-fluorotamoxifen for imaging breast tumors.
Yang DJ, Li C, Kuang LR et al. (1994) Imaging, biodistribution and therapy potential of halogenated tamoxifen analogues. Life Sci 55: 53–67
Zincke M, Avril N, Dose J et al. (1997) PET imaging of breast cancer: comparison between FDG uptkae vs. histology and expression of the glucose transporter protein GLUT-1. J Nucl Med 38: 250 A

5.6 Pancreatic Cancer

C. G. Diederichs

5.6.1 Clinical Principles

Approximately 10,000 new cases of pancreatic cancer are diagnosed annually in the Federal Republic of Germany. They represent approximately one-fifth of all gastrointestinal cancers. More than 97 % of these patients will die of the disease. The incidence of pancreatic cancer is highest between ages 50 and 70, men are more likely to develop it than women, and patients from disadvantaged social classes are more frequently affected.

The etiology of pancreatic cancer is unclear, but some risk factors have been well known for a long time. Probably the most important risk factor is smoking; the risk is proportional to the amount of tobacco smoked. Experimental animal studies give rise to speculation that an increased ratio of meat, fat and nitrosamines in the patient's diet can favor the development of pancreatic cancer. Studies concerning the influence of alcohol and coffee on the genesis of pancreatic cancer are contradictory. Environmental toxins can also contribute to the pathogenesis of pancreatic cancer. A higher risk has also been established for patients with chronic pancreatitis.

The majority of pancreatic cancers arise from the exocrine glands of the pancreas. 80 % of these carcinomas correspond histologically to an adenocarcinoma. These carcinomas are generally ductal in origin and are mostly localized in the head of the pancreas; however, an accurate histological work-up often reveals multicentricity. Cystadenocarcinomas arise from acinar cells and present macroscopically with large cysts of varying sizes. Papillary carcinoma, which originates in the papilla, appears less frequently, more often affects young women, and has a better prognosis.

In the molecular-biological work-up, a high proportion of patients with pancreatic carcinoma (approximately 70–80 %) presents with a mutated K-ras oncogene and p53 suppressor gene. But these mutations can also appear in some patients with chronic pancreatitis or cell hyperplasias.

Unfortunately, most newly diagnosed pancreatic cancers have already spread beyond the boundaries of the organ. Direct invasion of neighboring organs such as the stomach, duodenum, the larger blood vessels, the retroperitoneum, bile ducts and colon can influence surgical resectability. Early metastatic spread in the local-regional lymph nodes, peritoneum and liver are also very frequent. Pancreatic cancer also metastasizes in the lung, bones, and brain.

The clinical picture of a patient with pancreatic cancer is unfortunately very non-specific. The most commonly reported symptoms include stomach malaise, abdominal pain, and weight loss. Painless jaundice, a reoccurrence of diabetes mellitus, ascites, hepatomegaly, and a palpable abdominal mass are compelling reasons for an examination of the pancreas. Occasionally a migratory superficial thrombophlebitis can indicate pancreatic cancer.

5.6.2 Current Therapy

A curative surgical approach is an option for only a minority of patients with pancreatic cancer since only a relatively small percentage of patients are diagnosed at an early stage of the disease. The pancreaticoduodenectomy or Whipple operation necessitated by the presence of a tumor in the head of the pancreas is a technically difficult operation with significant morbidity and mortality. However, mortality has dropped to less than 5 % at the major medical centers thanks to better surgical techniques and intensive-care methods, and the five-year survival probability of patients treated with a curative therapy approach has risen to 14–33 % (Beger et al. 1995). The prognosis for patients with tumors in the tail of the pancreas is significantly worse. Total pancreatectomy is now performed at many medical centers because of the high frequency of multicentricity. However, it has not been accepted as a routine method due to the high rate of complications and is generally reserved for a few individual cases. Recent therapeutic approaches combine the radical surgical removal of the tumor with adjuvant regional chemotherapy in combination with local radiation therapy. Initial results exhibit significantly longer survival times for certain groups of patients (Ozaki et al. 1988). The exclusive use of either chemotherapy or radiation therapy has no value for pancreatic cancer therapy at the present time.

Palliative measures consist of decompression of intestines affected by pancreatic cancer (gastrointenstinal anastomosis). A bilary obstruction is treated either surgically with biliodigestive anastomosis or by means of an endoscopic stent insertion. The latter procedure is less traumatic but has a higher risk of complication: stent obstruction can lead to cholangitis or jaundice, for example. The value of prophylactic gastroenterostomy is controversial and the procedure is generally reserved for patients whose tumor stage has not yet progressed very far. Severe pain that cannot be controlled by conservative methods can be treated successfully in a majority of cases by chemical ablation of the celiac plexus (intraoperatively or percutaneously) or by radiation therapy.

5.6.3 PET

A normal pancreas can be effectively imaged by modern PET scanners using H_2O-15 (because of the relatively high perfusion of the pancreas) or labeled amino acids (because of the high protein synthesis rate of the pancreas). But pancreatic tumors exhibit a non-specific uptake defect in the pancreatic parenchyma during imaging. The greatest amount of clinical data – more than 300 published cases – has been acquired using ^{18}F-fluorodeoxyglucose (FDG). For this reason, the following discussion will focus exclusively on FDG PET (Bares et al. 1994; Friess et al. 1995; Higashi et al. 1995; Ho et al. 1996; Inokuma et al. 1995; Kato et al. 1995; Teusch et al. 1996; Zimny et al. 1997; Diederichs et al. 1997, 1998). FDG imaging of pancreas malignancies succeeds because a glucose transporter and glycolytic key enzymes are definitely overexpressed in these tumors compared with benign tumors or chronic pancreatitis (Reske et al. 1997).

Scanning Technique (FDG PET)

Since the PET scan is based on glucose metabolism, it is important that patients fast at least six – and if possible, twelve – hours before the scan, as for other FDG scans. Patients should drink sufficient quantities of beverages that do not contain glucose, however. As a rule, patients can continue to take any medication. Blood glucose levels should be lower than 130 mg/dl at the time of FDG administration, if at all possible, since otherwise tumor FDG uptake can be reduced (Zimny et al. 1997; Diederichs et al. 1998; Langen et al. 1993). Glucose should be well regulated in diabetics (less than 130 mg/dl, if possible). The usual intravenously administered dose used for full ring PET scanners varies from 200 to more than 600 MBq. Emission scanning should begin approximately 45 – 60 minutes after the injection at the earliest. With a modern PET scanner emission scanning takes approximately 15-30 minutes for an abdominal scan and up to an hour or longer for a whole-body scan, if indicated. The emission scan can take place in two stages, if necessary, with a short pause in between for the purpose of emptying the bladder.

For better anatomic imaging of the pancreas, the emission scan can take place with the patient in a right-lateral position after intravenous application of an intestinal relaxant, e.g. butylscopolamine methylbromide [Buscopan(R)] and oral contrasting of the stomach and duodenum using water (Hydro-PET). The patient must be well hydrated for this procedure and must drink another 0.2 – 0.4 liters of water immediately before the emission scan. At this point 20 – 40 mg of Buscopan® are injected intravenously to relax the intestines.

In principle we recommend the additional performance of a attenuation scan for attenuation correction of the emission scan, since attenuation-corrected images are simpler to record and evaluate. However, the additional diagnostic information that may result from the attenuation scan has not yet been scientifically substantiated. For a whole-body examination the attenuation scan currently takes up to one additional hour with some older scanners. This scan can be performed before, during or after the emission scan, depending on scanner type. A body position as identical as possible to that of the emission scan is of great importance in order to avoid artifacts. This poses difficulties if the patient is examined in a right-lateral position, since this position is not as stable as a supine position. One advantage of attenuation correction of emission data is the possibility of a more a precise semiquantitative evaluation of the lesions based on the standard uptake value (SUV). The advantage of these SUV measurements is a matter of dispute. Visual evaluation of an FDG PET scan of pancreatic tumors probabely has at least equal value (Zimny et al. 1997; Stollfuss et al. 1995). A more recent comparison of two groups of patients (with and without attenuation correction) was not able to show any difference in the accuracy of PET (Diederichs et al. 1998). In our experience, the fasting glucose value and an acute-phase protein (C-reactive protein CRP, for example) should also be determined and recorded for every examination in order to possibly identify patients that may have acute inflammatory pancreatic disease with false positive FDG-accumulation (see "Results" below).

Evaluation Criteria

The typical finding of pancreatic malignancy is a circumscribed focally increased FDG-uptake within the pancreas. For attenuation-corrected images, standard uptake value (SUV) cut-offs between 2 and 3 are valid as a quantitative criterion, depending on the literature. For non-attenuation-corrected images, lesions are considered suspicious for malignancy when they exhibit an uptake higher than that of the liver in a segment suitable for comparison (Fig. 5.6.1). This liver segment must have attenuation conditions similar to those of the pancreas lesion being evaluated; that is, the same distances to the surface of the body. All extra-pancreatic focal excess accumulations should be regarded initially as suspicious for metastases. The liver, peripancreatic lymph node stations, the abdominal cavity (peritoneum), the imaged bones and the lung should be evaluated in particular (Fig. 5.6.2). False positive liver findings can appear in patients with markedly dilated bile ducts. This

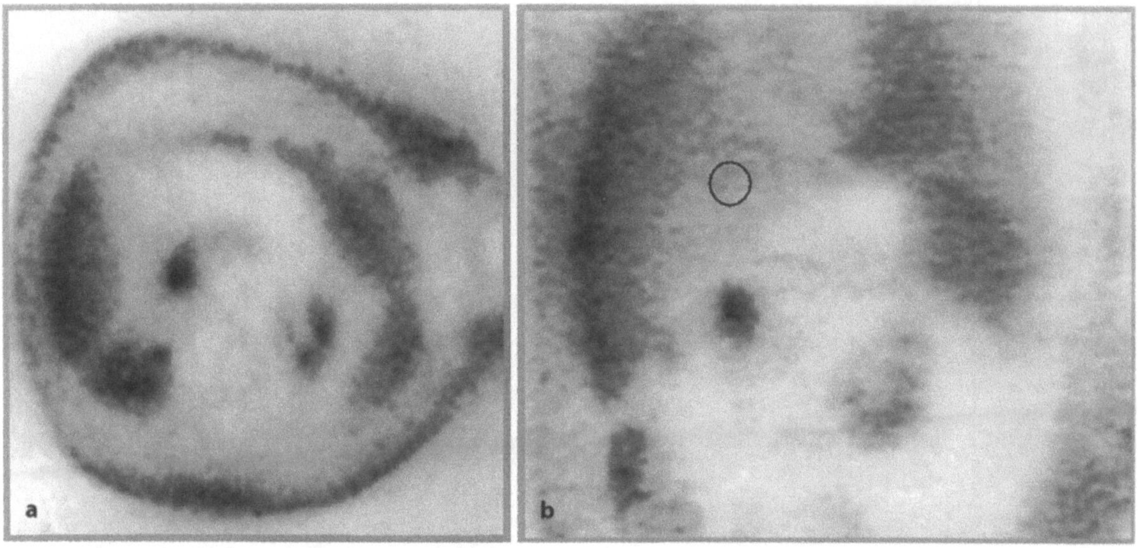

Fig. 5.6.1a,b. Representative transverse and coronal emission images of the abdomen of a 64 year-old patient one hour after i.v. administration of 440 MBq of F^{18}-FDG and oral hypotonic stomach-intestinal constrasting using water (Hydro-PET). A focally increased FDG-accumulation in the head of the pancreas is visible as a typical finding of a small ductal adenocarcinoma. Uptake in the lesion is significantly higher than uptake in the liver at a point comparably distant from the surface of the body (*circle* in **b**). Corpus and cauda are easily recognized owing to the water-distended stomach and the hypotonic duodenum and have a slightly elevated FDG uptake as the expression of a subsequent pancreatitis

could be checked with a recent CT (Fröhlich et al. 1997). Peritoneal carcinomatosis can be erroneously diagnosed if there is infrequent, atypically patchy, non-specific intestinal accumulation of FDG. Trials of routine intestinal distension to eliminate unspecific intestinal FDG-uptake are currently being undertaken.

Results to Date

A number of studies have detected significantly increased FDG uptake in pancreatic malignancies (Bares et al. 1994; Friess et al. 1995; Higashi et al. 1995; Ho et al. 1996; Inokuma et al. 1995; Kato et al. 1995; Teusch et al. 1996; Zimny et al. 1997; Diederichs et al. 1997, 1998a,b,c,d; Reske et al. 1997; Stollfuss et al. 1995). FDG PET was able to differentiate pancreatic malignancies from chronic pancreatitis: whereas malignancy is characterized by a high, focally increased glucose uptake, chronic pancreatitis normally exhibits only a very low and indistinctly contoured glucose uptake or no pathological findings at all. In a statistical survey encompassing a total of 361 patients, there was a sensitivity of 89 % and a specificity of 80 % in the differentiation of benign from malignant pancreas disease using FDG PET (Table 5.6.1).

False positive findings obtained using FDG PET are described mainly in conjunction with acute inflammatory pancreas changes (Diederichs et al. 1997). Figure 5.6.3 shows a pathologically elevated FDG uptake in a female patient with diffuse florid pancreatitis. The focal inflammatory processes include acute episodes of pre-existing chronic pancreatitis caused by inflammatory pseudotumors and the formation of abscesses in the pancreas as a late complication of chronic pancreatitis. The serum of such patients frequently exhibits an elevated level of acute phase proteins, however, for which reason levels of C-reactive protein, for example, should also be determined (Diederichs et al. 1997). In individual cases false positive find-

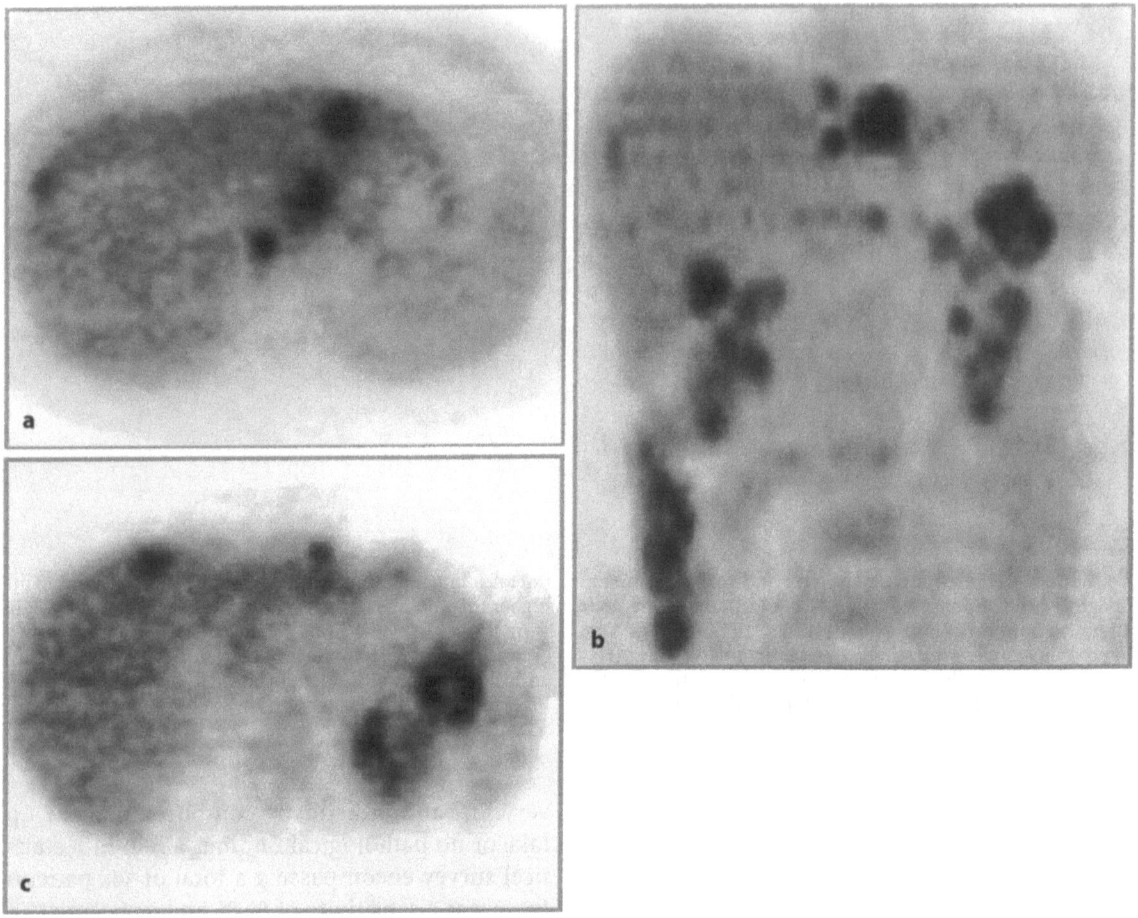

Fig. 5.6.2a-c. A 56 year-old patient with ductal pancreatic carcinoma of the tail. The attenuation corrected FDG PET scan shows a large FDG-accumulation in the tail with a photopenic defect indicative of a central necrosis. In addition, there are multiple foci of increased uptake in the liver which in the absence of dilated bile ducts are highly suggestive of hepatic metastasis. Also of note is physiologic uptake of FDG in the kidneys and in the ascending colon

ings are encountered in cases of portal vein thrombosis, after a Billroth-II gastroenterostomy, and with horizontal nasobiliary drainage (Friess et al. 1995). False negative FDG PET findings have been reported with very small tumors (< 1 cm), such as frequently exist in periampullary carcinomas; in highly differentiated G1 tumors (which are rare), and in patients with diabetes mellitus and a blood glucose level > 130 mg/dl (Zimny et al. 1997; Diederichs et al. 1997, 1998a).

The available data for N-staging are still quite limited. In a prospective multidisciplinary diagnostic study hopes of achieving improved lymph node staging with PET have not been fulfilled as compared with spiral-CT and endosonography.

Based on our own data, metastases in the liver, bone, lung, and peritoneum can be diagnosed when staging distant metastases (see Fig. 5.6.2). Pancreatic cancer liver metastases > 1 cm in diameter can be detected with a sensitivity of 97 % and a specificity of 95 % (Fröhlich et al. 1997). Ex-

Table 5.6.1. Literature survey regarding the accuracy of FDG PET for differentiation between benign and malignant pancreatic masses. (Accuracy 86 %, sensitivity 89 %, specificity 80 %, positive predictive value 89 %, negative predictive value 79 %.)

	Correct positive	Correct negative	False positive	False negative	N
Bares (1994)	25	11	2	2	40
Inokuma (1995)	24	–	–	1	25
Kato (1995)	14	7	2	1	24
Ho (1996)	8	4	2	–	14
Zimny (1997)	63	27	5	11	106
Diederichs (1998a)[a]	76	50	14	12	152
Summen	210	99	25	27	361

[a] Only patients with a blood glucose level <130 mg/dl.

clusion of metastases with a diameter of only a few mm to 1 cm appears unreliable with PET, at least with our clinical and technical settings. With the current technique and equipment, detection of lesions < 1 cm is possible using FDG PET in 43 % of cases with a remarkable specificity of 95 % (Fröhlich et al. 1997). False positive findings were observed only with preexisting marked cholestasis. These false positives are probably attributable to inflammatory cholangitic granulomas.

Our group's initial data show very promising possibilities for using FDG PET in diagnosing recurrence of pancreatic cancer. FDG PET can generally detect a recurrent carcinoma even when conventional imaging is difficult due to scar formation.

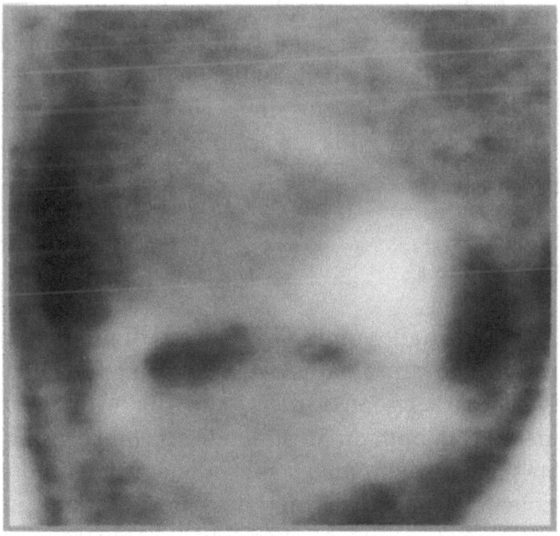

Fig. 5.6.3. A 42 year-old patient with an indeterminate mass in the head of the pancreas and chronic pancreatitis. The coronal slice shows nearly the entire organ with a diffuse, significantly elevated FDG uptake. The postoperative diagnosis was pronounced florid chronically sclerosing pancreatitis. Of note is the hypotony of the stomach and duodenum using oral water and intravenous intestinal relaxation (Hydro-PET)

5.6.4 Other Diagnostic Methods

The diagnostician faces the following questions in the case of a patient with an indeterminate pancreatic mass:

- Status: is the mass benign or malignant?
- If it is malignant, is it resectable?

The second point encompasses the question of distant metastases. The correct answer to both questions determines whether a curative or palliative approach to therapy is indicated.

A pancreas malignancy is suspected when a patient presents with symptoms such as obstructive jaundice, back pain, weight loss, a new onset of diabetes or elevated alkaline phosphatase in combination with a palpable or sonographically visible abdominal tumor. Unfortunately, these symptoms are non-specific and appear relatively late. Often the tumor marker CA 19–9 is not significantly elevated, especially when the tumor is small. High CA 19-9 levels have also been described for cases of acute inflammatory processes.

Subsequent diagnostic procedures include ERCP, which exhibits an accuracy of 80–90 % in diagnosing status and is regarded by many as the most important diagnostic examination. False negative ERCP findings occur, on the one hand, with malignancies that do not originate in the pancreatic duct and, on the other hand, with inflammatory pseudotumors. The examination demands considerable experience and is not successful technically in 3–10 % of cases. An iatrogenic pancreatitis occurs subsequently in 1–8 % of patients and can lead to death in approximately 0.2 % of cases. On the other hand, it is possible in conjunction with an ERCP to biopsy tissue, selectively acquire duodenal juice for gene mutation analysis, or perform decompression of the bile ducts by means of stent insertion.

Spiral CT has been gaining in importance recently in the diagnosis of pancreas tumors. Spiral CT is therefore viewed by some as the gold standard of imaging techniques in pancreas diagnostics. In a recent prospective study by the authors, the accuracy of this procedure was 80–85 % (Diederichs et al. 1998c,d). Accuracy in differentiating between benign and malignant disease is lower in older studies that relied on computer tomography without spiral technique. With CT, the primary differential diagnosis is the inflammatory pseudotumor that can look exactly like a malignancy. However, the great significance of spiral CT does not lie in tissue diagnosis, but rather in the determination of operability and the exclusion of liver metastases. As regards operability, PET can probably contribute very little to local resectability because of its relatively low spatial resolution. Important in this context is the detection of distant metastasis which alleviates curative resection of the tumor. Lesions > 1 cm can be detected with great sensitivity and specificity using PET (Fröhlich et al. 1997). The sensitivity of FDG PET is admittedly lower for smaller lesions, but the great advantage of the method appears to be its high specificity of nearly 100 %. FDG PET should therefore be nicely complementary to sensitive but less specific spiral CT.

Endosonography has also become increasingly more important in recent years. According to some studies it is even superior to conventional CT for status diagnosis and local staging. In a current comparative study that has not yet been published, the accuracy of endosonography is about the same as spiral CT as regards status diagnosis and local staging.

The significance of MRI in pancreas tumor diagnostics has also increased. A claim can be made for 'one-stop shopping' with MRI: imaging of the upper abdomen can be performed in several planes and with several sequences in one sitting of approximately 40 minutes. Local staging, liver staging, and imaging of the common bile and pancreatic ducts can also be undertaken in addition to status evaluation. No published results of detailed prospective comparative studies involving a direct comparison with other techniques are available at the present time.

All conventional imaging techniques can be supplemented by fine needle biopsy. However, this means an invasive removal of tissue. A negative finding does not rule out malignancy (sampling error). In summary, it should be noted that the status of a pancreatic mass cannot be reliably evaluated by any single clinical or imaging technique, i.e., with an accuracy of more than 85 %.

5.6.5 Indications

Available studies on FDG PET scans of pancreatic masses show that status diagnosis using FDG PET is at least as good – if [illegible] superior – to other methods in both direct and indirect comparisons. Staging of distant metastases in one sitting is possible for almost all metastasis localizations in question ("one-stop shopping"; compare Fig. 5.6.2). In a recently completed prospective trial comprising 95 patients, PET of the abdomen found more metastasis than spiral CT and MRI together, however the numbers are presently too small to be statistically significant. There is too little data on diagnostics of recurrencies and therapy monitoring. The shortcomings of individual methods mean that pancreas diagnostics must be undertaken with a multimodal approach. At the present time it is difficult to assess the importance of individual procedures with respect to one other or to produce a diagnostic algorithm because of qualitative differences in equipment from place to place, differences in the experience of diagnosticians, and the limited number of published multimodal direct comparisons. On the basis of previously published results, FDG PET should always be performed for pancreas masses when the gold standards of conventional diagnostics (spiral CT, ERCP, endosonography) produce inconclusive or contradictory results or when distant metastases must be ruled out or confirmed with greater certainty. All other indications currently require careful individual testing and should as a rule be performed under clinical trial conditions.

References

Bares R, Klever P, Hauptmann S et al. (1994) F-18 fluorodeoxyglucose PET in vivo evaluation of pancreatic glucose metabolism for detection of pancreatic cancer. Radiology 192: 79–86

Beger HG, Birk D, Bodner E, Fritsch A, Gall FP, Trede M (1995) Ist die histologische Sicherung des Pankreaskarzinoms Voraussetzung für die Pankreasresektion? Langenbecks Arch Chir 380/1: 62–66

Diederichs CG, Staib L, Glatting G, Vogel J, Brambs H-J, Beger HG, Reske SN (1997) Differentiation of malignant and benign pancreatic disease. J Nucl Med 38/5: 257P (abstr)

Diederichs CG, Staib L, Glatting G, Beger HG, Reske SN (1998a) FDG-PET: elevated plasma glucose reduces both uptake and detection rate of pancreatic malignancies. J Nucl Med, im Druck

Diederichs CG, Sokiranski R, Pauls S, Schwarz M, Guhlmann CA, Glatting G (1998b) FDG-PET von pankreatischen Tumoren: Transmission obligat? Nuklearmedizin, im Druck

Diederichs CG, Sokiranski R, Pauls S et al. (1998c) Prospective comparison of FDG-PET of pancreatic tumors with high end Spiral-CT and MRI. J Nucl Med (abstr), im Druck

Diederichs CG, Pauls S, Schwarz M, (1998d) Dreiphasiges Spiral-CT und Multisequenz MRT von Pankreaskopf-Tumoren: Wozu noch FDG-PET? Rofo Fortschr Geb Rontgenstr Neuen Bildgeb Verfahr (abstr), im Druck

Friess H, Langhans J, Ebert M, Beger HG, Stollfuss J, Reske SN, Büchler MW (1995) Diagnosis of pancreatic cancer by 2[18F]-fluoro-2-deoxy-D-glucose positron emission tomography. Gut 36/5: 771–777

Fröhlich A, Diederichs CG, Staib L, Beger HG, Reske SN (1997) FDG-PET in the detection of pancreatic cancer liver metastases. J Nucl Med 38/5: 145P (abstr)

Higashi T, Tamaki N, Torizuka T et al. (1995) Differentiation of malignant from benign pancreatic tumors by FDG-PET: comparison with CT, US, and endoscopic ultrasonography. J Nucl Med 36: 224P (abstr)

Ho CL, Dehdashti F, Griffeth LK, Buse PE, Balfe DM, Siegel BA (1996) FDG-PET evaluation of indeterminate pancreatic masses. J Comput Assist Tomogr 20/3: 363–369

Inokuma T, Tamaki N, Torizuka T et al. (1995) Value of fluorine-18-fluorodeoxyglucose and thallium-201 in the detection of pancreatic cancer. J Nucl Med 36/2: 229–235

Kato T, Fukatsu H, Ito K, et al. (1995) Fluorodeoxyglucose positron emission tomography in pancreatic cancer: a unsolved problem. Eur J Nucl Med 22: 32–39

Langen KH, Braun U, Kops ER, Herzog H, Kuwert T, Nebeling B, Feinendegen LE (1993) The influence of plasma glucose levels on fluorine-18-fluorodeoxyglucose uptake in bronchial carcinomas. J Nucl Med 34: 355–359

Ozaki H, Hojo K, Kato H, Kinoshita T, Egawa S, Kishi K (1988) Multidisciplinary treatment for resectable pancreatic cancer. Int J Pancreatol 3: 249–260

Reske SN, Grillenberger KG, Glatting G, Port M, Hildebrandt M, Gansauge F, Beger H-G (1997) Overexpression of glucose transporter-1 and increased FDG-uptake in pancreatic carcinoma. J Nucl Med 38: 1344–1347

Stollfuss JC, Glatting G, Friess H, Kocher F, Beger HG, Reske SN (1995) 2-(fluorine-18)-fluoro-2-deoxy-D-glucose PET in detection of pancreatic cancer: value of quantitative image interpretation [see comments]. Radiology 195/2: 339–344

Teusch M, Buell U (1996) Classification of pancreatic tumors by FDG-PET: comparison of visual and quantitative image interpretation by ROC-analysis. J Nucl Med 37/5: 140P (abstr)

Zimny M, Bares R, Faß J et al. (1997) Fluorine-18 fluorodeoxyglucose positron emission tomography in the differential diagnosis of pancreatic carcinoma: a report of 106 cases. Eur J Nucl Med 24: 678–682

5.7 Colorectal Cancer

J. Ruhlmann and P. Oehr

5.7.1 Incidence, Etiology and Risk Factors

Colorectal cancers are among the most common tumors in the western world with an incidence of approximately 12–13 %. Colon cancer is second only to lung cancer as the most frequent cause of cancer mortality in the U.S. The majority of individuals affected by it are 50 years of age or older.

Environmental factors appear to influence the etiology of most colon cancers. The disease more frequently affects members of upper-level socioeconomic urban classes. Epidemiological studies have shown that there is a direct correlation between colorectal cancer and the per capita consumption of calories, dietary fats and oils, and animal protein, as well as elevelated cholesterol levels and a predisposition to coronary artery diseases. It is well known that certain population groups such as Mormons and Seventh Day Adventists, whose dietary habits and way of life differ somewhat from those of their neighbors, exhibit a significantly lower incidence and mortality rate than expected. On the other hand, incidence of the disease has increased in Japan since that country has adopted a more "western" diet. One can conclude that eating habits influence the development of colorectal cancers.

Nonetheless, 25 % of all patients with colorectal cancer have a positive family medical history; one could therefore assume a heritable predisposition. These genetically influenced cancers can be divided into two main groups: familial adenomatous polyposis, which has been sufficiently researched but occurs infrequently; and hereditary non-polyposis colorectal cancer, which is less well defined. The former is an autosomal dominant disorder, but in patients with no relevant family history (this occurs occasionally) a spontaneous mutation is presumed to be responsible. The proximal colon is involved with unusual frequency in the form known as hereditary non-polyposis colorectal cancer. Patients with multiple primary carcinomas are often observed in these families, and in women colorectal adenocarcinomas appear sometimes in combination with endometrial carcinomas. A predisposition to malignant disease appears to be autosomal dominant, which may possibly be attributable to an anomaly on chromosome 2.

Colon cancer is a frequent complication of long-standing inflammatory bowel disease. Patients with ulcerative colitis appear to develop a neoplasm more often than patients with granulomatous colitis. However, this impression could also easily arise from the difficulty of distinguishing between these two clinical pictures. For these patients, the risk of developing a colorectal cancer is relatively low within the first ten years after the onset of colitis, but after this point it appears to increase at the rate of 0.5 – 1.0 % per year. Purely mathematically, the rate of cancer increases from 8 % to 30 % after 25 years. Preventive examinations for these patients are unsatisfactory because symptoms such as diarrhea, abdominal cramps and obstruction can resemble the complaints associated with a flare-up of the original disease and also signal a tumor. The value of follow-up examinations (colonoscopy with mucosal biopsy and brush biopsies) is doubtful. The goal of these tests is to differentiate between inflammatory changes and premalignant mucosal dysplasia and thus provide an indication for surgery. Unfortunately, this costly approach has become controversial due to a lack of agreement on the pathological criteria for dysplasia and the absence of corresponding data demonstrating that the follow-up examinations reduce the rate of development of fatal cancer.

The majority of all colorectal cancers, regardless of etiology, are presumed to develop from adenomatous polyps. A polyp can be described histologically as a non-neoplastic hamartoma, hyperplastic mucosal proliferation or an adenomatous polyp. Adenomas are clearly premalignant, but they represent only a minority of the lesions that develop into cancer. Adenomatous polyps in the colon occur in approximately 30 % of all persons during middle age or old age. If one analyzes these findings in conjunction with the known rate of development of colon cancer, then fewer than 1 % of all polyps appear ever to degenerate. Occult blood is found in the stools of fewer than 5 % of patients; the polyps remain asymptomatic. The probability of an invasively growing cancer is also dependent on the size of the polyp. Probability is low with lesions smaller than 1.5 cm (< 2 %); fair (2 – 10 %) with lesions 1.5 – 2.5 cm in size; and very great (> 10 %) with lesions larger than 2.5 cm.

Detection of lesions is only possible when the entire colon is examined endoscopically and radiologically, since synchronous lesions are present in approximately one third of all cases. Colonoscopy must be repeated periodically thereafter, since there is a probability of 30–50 % that these patients will develop a new adenoma. Their risk of developing colorectal cancer is therefore higher than average.

Since adenomatous polyps have a growth period of more than five years before they are clinically detectable, colonoscopy does not need to be performed more frequently than every three years.

5.7.2 Diagnostics

Screening Procedures

For a superficial neoplasm that has been localized early, the chance of a cure is increased through surgery. A colorectal screening program is therefore advisable. For inexplainable reasons, colon cancers in the vicinity of the rectum have decreased in number in recent decades, while those of the proximal descending colon have increased. This means that rigid rectosigmoidoscopy no longer suffices: a flexible fiberoptic sigmoidoscopy must be performed at a minimum. A well-trained diagnostician can observe up to 60 cm of the colon with this procedure. A digital examination should be performed as a routine measure on all adults over 40 years of age; it also serves as an effective preventive test for prostate cancer in men and is a part of the pelvic examination in women. It is a cost-effective method for discovering possible tumors in the rectum. The development of the fecal occult blood test is a far-reaching, simplified solution for finding occult blood in stools. But this test has its limits as a preventive examination even under optimum conditions since an average of 50 % of patients with colorectal cancer have a negative fecal occult blood test result despite intermittent bleeding from these tumors. A colorectal neoplasm is *not* found in the majority of asymptomatic individuals who have occult blood in their stools. However, additional examinations are performed on patients with occult blood in their stools, including sigmoidoscopy, contrast enema and/or colonoscopy. These procedures are not merely unpleasant and expensive, they also involve the risk of serious complications, even if that risk is very limited.

Screening procedures for detecting colon cancers in asymptomatic patients have been unsatisfactory to date. There is a need for more effective screening procedures (Mayer 1995).

Clinical Symptoms

Symptoms of colorectal cancer vary according to the anatomic localization of the tumor.

Because stools have a fluid consistency, neoplasms developing in the cecum or ascending colon can become fairly large and constrict the lumen without causing symptoms of obstruction or a relevant change in bowel function. But in the right colon, lesions usually ulcerate and lead to chronic occult blood loss that is not detected positively by a fecal occult blood test. Thus, patients with a tumor in the ascending colon often exhibit symptoms such as fatigue and heart palpation or have hypochromic microcytic anemia as an indicator of iron deficiency. However, since an incidental fecal occult blood test can be negative because the cancer only bleeds intermittently, any unexplained iron deficiency anemia in an adult (with the possible exception of pre-menopausal multiparous women) is cause for a thorough examination of the entire colon.

Tumors in the transverse and descending colon quickly obstruct the stool, which increases in consistency at that point in the intestine. The result is abdominal cramping and occasionally obstruction or even perforation. Malignancies in the rectosigmoid often lead to tenesmus and a reduced stool diameter. An immediate digital rectal examination and a proctosigmoidoscopy are particularly necessary in conjunction with rectal bleeding and/or a change in bowel function (Mayer 1995).

5.7.3 Prognosis, Staging and Tumor Spread

The prognosis for colorectal cancer is closely connected to the tumor's depth of penetration into the bowel wall, the involvement of regional lymph nodes, and the presence of distant metastases. The Dukes staging system reflects these possibilities (Table 5.7.1).

Unless metastases can be diagnosed (i.e., detected or ruled out), it is impossible to define the stage of disease accurately. For this reason, an optimal diagnosis is also necessary for determining prognosis. Criteria for a bad prognosis after a total resection include regional lymph nodes (number) involved with tumor, tumor invasion through the bowel wall, poorly differentiated histology, perforation, infiltrative growth to adjacent organs, venous infiltration, preoperative increase in CEA levels (> 5.0 ng/ml), aneuploidy, and specific chromosome deletion.

Colon cancer normally involves regional lymph nodes and/or spreads by way of the portal circulatory system to the liver. The liver is the organ most frequently affected by distant metastases and the primary organ site in 33 % of all recurrences. It is possible that it is involved with tumor in more than 66 % of patients at the time of death. Colorectal cancer rarely metastasizes in the lungs, subclavicular lymph nodes, bones or brain without first having invaded the liver. The exception is patients with a primary tumor in the distal rectum; from this site tumor cells spread by way of the paravertebral venous plexus and bypass the portal circulatory system. After distant metastases are detected, the mean survival time can range from 6–9 months (hepatomegaly, liver changes) to 24–30 months (small liver nodules can be detected initially by elevated CEA and confirmed by subsequent CT) (Mayer 1995).

Table 5.7.1. Modified Dukes classification of colorectal cancer

Stage	Pathologic description	Approximate 5-year-survival rate [%]
A	Cancer confined to mucosa and submucosa	>90
B1	Cancer spreads into the muscularis	85
B2	Cancer spreads into or penetrates the serosa	70–85
C	Cancer involves regional lymph nodes	30–60
D	Distant metastases (liver, lung, etc.)	5

5.7.4 Therapy

The optimal treatment of colorectal cancer appears to be the total resection of the tumor. Metastatic spread should be diagnosed preoperatively as completely as possible, since the discovery of metastases in patients with tumor-causing symptoms (gastrointestinal bleeding or obstruction) does not preclude surgery but often brings about a decision in favor of a less radical surgical invasion.

Radiation of the pelvis is generally necessary for patients with rectal cancer since there is a 30–40 % risk of local recurrence after total resection of stage B or C tumors, especially if the tumor has already penetrated the serosa. Preoperative radiation is clearly indicated for patients with large, potentially inoperable rectal cancers since the tumors will shrink sufficiently under irradiation to permit subsequent surgery.

Chemotherapy has only proven to be marginally useful for patients with advanced colorectal cancer. The most effective treatment for this disease is therapy with 5-fluorouracil. Recent studies have shown that the additional administration of folic acid increases the effectiveness of this chemotherapy in patients with advanced colorectal cancer. However, its effect for the duration of life remains questionable, and the optimal dose/time relationship has yet to be determined. Postoperative chemotherapy and/or radiation therapy for stage B and C patients are used to destroy clinically undetectable mirometasases and thus improve the chances of a cure. The administration of these therapies simultaneously with the supporting anthelmintic agent levamisole in stage C patients led to a reduction in the probability of a recurrence and a modest extension of survival time. In contrast, controlled studies have shown that when patients received postoperative radiation therapy combined with chemotherapy after resection of a rectal tumor, the probability of a local recurrence was reduced and the chances of cure were improved. It is assumed that chemotherapy is an ineffective prophylaxis for patients with colon lesions, but on the other hand it has a sensitizing effect for radiation therapy so that the biological effect of radiation is heightened.

Table 5.7.2. Representative studies regarding sensitivity and specificity of CT, MRI, and PET for colorectal cancer

Author	Patients (n)	Sensitivity [%]	Specificity [%]
Abdel-Nabi	14	100	100
Falk	16	87 (CT 47)	67 (CT 100)
Ito	15	100 (MRT 75)	100
Pounds	-	51 (CT 68) 96 (CT 53)	-
Ruhlmann	59	100 (MRT 77)	67
Schiepers	74	93 (CT 60)	97 (CT 72)
Strauss	29	100 (MRT 77)	100
Vitola	24	90	100

5.7.5 Positron Emission Tomography

As noted, positive detection of lymph node, liver, and/or other distant metastases is important for planning the therapeutic approach (palliative surgery vs. resection in a healthy patient) (Strauss et al. 1989; Ito et al. 1992; Ruhlmann et al. 1996, 1997; Schiepers et al. 1995). Bone and lung metastases are evidence of systemic disease, for which – according to the current state of knowledge – only palliative measures are possible. On the other hand, local lymph node and liver metastases can be resected if necessary. Our own data (see Table 5.7.3) and the data reported in the literature (Falk et al. 1994; Haberkorn et al. 1991; Ito et al. 1992; Strauss et al. 1989; Vitola et al. 1996; Ruhlmann et al. 1996 and 1997; Delbeke 1999) substantiate the suitability of FDG PET for detecting primary tumors, recurrences and metastases. It is well known that a significant advantage of PET over other imaging techniques is that PET is basically a whole-body examination method and is capable of imaging recurrences and metastases with very good contrast, largely independent of localization. Even atypical localizations of metastases (breast metastases, for example) can be detected, as our own data show. No other imaging technique makes examination of the entire body so simple and offers the possibility of such high sensitivity and specificity than PET, especially not CT and MRI (Tables 5.7.2 and 5.7.3).

Primary Tumor Diagnosis

Although there are few published reports on the use of PET for primary tumor diagnosis, our data and the data of other researchers (Valk et al. 1996; Gupta et al. 1993; Thoeni 1997) show that a diagnosis of the primary tumor using PET is very possible, especially when there is strong clinical suspicion of tumor and when conventional diagnostic techniques yield unclear results (Fig. 5.7.1 and 5.7.2). Naturally this also depends on the stage of the disease, since as a measurement of metabolism PET can detect malignant changes before more pronounced anatomic changes have occurred. Whole-body PET is thus clearly indicated for primary tumor diagnosis if there is an increase

Table 5.7.3. Author's results regarding sensitivity, specificity and predictive value of PET for colorectal carcinoma

	Patients (n)	Sensitivity	Specificity	Negative predictive value	Positive predictive value
PET	114	96	64	86	88

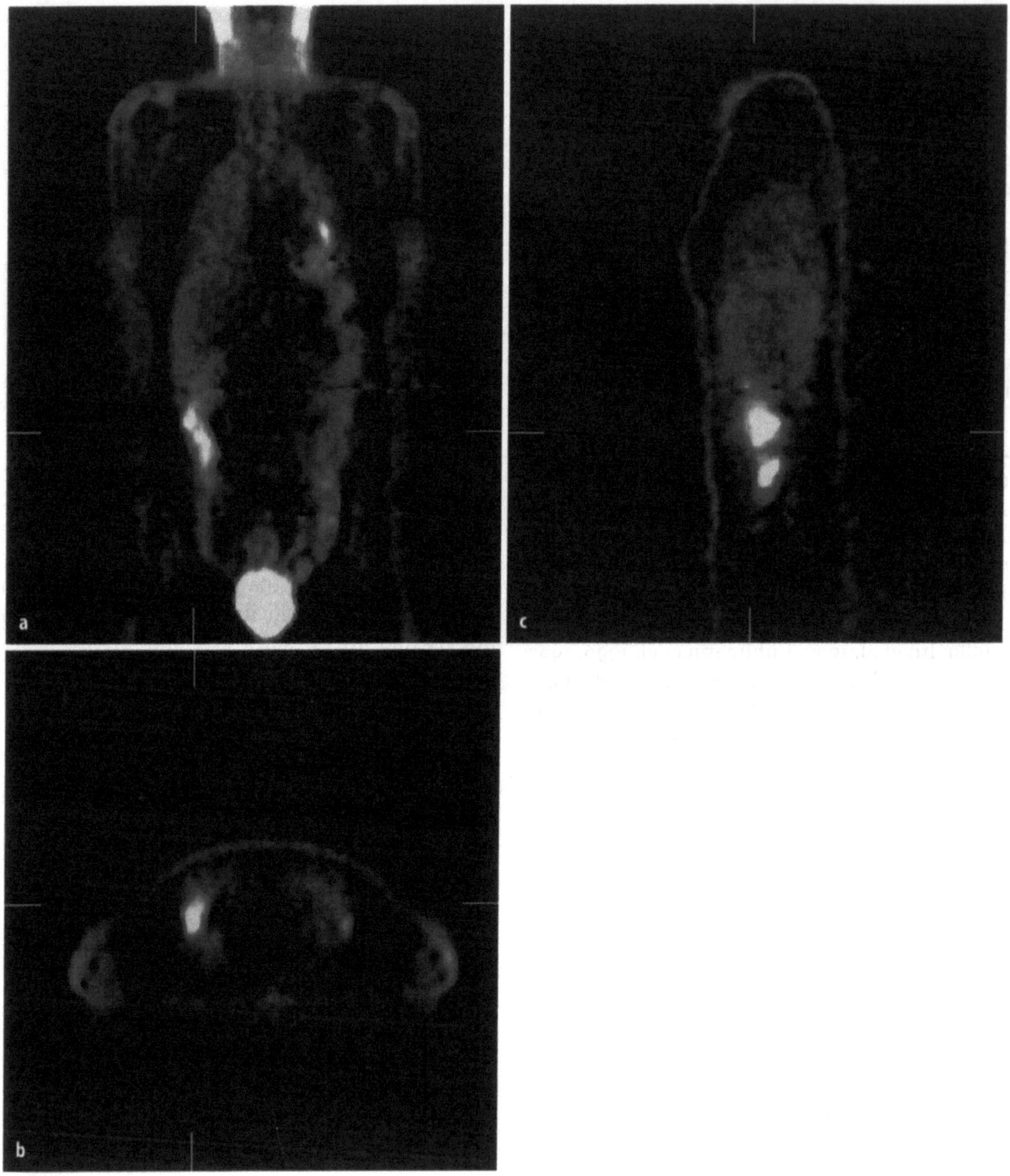

Fig. 5.7.1. Coronal (**a**), transaxial (**b**) and sagittal (**c**) emission tomogram. Cancer in the ascending colon, primary tumor without metastases

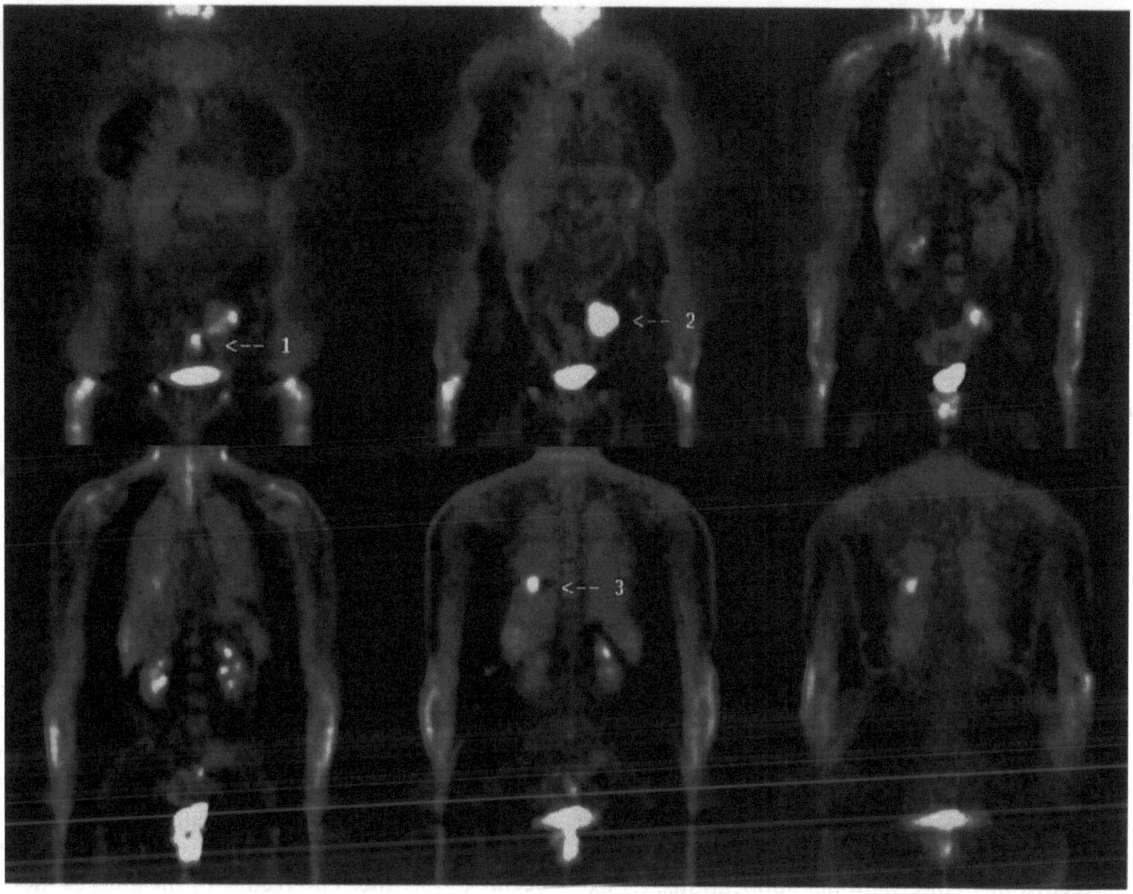

Fig. 5.7.2. Coronal emission tomogram, from ventral to dorsal. Colon cancer, primary tumor (*arrow 2*) with local metastasis (*arrow 1*) and lung metastasis (*arrow 3*)

in tumor marker concentration (CEA, CA 19–9) in the serum (Moser 1997).

Detection of Presacral Changes

Most publications show the superior capability of PET for detecting viable tumor tissue in presacral changes and differentiating between tumor and changes involving scar tissue (Fig. 5.7.3). Even the close anatomic proximity of a bladder filled with FDG-labeled urine does not materially restrict the evaluative usefulness of a presacral scan (Ruhlmann et al. 1997); however, the administration of furosemide and the use of a bladder catheter, if necessary, can be advisable (Miraldi et al. 1997).

Diagnosis of Recurrence and Metastases, Especially with Elevated Tumor Marker

Representative studies regarding the sensitivity and specificity of CT, MRI and PET to colorectal cancer show clearly that PET is superior to CT and MRI when a tumor is suspected and when that suspicion is based on increased levels of tumor marker such as CEA or CA 19-9. Even patients who appeared to be positive for tumor as a result of the PET scan but in whom a tumor could not be

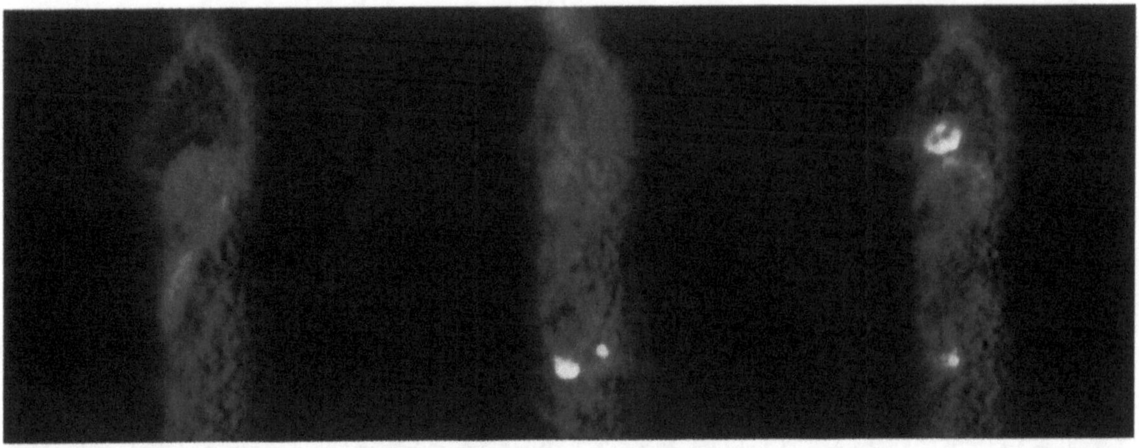

Fig. 5.7.3. Transmission-corrected sagittal tomogram. Condition after resection of rectal cancer. Presacral recurrence

detected during subsequent diagnosis exhibited positive findings with conventional diagnostic techniques during follow-up several months later (Ruhlmann et al.; Fig. 5.7.4). The 67 % specificity that was initially calculated in the above-mentioned study increased to 75 % with a sensitivity of 96 % with the larger patient group referred to in Table 5.7.2 and longer follow-up time (see authors' results in Table 5.7.3).

According to international publications, CT exhibits a much lower sensitivity of between 47 % and 68 % at the most. MRI also shows a clearly lower sensitivity of 77 % at best.

PET is suitable for detecting or ruling out recurrence or metastases even in patients who exhibit only a slight increase in tumor marker. In this context, special consideration should be given to the fact that diseases such as salivary gland inflammation can exhibit false positive tumor marker levels (CEA, CA 19-9).

The results of international studies show that we must now take a very critical view of the common assumption to date that CT, MRI, sonography and colonoscopy are the gold standards of colorectal screening (Delbeke 1999).

Assessment of Operability

It is important to select patients carefully for surgical therapy for a neoplastic disease that may be accompanied by metastatic spread. This is not only true from the point of view of treatment cost but also from the important perspective of quality of life. Only those patients will profit from surgical therapy whose disease has not yet become systemic. The results of the studies mentioned here substantiate PET's superiority over all other imaging techniques for detecting metastases, evaluating patterns of involvement, and determining the status of indeterminate focal changes in the liver and lung. The evaluation of lymph node status in particular is also a significant prognostic parameter. Established imaging modalities have an insufficient sensitivity and specificity with respect to the detection of metastases, since the size of the lymph nodes (principal criterion for radiology) correlates unsatisfactorily with tumor involvement.

Therapy Monitoring

The indication for chemotherapy after surgery is a function of the presence of viable residual tumor tissue in the remaining scar tumor tissue. FDG

PET can evaluate the viability of residual tumor and the results of previous therapeutic intervention and influence the modality of further treatment strategies. International studies overwhelmingly express support for the clinical value of therapy monitoring (Moser 1997; Ruhlmann et al.1996, 1997; Strauss et al. 1989; Ito et al. 1992; Schiepers et al. 1995; Pounds et al. 1995; Falk et al. 1994; Delbeke 1999).

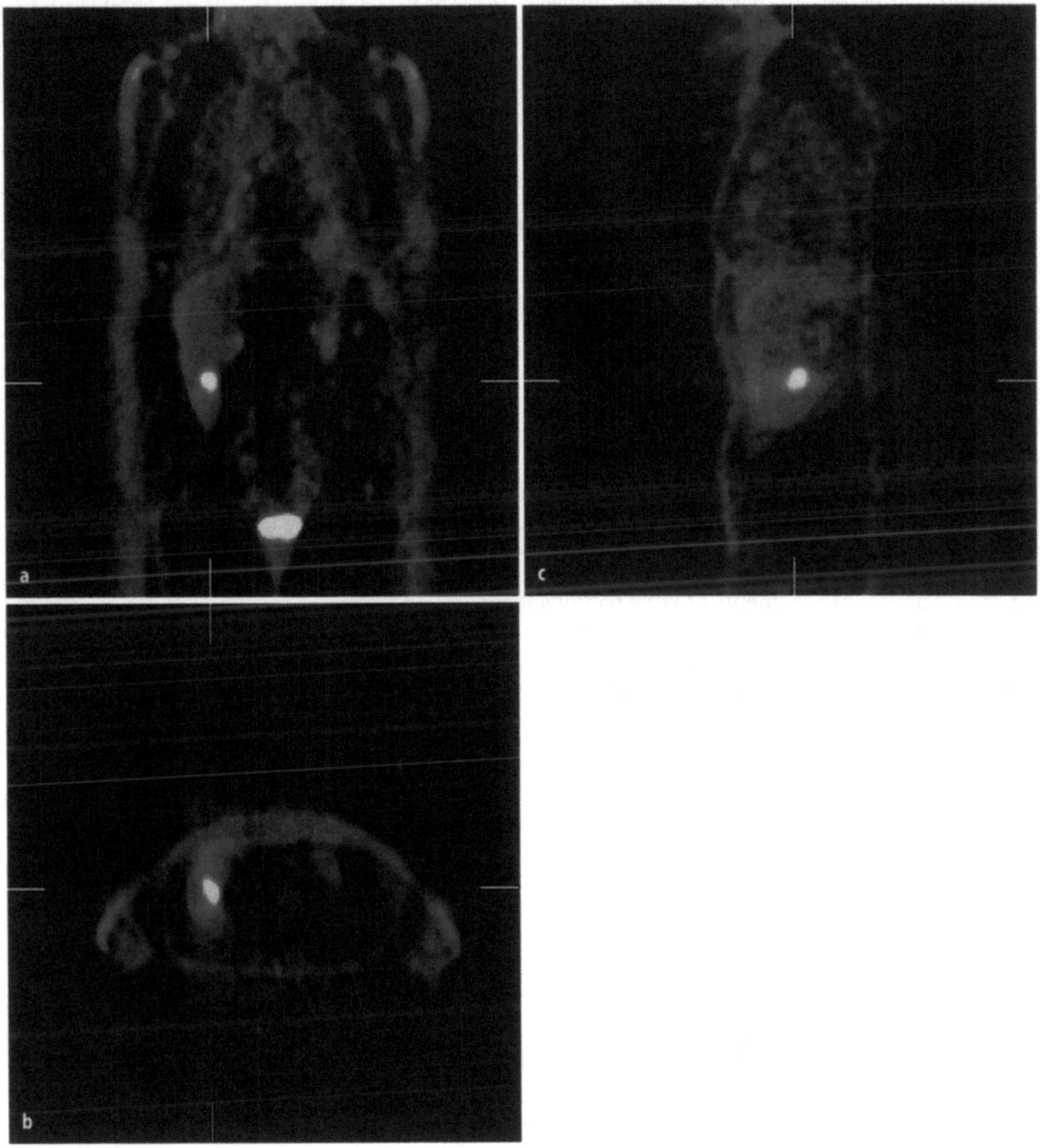

Fig. 5.7.4. Condition after resection of colon cancer. Single metastasis in the liver, (**a**) coronal, (**b**) transaxial, (**c**) sagittal images

Limits of PET

PET is a functional diagnostic technique and offers only limited anatomical information. For this reason, a supplementary sectional imaging technique is often necessary. Programs are under development that permit an overlay of PET images (function, metabolism) and CT/MRI images (morphology) as a matter of routine.

A PET scan and the associated image reconstruction currently require a total of 1.5 – 2.0 hours per patient, which limits the number of patient scans possible. A reduction in these durations can surely be expected in the near future through improvements in scanning and evaluation possibilities.

Since inflammatory changes are shown as positive findings on a PET scan (macrophages take up FDG), additional information (clinical data, other imaging techniques, etc.) must often also be considered during evaluation in order to avoid false positive results. A more exact differentiation may be possible through the use of other radiopharmaceuticals (such as amino acids like ACBC).

Our own experience with aftercare examinations shows that a considerable FDG accumulation can often occur in segments or large sections of the colon after colonoscopy, most often in terms of an unspecific inflammatory reaction. For this reason, the chronological relationship between colonoscopy and the PET scan should be considered carefully, and the PET scan may need to be performed before or at least three weeks after colonoscopy. Otherwise, there is danger of false positive findings.

References

Delbeke D (1999) Oncological applications of FDG PET imaging: brain tumors, colorectal cancer, lymphoma and melanoma. J. Nucl Med 40: 591–603

Falk PM, Gupta NC, Thorson AG et al. (1994) Positron emission tomography for preoperative staging of colorectal carcinoma. Dis Colon Rectum 37: 153–156

Gupta NC, Falk PM, Frank AL, Thorson AM, Frick MP, Bowman B (1993) Pre-operative staging of coloretal carcinoma using positron tomography. Nebr Med J 78/2: 30–35

Haberkorn U, Strauss LG, Dimitrakopoulou A (1991). PET Studies of FDG metabolism in patients with recurrent colorectal tumors receiving radiotherapy. J Nucl Med 32: 1485–1490

Ito K, Kato T, Tadokoro M (1992) Recurrent rectal cancer and scar: differentiation with PET and MR imaging. Radiology 182: 549–552

Mayer RJ Tumoren des Dünn- und Dickdarms (1995) In: Schmailzl KJG (Hrsg) Harrisons Innere Medizin Bd 2, 13. Aufl. Blackwell Wiss. Verlag, S 1669–1676

Miraldi F, Vesselle H, Faulhaber PF et al. (1989) Elimination of artifactual accumulation of FDG in PET imaging of colorectal cancer. Clin Nucl Med 23: 3–7

Ruhlmann J, Kozak B, Biersack HJ (1996). Sensitivität des PET beim frühen Nachweis des kolorektalen Karzinoms. Tumor Diagn Ther 17: 93–96

Ruhlmann J, Schomburg A, Bender H, Oehr P et al. (1997) Dis Colon Rectum 40/10: 1195–1204

Schiepers C, Penninckx F, De Vadder N et al. (1995). Contribution of PET in the diagnosis of recurrent colorectal cancer: comparison with conventional imaging. Eur J Surg Oncol 21: 517–522

Strauss LG, Corius JH, Schlag P (1989). Recurrence of colorectal tumors: PET evaluation. Radiology 170: 329–332

Thoeni RF (1997) Colorectal cancer. Radiologic staging. Radiol Clin North Am 35: 457–485

Valk PE, Pounds TR, Tesar RD, Hopkins DM, Haseman MK (1996). Cost-effectiveness of PET imaging in clinical oncology. Nucl Med Biol 23: 737–743

Vitola JV, Delbeke D, Sandler MP et al. (1996). Am J Surg 171: 21–26

5.8 Ovarian Cancer

M. Zimny, U. Cremerius, and U. Büll

5.8.1 Epidemiology

Ovarian epithelial cancer is one of the leading causes of cancer deaths in women, with age peaks for incidence and mortality in older patients. Ovarian carcinoma is the most common ovarian malignancy (>90 %). Less frequent malignancies include mixed tumors (mixed Mullerian tumor, carcinosarcoma and malignant fibroepithelial tumors), stromal tumors, germ cell tumors, and sarcomatous tumors. Germ cell tumors, however, predominate among patients under 45 years of age (Yancik 1993).

The most important risk factor for the development of ovarian cancer is the occurrence of ovarian cancer in 2 or more first-degree relatives. A hereditary syndrome characterized by predisposition to breast cancer and ovarian cancer has been linked to mutation of the BRCA1 gene on chromosome 17 (Steichen-Gersdorf et al. 1994). However, the familial forms account for only 5–10 % of all ovarian cancer. A higher risk of spontaneous forms is associated with late birth of the first child or nulliparity; a lower risk is associated with early birth of the first child and the use of oral contraceptives (Cannistra 1993).

5.8.2 Pathophysiology and Tumor Spread

Ovarian cancer begins in the surface epithelium (germinal epithelium) and spreads locally into adjacent structures such as fallopian tube, uterus and contralateral ovary. The pelvic wall, bladder, rectum, and Douglas' pouch can be involved both continuously and by drop metastases. Exfoliation of tumor cells into the peritoneal cavity occurs when the tumor breaks through the capsule of the ovary. The tumor cells can then be distributed in the abdominal cavity by the peritoneal fluid and result in metastases – especially in the paracolic gutters, along the subphrenic spaces, and in the omentum. Tumor cells can reach the surface of the pleura by way of lymph vessels in the diaphragm and give rise to malignant pleural effusion. Another path of spread involves the lymph tract. Metastases of the pelvic and paraaortic lymph nodes develop in as many as 75 % of all patients, depending on tumor stage (Burghardt et al. 1991); inguinal lymph nodes can also be involved. Hematogenic seeding is possible but rare (Hoskins 1993). Another characteristic of ovarian cancer is ascites formation, although genesis is indeterminate.

5.8.3 Histology

Histologically we differentiate between four main types of ovarian epithelial cancer: serous-papillary ovarian carcinoma, which is the most common type and affects both ovaries in approximately 50 % of all cases; mucinous ovarian carcinoma, which is frequently associated with a normal serum level of the tumor marker CA-125, endometrioid carcinoma, and clear-cell carcinoma. Clear-cell carcinoma has the worst prognosis in all stages (Cannistra 1993). This histologic variety is explained by the fact that the epithelial tumors can imitate all differentiation directions of Mullerian epithelium. All differentiation directions are associated with both malignant and benign tumors (e.g. serous cystademona) as well as an intermediate group of tumors of low malignant potential (borderline tumors).

5.8.4 Tumor Staging

Staging is based on the TNM and FIGO classifications (Sobin and Wittekind 1997). The definitions are as follows: T1 or FIGO I = carcinomas limited to the ovaries, T2 or FIGO II = carcinomas involving one or both ovaries with pelvic extension, T3 or FIGO III = peritoneal metastasis, and T4 or FIGO IV = distant metastases. Lymph node metastases are defined as TxN1 or FIGO III. Metastases of the liver capsule are classified as T3 or FIGO III, while intrahepatic metastases are assigned to Stage T4 or FIGO IV. Subgroups are also defined for each stage; these subgroups include regional spread, cytologic detection of tumor cells by peritoneal washings, and the size of peritoneal metastases.

The tumor stage is a crucial prognostic factor. For example, the percentage of patients free of disease for 5 years decreases with an increase in tumor stage and drops from over 90 % in Stage I without peritoneal carcinomatosis to less than 10 % in Stages III and IV (Cannistra 1993). The tumor stage is determined primarily during surgery. For the early stages especially, an extensive surgical procedure is required for correct staging. This will normally include a bilateral adnexectomy and a hysterectomy. In addition, multiple biopsies in the pelvic and abdominal regions up to the subphrenic area and a lymph node sampling of the pelvic and paraaortic lymph node groups are also required (Hoskins 1993).

5.8.5
Therapy

The tumor stage is critical for therapy. Whereas an exclusively surgical procedure is justified in Stage I, advanced tumor stages require extensive cytoreductive surgery along with tumor debulking and chemotherapy. The surgical procedure is determined by the spread of the tumor to other organs. Frequently an omentectomy is required, and occasionally also resection of intestinal segments (Hoskins 1993).

Chemotherapy generally involves the platinum analogues cisplatin or carboplatin in combination with cyclophosphamide or even taxol, which has been used more recently (Cannistra 1993).

5.8.6
Diagnosis

Since ovarian cancer in the early stages generally exhibits only unspecific symptoms, diagnosis generally occurs in advanced tumor stages (Soper 1996). Despite promising results of individual studies on screening by transvaginal sonography (De Priest et al. 1997), an established screening procedure for early detection of ovarian cancers is not yet available (Karlan and Platt 1995). Although the CA-125 tumor marker is elevated in the majority of patients with advanced tumor stages, it is not suitable for use as a screening method. This is because the marker can also be elevated for many benign changes such as ovarian cysts, especially in premenopausal women (Brooks 1994). Conversely, it can even be within the normal range, especially in the case of mucinous ovarian carcinoma (Cannistra 1993).

Although a mass lesion of the ovaries is usually detected by gynecological examination, imaging techniques will make it possible to evaluate tumor status and tumor spread. The available imaging modalities include transabdominal and transvaginal sonographic techniques, CT, MRI, immunoscintigraphy, and now PET.

Individual groups report a rather high diagnostic certainty of about 90 % for transvaginal color Doppler ultrasonography when used to differentiate between benign and malignant ovarian processes (Chou et al. 1994), but a review article by Tekay and Jouppila (1996) concludes that the pulsatility and resistance indices that are generally used do not permit a definitive status determination.

CT and MRI are not very reliable in evaluating tumor spread since lymph node metastases and smaller peritoneal implants may be missed (Forstner et al. 1995). Immunoscintigraphy, which is thought to be the most specific imaging technique, has not yet been accepted as a routine method. Immunoscintigraphy with ^{111}In-Cyt-103, an antibody directed against the tumor-associated antigen TAG72, demonstrated a somewhat higher sensitivity than CT in a multicenter study of 103 patients, but it had a much lower specificity (69 vs. 44 % and 57 vs. 79 %, respectively) (Krag 1993).

Since the introduction of whole-body scanners and ^{18}F-FDG in oncologic nuclear medicine a new imaging tool is available. However, up to now published data on PET and ovarian cancer are rare. The first report on FDG-accumulation in ovarian cancer cells was by Wahl et al. 1991 using an animal model. The first promising results in patients were reported by Hubner et al. (1993). Studies published to date have investigated the value of PET for differential diagnosis of primary ovarian tumors and for the detection of local recurrences (Hübner et al. 1993; Karlan et al. 1993; Casey et al. 1994; Römer et al. 1997; Zimny et al. 1997a), whereas only limited data is available regarding diagnosis of tumor spread (Zimny et al. 1997b).

5.8.7
Positron Emission Tomography

Procedure

The scan is performed either as a whole-body scan or as PET scan of the abdomen and the pelvis. The scanning field should extend at least from the dome of the liver into the inguinal region. However, since metastases outside this scanning field are also possible in principle and since hereditary forms may involve simultaneous existence of breast cancer, a whole-body scan is recommended. The necessity of a transmission scan for attenuation correction has not yet been demonstrated, but transmission scans have been performed in the majority of studies published to date. Patient preparation should involve a fasting period of at least 6 hours, as is recommended for all oncological PET scans. Catheterization of the bladder for the duration of the emission scan is advisable in order to facilitate evaluation of the pelvic region. In order to reduce the tracer concentration in the kidneys and the urinary tract a forced diuresis is recommended (i.e. 500 ml NaCl + 20 mg furosemide IV). At our center we begin the 2D emission scan approximately one hour after administration of 200–300 MBq [^{18}F]FDG. Depending on the patient's body size, the total scanning time is 2–3 hours, including a "classic" transmission scan with germanium sources without segmentation. Because of the better image quality, we recommend iterative reconstruction of the image data and documentation in at least 2 orthogonal slice planes.

Findings

Fig. 5.8.1 shows the typical findings of an extended ovarian carcinoma. In most cases the tumor shows a mixture of regions with high and with low or lacking glucose consumption; corresponding to solid or cystic parts of the tumor. Because of the tumor size, lateral assignment of the findings is usually not possible. Recurrences in the pelvic region are generally found in Douglas' pouch, the region of the bladder peritoneum, and the wall of the pelvis. Evaluation should address not only primary or recurrent tumor but also include an opinion about any peritoneal and/or lymph node metastasis that might be present. Peritoneal seeding is usually demonstrated by circumscribed foci dissiminated throughout the abdomen and Douglas' pouch as well as more diffuse FDG uptake on the liver surface and in the paracolic gutters (Fig. 5.8.2). Lymph node metastases are shown as circumscribed and partly confluent foci along the iliac vessels, paravertebral on both sides and less frequently also inguinal (Fig. 5.8.3).

Problems

Several possible pitfalls must be taken into consideration when evaluating the scans. Low malignant potential tumors and highly differentiated ovarian carcinomas often exhibit only slightly elevated glucose consumption. In addition, there are some benign changes that can exhibit elevated glucose metabolism. Foremost among these are inflammatory changes such as tubo-ovarian abscesses, followed by corpus luteum cysts, hemorrhaged follicular cysts, endometriosis, and endosalpingiosis.

In evaluating tumor spread it is necessary to differentiate peritoneal seeding from increased bowel activity in projection on intestinal structures (Bischof-Delaloyle and Wahl 1995). Based on our experience this is possible if the configura-

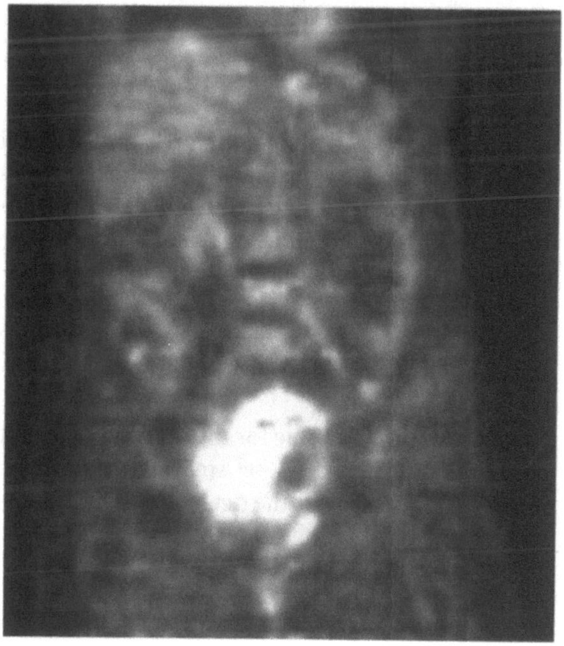

Fig. 5.8.1. FIGO IIIc: 60 year-old patient with serous/mucinous ovarian cancer

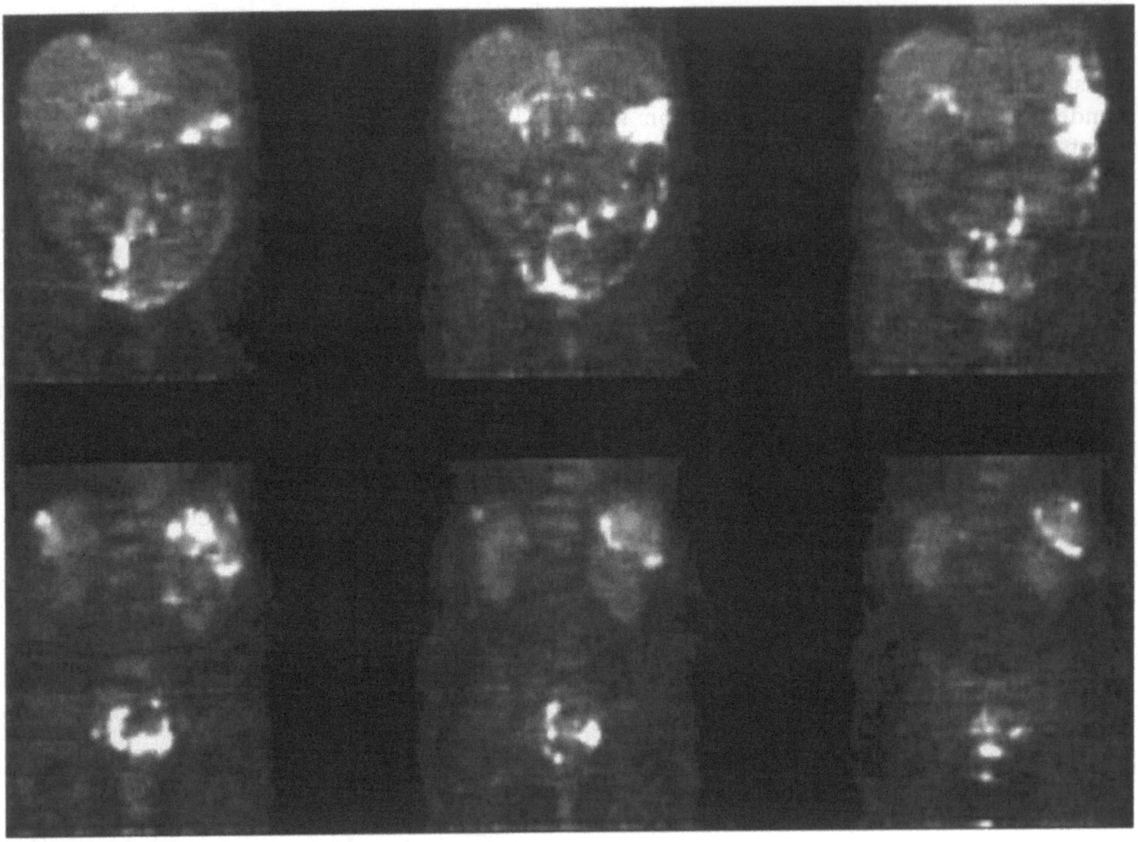

Fig. 5.8.2. 70 year-old patient with FIGO IIIc ovarian cancer; extended peritoneal carcinomatosis

tion of findings within the three-dimensional orthogonal slices is considered. Extended longish lesions along the colon usually indicate "unspecific" FDG uptake and argue against peritoneal carcinomatosis. Preparation of the patient with iso-osmotic solutions, as in the case of colonoscopy, was recently recommended in order to reduce radioactivity accumulation in the intestine (Miraldi et al. 1998).

PET is of limited value for the detection when it comes to the detection of small-node or even microscopic seeding or the detection of microscopically involved lymph nodes.

5.8.8 Results

In our patient population (Zimny et al. 1997a,b; see Tables 5.8.1 and 5.8.2) we obtained a sensitivity, specificity and diagnostic accuracy of 88, 80 and 85 %, respectively, for primary tumor diagnosis; 72, 93 and 81 %, respectively, for evaluation of peritoneal metastasis; and 50, 95 and 80 % for lymph node staging. All local recurrences have been detected to date.

Hubner (1993) reports comparable results for primary diagnosis (sensitivity 93 %, specificity 82 %). The results obtained by Römer et al. (1997) exhibit a sensitivity of 83 % but a much lower specificity of only 54 %; this is attributed to a high proportion of inflammatory processes in the patient population.

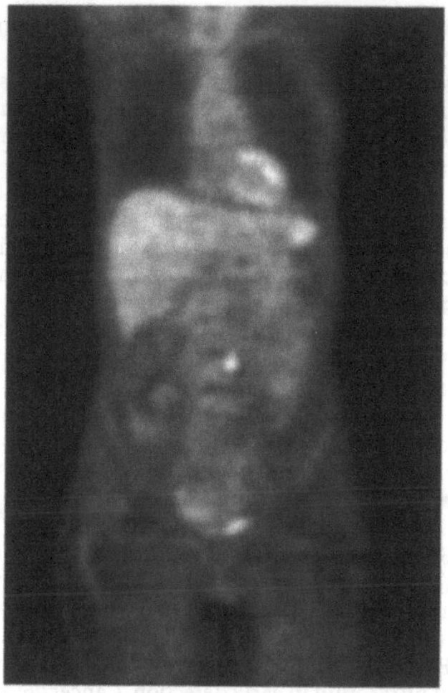

Fig. 5.8.3. 57 year-old patient with paraaortic lymph node metastasis 2 years after cytoreductive surgery and 6 cycles of chemotherapy with carboplatin and taxol for ovarian cancer (FIGO IV)

Table 5.8.1. Comparison of various techniques used in diagnosing primary and recurrent ovarian carcinoma. (*RIS* radioimmunoscintigraphy, *TV-US* transvaginal ultrasound)

	Sensitivity [%]	Specificity [%]	References
CT	80–88	53–96	Buy et al. (1991) Ghossain et al. (1991) Tibben et al. (1992)
MRT	67–85	37–97	Buist et al. (1994) Ghossain et al. (1991) Hata et al. (1992)
TV-US	81–94	53–92	Chou et al. (z) Tekay u. Jouppila (1996) Hata et al. (1992)
RIS	69–90	25–>90	Krag (1993) Granowska et al. (1991) Tibben et al. (1992)
PET	83–93	54–82	Hübner et al. (1993) Römer et al. (1997) Zimny et al. (1997 a)

The only existing direct comparison of PET with other imaging techniques for use in primary diagnosis relates only to CT (Hubner et al. 1993). Although sensitivity was comparable at about 80 %, PET exhibited a higher specificity (80 % vs. 53 % for CT). The data given in the literature for CT, MRI, immunoscintigraphy, and transvaginal ultrasound do not permit a conclusive comparison due to the very heterogeneous results (Table 5.8.1). Even more difficult is a comparison with regard to peritoneal carcinomatosis. For example, a sensitivity ranging between 53 % and 100 % and a specificity covering an even wider range from 17 % to 100 % are reported for immunoscintigraphy (Table 5.8.2). The divergent results for the different modalities are primarily due to small groups of patients selected on the basis of different criteria. Only comparative studies of larger patient groups will be able to clarify this issue.

No study comparing PET and immunoscintigraphy directly has been carried out yet, to the best of our knowledge. However, PET should be superior to immunoscintigraphy because of its higher spatial resolution, better image contrast in the liver and kidney regions, and lack of induction from human anti-mouse antibodies, which make follow-up immunoscintigraphy impossible. For one thing, it has been shown that even "more specific" immunoscintigraphy has problems differentiating inflammatory changes from malignant processes (Method et al. 1996).

Table 5.8.2. Comparison of different techniques for the detection of peritoneal carcinomatosis in ovarian cancer. (*RIS* radioimmunoscintigraphy, *TV-US* transvaginal ultrasound)

	Sensitivity [%]	Specificity [%]	References
CT	16–66	67–88	Forstner et al. (1995) Method et al. (1996) Giunta et al. (1994)
MRT	81	88	Forstner et al. (1995)
RIS	53–100	17–100	Method et al. (1996) Carrasquillo et al. (1988) Barzen et al. (1990)
PET	72	93	Zimny et al. (1997a)

In summary, PET has advantages over established techniques, especially since the introduction of whole-body technique. Even this technique, however, reaches its limits in the evaluation of minimal disease. We see the future for this method not in primary diagnosis of ovarian tumors but in therapy management and in early diagnosis of recurrences when there is tumor marker elevation.

References

Barzen G, Cordes M, Langer M, Friedmann W, Mayr AC, Felix R (1990) Wertigkeit der Radioimmunszintigraphie im Vergleich zur CT in der Diagnostik und Verlaufskontrolle des primären Ovarialkarzinoms. Fortschr Röntgenstr 153: 85–91

Bischof-Delaloyle A, Wahl R (1995) How high a level of FDG abdominal activity is considered normal? J Nucl Med 36: 106 (abstr)

Brooks SE (1994) Preoperative evaluation of patients with suspected ovarian cancer. Gynecol Oncol 55: 80–90

Buist MR, Golding RP, Burger CW et al. (1994) Comparative evaluation of diagnositc modalities in ovarian carcinoma with emphasis on CT and MR. Gynecol Oncol 52: 191–198

Burghardt E, Girardi F, Lahousen M et al. (1991) Patterns of pelvic and paraaortic lymphnode involvement in ovarian cancer. Gynecol Oncol 40: 103–106

Buy JN, Ghossain MA, Sciot C et al. (1991) Epithelial tumors of the ovary: CT findings and correlation with US. Radiology 178: 811–818

Cannistra SA (1993) Cancer of the ovary. N Engl J Med 329: 1550–1559

Carrasquillo JA, Sugarbaker P, Colcher D et al. (1988) Peritoneal carcinomatosis: imaging with intraperitoneal injection of I-131-labeled B72.3 monoclonal antibody. Radiology 167: 35–40

Casey MJ, Gupta NC, Muths CK (1994) Experience with positron emission tomography (PET) scans in patients with ovarian cancer. Gynecol Oncol 53: 331–338

Chou CY, Chang CH, Yao BL, Kuo HC (1994) Color Doppler ultrasonography and serum Ca 125 in the differentiation of benign and malignant ovarian tumors. J Clin Ultrasound 22: 491–496

DePriest PD, Gallion HH, Pavlik EJ, Kryscio RJ, Nagell JR (1997) Transvaginal sonography as a screening method for the detection of early ovarian cancer. Gynecol Oncol 65: 408–414

Forstner R, HricakH, Icchipinti KA, Powell CB, Frankel SD, Stern JL (1995) Ovarian cancer: staging with CT and MR imaging. Radiology 197: 619–626

Ghossain MA, Buy JN, Lignères C et al. (1991) Epithelial tumors of the ovary: comparison of MR and CT findings. Radiology 181: 863–870

Giunta S, Venturo I, Mottolese M et al. (1994) Noninvasive monitoring of ovarian cancer: improved results using CT with intraperitoneal contrast combined with immunocytology. Gynecol Oncol 53: 103–108

Granowska M, Mather SJ, Britton KE (1991) Diagnostic evaluation of 111In and 99mTc radiolabelled monoclonal antibodies in ovarian and colorectal cancer: correlations with surgery. Nucl Med Biol 18: 413–424

Hata K, Hata T, Manabe A, Sugimura K, Kitao M (1992) A critical evaluation of transvaginal Doppler studies, transvaginal sonography, magnetic resonance imaging, and CA 125 in detecting ovarian cancer. Obstet Gynecol 80: 922–926

Hoskins WJ (1993) Surgical staging and cytoreductive surgery of epithelial ovarian cancer. Cancer 71 [Suppl]: 1534–1540

Hubner KF, McDonald TW, Niethammer JG, Smith GT, Gould HR, Buonocore E (1993) Assessment of primary and metastatic ovarian cancer by positron emission tomography (PET) using 2-[18-F]deoxyglucose (2-[18F]FDG). Gynecol Oncol 51: 197–204

Karlan BY, Hoh C, Tse N, Futoran R, Hawkins R, Glaspy J (1993) Whole-body positron emission tomography with (fluorine-18)-2-deoxyglucose can detect metastatic carcinoma of the fallopian tube. Gynecol Oncol 49: 383–388

Karlan BY, Platt LD (1995) Ovarian cancer screening. The role of ultrasound in early detection. Cancer 76: 2011–2015

Krag DN (1993) Clinical utility of immunoscintigraphy in managing ovarian cancer. J Nucl Med 34: 545–548

Lapela M, Leskinen-Kallio S, Varpula M et al. (1995) Metabolic imaging of ovarian tumors with carbon-11-methionine: a PET study. J Nucl Med 36: 2196–2200

Method MW, Serafini AN, Averette HE, Rodriguez M, Penalver MA, Sevin BU (1996) The role of radioimmunoscintigraphy and computed tomography scan prior to reassessment laparotomy of patients with ovarian carcinoma. Cancer 77: 2286–2293

Miraldi F, Vesselle H, Faulhaber PF, Adler LP, Leisure GP (1998) Elimination of artifactual accumulation of FDG in PET imaging of colorectal Cancer. Clin Nucl Med 23: 3–7

Römer W, Avril N, Dose J et al. (1997) Metabolische Charakterisierung von Ovarialtumoren mit der Positronen-Emissions-Tomographie und F-18-Fluordeoxyglukose. Fortschr Röntgenstr 166: 62–68

Sobin LH, Wittekind CH (1997) TNM classification of malignant tumours. Wiley-Liss, New York, pp 152–156

Soper JT (1996) Malignancies of the ovary and Fallopian tube. In: Sevin BU (ed) Multimodality therapy in gynecologic oncology. Thieme, Stuttgart New York pp 135–190

Steichen-Gersdorf E, Gallion HH, Ford D et al. (1994) Familial site-specific ovarian cancer is linked to BRCA1 on 17q12–21. Am J Hum Genet 55: 870–875

Tekay A, Jouppila P (1996) Controversies in assessment of ovarian tumors with transvaginal color Doppler ultrasound. Acta Obstet Gynecol Scand 75: 316–329

Tibben JG, Massuger LF, Claessens RA et al. (1992) Tumour detection and localization using 99Tcm-labelled OV-TL 3 Fab' in patients suspected of ovarian cancer. Nucl Med Commun 13: 885–893

Wahl RL, Hutchins GD, Buchsbaum DJ, Liebert M, Grossmann HB, Fisher S (1991) 18F-2-Deoxy-2-Fluoro-D-Glu-

cose uptake into human tumor xenografts. Cancer 67: 1544–1550
Yancik R (1993) Ovarian cancer: age contrasts in incidence, histology, disease stage at diagnosis, and mortality. Cancer 71: 517–523
Zimny M, Schröder W, Wolters S, Cremerius U, Rath W, Büll U (1997a) 18F-Fluordeoxyglukose PET beim Ovarialkarzinom: Methodik und erste Ergebnisse. Nuklearmedizin 36: 228–233
Zimny M, Schröder W, Wolters S, Cremerius U, Rath W, Büll U (1997b) F-18-FDG-PET to diagnose and to stage ovarian cancer: preliminary results. Eur J Nucl Med 24: 924 (abstr)

5.9 Testicular Tumors

U. Cremerius, M. Zimny, and U. Büll

5.9.1 Clinical Principles and Current Therapy

When compared internationally, Germany is one of the countries with the highest rate of new cases of testicular tumors (incidence: 6.5 in 100,000 men). Approximately 2,600 new cases of the disease are expected per year. Tumor of the testis is ranked first among the malignant diseases that affect men 20 to 40 years of age, accounting for 40 % of all cases (Schöffski et al. 1991). The age peak is 37 years for seminomas and 28 years for nonseminomas. 70 % of all testicular cancer patients are first affected by the disease between ages 20 and 40. Genetic disposition is being discussed as a risk factor. Both genetic risk and a significantly higher risk after undescended testis (also contralateral) indicate primary germinal dysgenesis (Dieckmann et al. 1986).

Staging after histological confirmation of diagnosis by removal of the involved testis is done to determine the macroscopic and, if possible, also the microscopic extension of cancer in the primary tumor, lymph nodes and other organs at the time of diagnosis. This allows an estimate of prognosis and facilitates optimal therapy planning.

Approximately 40 % of all testicular tumors (30 % of seminomas and 70 % of nonseminomas) have already metastasized by the time of diagnosis. The paraaortic lymph nodes are the primary and most frequent site of testicular tumor metastasis. They are involved in approximately 40 % of all nonseminomatous tumors and approximately 22 % of all seminomas. Involvement of the lungs is the second most frequent type of metastasis for nonseminomas (15 %); for seminomas the second most frequent type involves iliac and inguinal lymph node metastases (Schultz et al. 1984; Boring et al. 1993).

Cures can be achieved through modern therapy in 80–90 % of cases, even with metastasized tumors (Garnick 1994). This has become possible through a combination of surgical procedures (especially retroperitoneal lymphadenectomy = RLA), percutaneous radiation therapy, and combination chemotherapy. Combination chemotherapy generally employs the substances bleomycin, etoposide and cisplatin (BEP protocol). Seminomas are very sensitive to radiation, thus percutaneous irradiation of the infradiaphragmal lymph node stations is the standard therapy for seminomas of clinical stages I (limited to the testis) and IIA/B (involvement of retroperitoneal lymph nodes up to 5 cm in diameter). The recurrence rate for Stage I tumors is less than 3 % with this procedure (Wannenmacher et al. 1988). The majority of recurrences after radiation therapy can be cured by combination chemotherapy (Zagars 1991). The administration of 2 courses of carboplatin as a monochemotherapy is currently being investigated in comparison with radiation therapy as a part of randomized studies. Beginning with Stage IIB, chemotherapy is used primarily. Nonseminomatous tumors are much less sensitive to radiation, and for this reason chemotherapy is the most important form of therapy. Because of the higher rate of side effects and toxicity, however, chemotherapy is generally only carried out after detection of metastatic disease. Therefore, correct identification of the tumor stage is even more important for nonseminomatous tumors than for seminomas. The necessity of a retroperitoneal lymphadenectomy (RLA) in Stage I is currently being discussed (Donohue et al. 1993). Alternative concepts for nonseminomas in clinical Stage I include tightly controlled follow-up and combination chemotherapy only if recurrence is detected (surveillance or wait-and-see strategy) primary administration of 2 cycles of combination chemotherapy (Read et al. 1992).

The usual procedure for noninvasive staging after removal of the testis involves physical examination, CT of the abdomen and thorax, and determination of the tumor markers AFP (alpha-fetoprotein), hCG (human chorionic gonadotropin) and LDH (lactate dehydrogenase). Acquisition of tumor-involved paraaortic lymph nodes by abdominal computer tomography (CT) is difficult, however. The main criterion in CT is the size of the lymph nodes. Both false negative and false positive findings are frequent, depending on the size criterion selected. When lymph nodes larger than 1.5 cm in diameter were considered suspicious for metastases, a sensitivity of 58% and a specificity of 76% were obtained, but when a size greater than 1.0 cm was selected as the criterion for metastases, sensitivity was 73 % and specificity 60 % (Stomper et al. 1987). Even when CT, sonography, tumor markers and bipedal lymphography are used in combination, peritoneal lymph node metastases are not detected by these noninvasive diagnostic methods in 17–38 % of the cases (Seppelt 1988; Klepp et al. 1990). For this reason, researchers have looked for other prognostic factors that can be used to predict probability of metastatic spread, especially for patients in Stage I. The most important factors determined in current routine diagnosis were found to be the infiltration depth (extent of primary tumor) and the T stage in the TNM classification (UICC 1978). A progression rate of 29 % was described for Stage T1, compared with a rate of 58 % for Stages T2 to T4 (Klepp et al. 1990). Other authors consider a Stage pT $>$ 2 to be an additional risk factor (Fung et al. 1988). Univariate analysis showed that the following factors associated with the primary tumor are relevant for predicting metastatic spread: vascular invasion, percentage of embryonal carcinoma, lymphatic invasion and tunical invasion (Moul et al. 1994). An unfavorable prognostic factor is the existence of undifferentiated tumor (Freedman et al. 1987).

The uncertainty of noninvasive diagnostic techniques argues for performing a retroperitoneal lymphadenectomy (RLA) for all nonseminomatous tumors in clinical Stage I. It is used primarily as a diagnostic measure. Indication for combination chemotherapy depends on the RLA result. A mortality of 1 % and a complication rate of approximately 10 % are given for RLA. For this reason, two other strategies are currently being discussed and investigated in studies of patients in clinical Stage I: the primary administration of 2 cycles of (adjuvant) chemotherapy for all patients, and the wait-and-see or surveillance strategy (Donohue et al. 1993).

With the wait-and-see strategy, tumor recurrence can be expected in 25–30 % of the cases, and approximately 50 % of metastases will be localized in the retroperitoneum, 30 % in the lung, and 5 % in the mediastinal lymph nodes (Peckham et al. 1988; Mead et al. 1992). This means that when chemotherapy is carried out systematically for all patients in Stage I, an avoidable toxicity must be accepted in approximately 70 % of the cases. For cases involving combination chemotherapy after clinical determination of recurrent tumor in conjunction with the surveillance strategy, customarily within the first year of observation, five-year survival rates of 98 % have been reported (Mead et al. 1992). Even when no tumor is detected by the RLA (pathological Stage I), as many as 15 % of patients exhibit tumor recurrence in the course of disease. Recurrent tumors are found in the lungs in 70 % of cases (Donohue et al. 1993).

Another diagnostic problem involves findings of residual cancer in CT scans after chemotherapy for testicular tumor metastases, which occur in 15–75 % of patients. The surgical diagnosis that is usually carried out in residual masses results in findings of basic necroses or fibroses in 40–50 % of the cases, differentiated teratomas in 12–40 % of cases (i.e., differentiated tumor parts remaining after successful chemotherapy for undifferentiated tumor parts), and remaining undifferentiated testicular tumors in 20–40 % of cases (Garnick 1994; Otto et al. 1993). Although mature teratomas must also be resected due to their continued probability of malignant transformation (Borchers et al. 1991), approximately 40 % of the patients with residual masses after chemotherapy could be spared a laparotomy if it were possible to rule out residual viable tumor by noninvasive methods.

The development of noninvasive techniques of higher sensitivity and specificity for the determination of retroperitoneal, pulmonary and mediastinal metastatic disease or of viable residual metastases after therapy would be an important key to an individualized therapeutic strategy and therefore to reduction of therapy-related morbidity and toxicity.

5.9.2 Performing PET Scans

With a state-of-the-art PET scanner, whole-body scans from the neck region to the upper thighs should always be carried out for staging or restaging in patients with testicular tumors. As with all oncological problems, the patient should be scanned on an empty stomach after fasting for at least 6 hours. Since optimal assessment of the retroperitoneum plays a crucial role, forced diuresis with 20 mg furosemide and 500 ml Ringer's solution, for example, should be carried out to reduce the radioactivity concentration in the renal pelvis and urinary bladder. If long scanning times are involved, it is advisable to provide an urinal; bladder catheterization is generally not necessary. Scans for the purpose of primary staging can be carried out shortly after removal of the testis. The inguinal surgical scar is generally clearly visible at that point, but cannot be confused with metastasis. When restaging is done after chemotherapy, our results show that a minimum interval of 2 weeks after the last therapy cycle is required, since scanning immediately after chemotherapy can give a false negative result (Cremerius et al. 1998). Restaging after percutaneous radiation therapy is even more problematic. No published data are available yet for testicular tumors, but experience with other types of tumors would suggest waiting at least 2 months after irradiation.

With metastasized testicular tumors, PET places high demands on diagnostic technique and image quality since the FDG uptake is sometimes only slightly greater than that of the background tissue, depending on histologic type. Therefore, even small focal increases in accumulation must be considered suspicious in case of doubt.

Figures 5.9.1 to 5.9.3 show typical findings for staging or restaging of testicular tumors. All the examples show iteratively reconstructed image data, which were acquired using a Siemens-CTI ECAT Exact scanner at the Department of Nuclear Medicine, Aachen Technical University. The transverse slices were reoriented and displayed in a frontal sequence of 7 mm slices. Forced diuresis results in a clearly visible filling of the urinary bladder and dilution of bladder activity. The pelvocaliceal system and the ureters do not appear, and thus retroperitoneal lymph nodes cannot be confused with activity excreted.

5.9.3 Results of PET Scans

Initially the only reports concerning FDG PET in patients with testicular tumors were case reports (Bachor et al. 1995), but in 1995 the first major study was published by Wilson et al. who used PET on 21 patients with metastasized testicular tumors. The authors found a significantly higher FDG uptake in metastases of seminomas and teratocarcinomas, but not in necrotic residual masses after therapy and in differentiated teratomas. They also described how the clinical response of testicular tumor metastases can be predicted by comparative PET scans before and after chemotherapy. Stephens et al. (1996) reported the use of FDG PET for differentiating residual masses after chemotherapy for metastasized nonseminomatous testicular tumors in 30 patients. They found a significantly higher FDG uptake (ex-

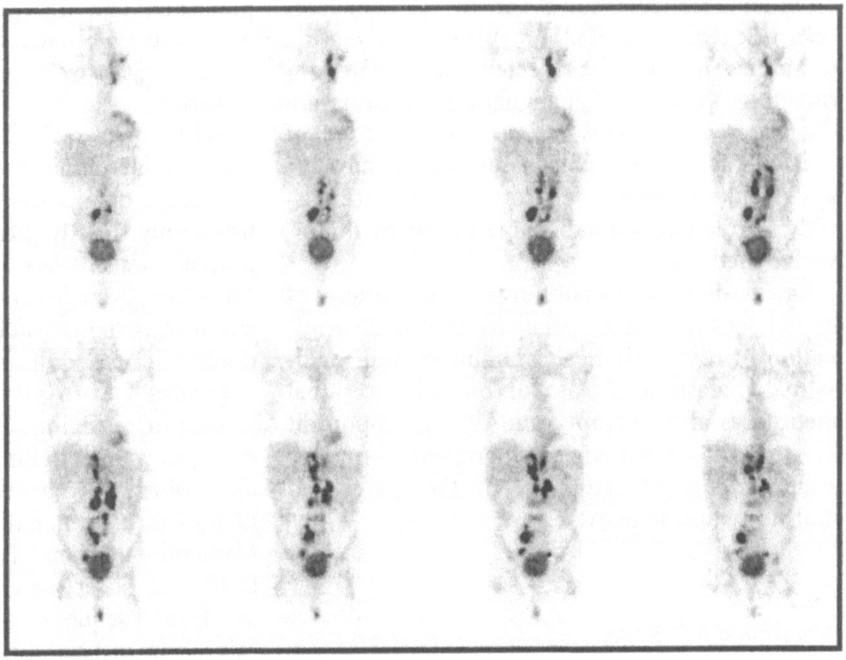

Fig. 5.9.1.
48 year-old man with retroperitoneal, mediastinal and supraclavicular metastasized seminoma before therapy

pressed as the standard uptake value or SUV) in residual viable carcinoma tissue than in complete necroses or fibroses or in residual differentiated teratomatous tissue. Differentiated teratomas and necroses or fibroses could not be distinguished from one another, however (see also

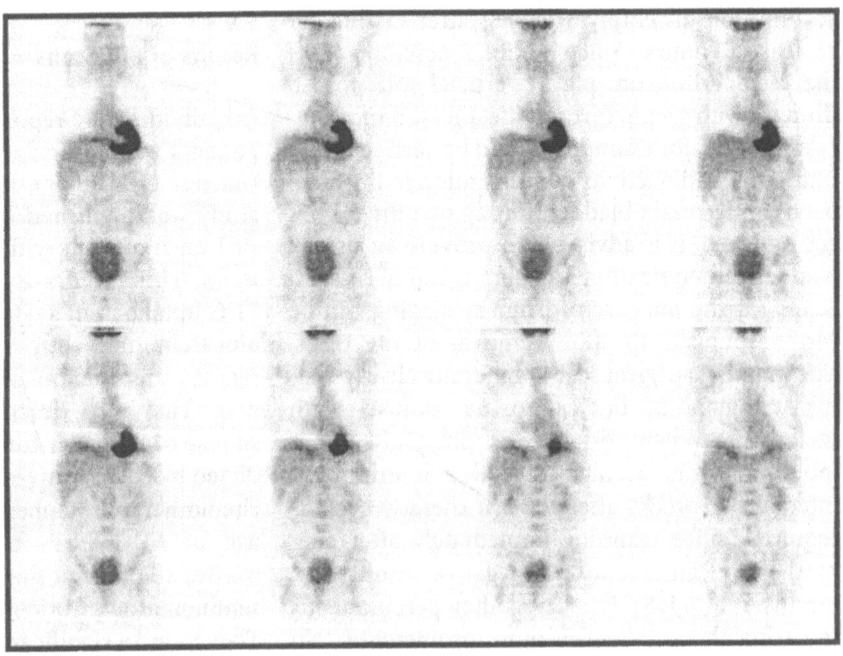

Fig. 5.9.2.
Follow-up after 4 cycles of chemotherapy for the patient shown in Fig. 5.9.1 – complete normalization of FDG uptake

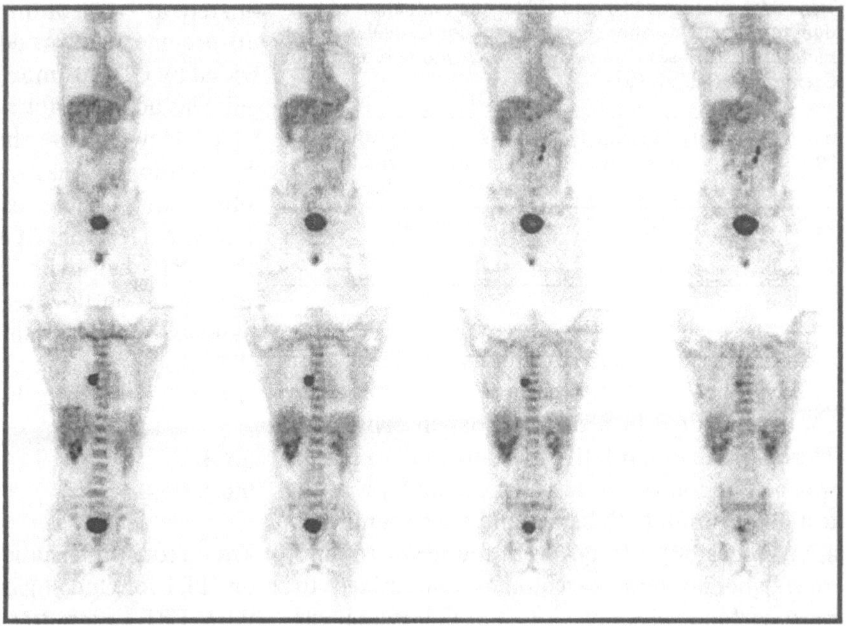

Fig. 5.9.3. 24 year-old patient, staging after removal of testis for embryonal testicular tumor (pT1). Indication of 2 lymph node filiae at left retroperitoneum and a pulmonary filia at right

Fig. 5.9.4). The authors concluded that FDG PET can be used as an additional diagnostic method in combination with CT in order to better identify those patients who can profit from post-chemotherapy resection. PET scanning should preferably be limited to patients in whom teratoma can be ruled out on the basis of primary histology. Reinhardt et al. (1997) arrived at a similar result and this group proposed that FDG PET should be used to identify the degree of differentiation of testicular tumor metastases. A study of 33 patients performed by our own group (Cremerius et al. 1998a) showed that in patients with metastasized testicular tumors, FDG PET was superior to CT in evaluating residual tumors if PET scans were made at least 14 days after completion of che-

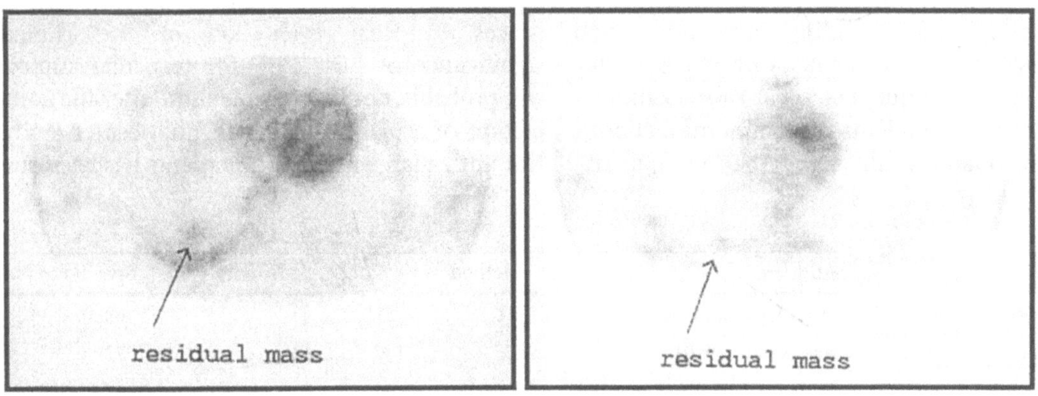

Fig. 5.9.4. At left a 25 year-old patient, residual mass after chemotherapy for pulmonary metastasized mixed testicular tumor, histologically mature teratoma. At right a 31 year-old patient with chorioncarcinoma after therapy for a lung metastasis, histologically complete necrosis. (Klinik für Nuklearmedizin der RWTH Aachen)

Table 5.9.1. Value of PET and CT for the evaluation of residual tumor activity after chemotherapy for testicular tumor metastases. PET scan > 14 days after chemotherapy. (After Cremerius et al. 1998 a)

n = 29	Sensitivity [%]	Specificity [%]	Positive Predictive Value [%]	Negative Predictive Value [%]
PET	78	90	78	90
CT	67	55	40	79

motherapy (Table 5.9.1). An interval of fewer than 14 days between chemotherapy and PET therapy control resulted in a definite loss in sensitivity. The SUV as a quantitative measure of FDG uptake was a function of the histological subtype of the testicular tumor both before and after chemotherapy. Values of 7.2 to 13.5 were found for seminomas, whereas teratocarcinomas and mixed tumors yielded values of 1.4 to 3.0. Embryonal carcinomas and choriocarcinomas exhibited a mean SUV of 3.5 to 5.0.

Only initial results have been published in abstract form regarding the use of PET for primary staging after removal of the testis. Bender et al. (1996) reported a relatively low PET sensitivity of only 50 % for acquisition of metastases of nonseminomatous testicular tumors in 23 patients; in these cases it was possible to check the PET result by retroperitoneal lymph node dissection. Reinhardt et al. (1997) examined a mixed group of 45 patients (16 seminomas and 29 nonseminomas); the PET and CT findings in the abdominal region were in agreement in 43 of 45 cases. Our own group (Cremerius et al. 1998b) also examined a group of mixed patients (19 seminomas, 12 nonseminomas) and could show that in approximately 10–15 % of the cases PET can be expected to provide relevant additional findings not provided by CT or tumor markers. A diagnostic benefit was achieved for seminoma patients in particular. However, we should qualify this statement by mentioning that validation of PET findings is often not possible, especially in seminoma patients, since today it is customary to follow up the PET scan with percutaneous radiation of the lymph outflow region without additional diagnosis. Table 5.9.2 shows a comparison of initial PET results for the staging of testicular tumors with CT data from the literature.

5.9.4 Indications

The second international consensus conference on "PET for Oncological Diagnosis" in September 1997 (PET Committee of the DGN 1997) termed the use of FDG PET "acceptable" (corresponding to a Ib indication) for monitoring the therapy of nonseminomatous germ cell tumors, except for differentiated teratomas. The use of FDG PET for lymph node staging and for restaging was viewed as "helpful" (corresponding to a IIa indication) for nonseminomatous germ cell tumors. The committee of experts found that at the present time a rating (corresponding to a IIb indication) is not yet possible for seminomas and teratomas. PET is considered unadvisable for evaluating primary testicular tumors or local recurrences. A final evaluation of the clinical significance of FDG PET for testicular tumors will probably not be possible until after the completion of a planned German multicenter study. Not until a large number of patients has been stu-

Table 5.9.2. Value of CT and PET for primary staging of nonseminomatous testicular tumors compared with pathologic staging

Authors	Method	n	Sensitivity [%]	Specificity [%]
Stomper et al. (1987)	CT	51	73	60
Aass et al. (1990)	CT	190	63	72
Carlsson-Farrelly et al. (1995)	CT	64	63	47
Bender et al. (1996)	PET	23	50	100
Cremerius et al. (1998 b)	PET	12	67	100

died will it be possible to differentiate the indication for PET according to the different histologic entities, which in FDG PET apparently exhibit heterogeneous uptake behavior.

References

Aass N, Fossa SD, Ous S, Lien HH, Stenwig AE, Paus E, Kaalhus O (1990) Is routine primary retroperitoneal lymph node dissection still justified in patients with low stage non-seminomatous testicular cancer? Br J Urol 65: 385–390

Arbeitsausschuß Positronen-Emissions-Tomographie der DGN (1997) Konsensus-Onko-PET. Nuklearmedizin 36: 45–46

Bachor R, Kocher F, Gropengiesser F et al. (1995) Positron emission tomography. Introduction of a new procedure in diagnosis of urologic tumors and initial clinical results. Urologe A 34: 138–142

Bender H, Schomburg A, Albers P et al. (1996) Grenzen von Ganzkörper-FDG-PET beim Staging von Hoden-Tumoren. Nuklearmedizin 35: A54

Borchers H, Sohn M, Müller-Leisse C, Fischer N, Jakse G (1991) Growing teratoma syndrome. Onkologie 14 [Suppl 4]: 13

Boring CC, Squires TS, Tong T (1993) Cancer statistics 1993. Ca Cancer J Clin 43: 7–26

Carlsson-Farrelly E, Boquist L, Ljungberg B (1995) Accuracy of clinical staging in non-seminomatous testicular cancer – a single center experience of retroperitoneal lymph node dissection. Scand J Urol Nephrol 29: 501–506

Cremerius U, Effert PJ, Adam G et al. (1998a) FDG-PET for detection and therapy control of metastatic germ cell tumor. J Nucl Med 39: 815–822

Cremerius U, Adam G, Zimny M, Jakse G, Büll U (1998b) Vergleich von FDG-PET, CT und Tumormarkern beim Hodentumor-Staging. Nuklearmedizin 37: A10

Dieckmann KP, Boeckmann W, Brosig W, Jonas D, Bauer HW (1986) Bilateral testicular germ cell tumors. Cancer 57: 1254

Donohue JP, Thornhill JA, Foster RS, Rowland RG, Bihrle (1993) Primary retroperitoneal lymph node dissection in clinical stage I nonseminomatous germ cell testis cancer. Br J Urol 71: 326

Freedman LS, Jones WG, Peckham MJ et al. (1987) Histopathology in the prediction of relapse of patients with stage I testicular teratoma treated by orchidectomy alone. Lancet 2: 294–298

Fung CY, Kalish LA, Brodsky GL, Richie JP, Garnick MB (1988) Stage I nonseminomatous germ cell testicular tumor: prediction of metastatic potential by primary histopathology. J Clin Oncol 6: 1467–1473

Garnick MB (1994) Testicular Cancer. In: Harrison's principles of internal medicine, 13th edition. McGraw-Hill, New York pp 1858–1861

Klepp O, Olsson AM, Henrikson H et al. (1990) Prognostic factors in clinical stage I non-seminomatous germ cell tumors of the testis: multivariate analysis of a prospective multicenter study. J Clin Oncol 8: 509–518

Mead GM, Stenning SP, Parkinson ML (1992) The second Medical Research Council Study of prognostic factors in nonseminomatous germ cell tumors. J Clin Oncol 10: 85–94

Moul JW, Melarthy WF, Fernendez EB, Sesterhenn JA (1994) Percentage of embryonal carcinoma and of vascular invasion predicts pathological stage I nonseminomatous testicular cancer. Cancer Res 54: 362–364

Otto T, Goepel M, Seeber S, Rübben H (1993) Delayed retroperitoneal lymph node excision in treatment of advanced nonseminomatous germinal cell tumors. I. Intraoperative findings in marker converted tumor. Urologe A 32: 189–193

Peckham MJ, Freedman LS, Jones WG et al. (1988) Der Einfluß der Histopathologie auf die Rezidivwahrscheinlichkeit bei Patienten mit nichtseminomatösen Hodenkarzinomen im Stadium I nach alleiniger Orchiektomie. In: Schmoll HJ, Weißbach L (Hrsg) Diagnostik und Therapie von Hodentumoren. Springer, Berlin Heidelberg New York Tokyo, S 152–160

Read G, Stenning SP, Cullen MH et al. (1992) Medical research council prospective study of survaillance for stage I testicular teratoma. J Clin Oncol 10: 1762

Reinhardt M, Müller-Mattheis V, Vosberg H, Ackermann R, Müller-Gärtner HW (1997) Staging retroperitonealer Lymphknoten bei Hodenkrebs mit FDG-PET. Nuklearmedizin 36: A33

Reinhardt MJ, Müller-Mattheis V, Gerharz CD, Vosberg HR, Ackermann R, Müller-Gärtner HW (1997) FDG-PET evaluation of retroperitoneal metastases of testicular cancer before and after chemotherapy. J Nucl Med 38: 99–101

Schöffski P, Bokemeyer C, Harstrick A, Schmoll HJ (1991) Ätiologie und Epidemiologie von Keimzelltumoren. Onkologie 14 [Suppl 4]: 1

Schultz HP, Arends J, Barlebo H et al. (1984) Testicular carcinoma in Denmark 1976–1980. Stage and selected clinical parameters at presentation. Acta Radiol Oncol 23: 249–253

Seppelt U (1988) Validierung verschiedener diagnostischer Methoden zur Beurteilung des Lymphknotenstatus. In: Weißbach L, Bussar-Maatz R (Hrsg) Die Diagnostik des Hodentumors und seiner Metastasen. Karger, Basel, S 154–169

Stephens AW, Gonin R, Hutchins GD, Einhorn LH (1996) Positron emission tomography evaluation of residual radiographic abnormalities in postchemo-therapy germ cell tumor patients. J Clin Oncol 14: 1637–1641

Stomper PC, Fung CY, Socinsky MA, Garnick MB, Richie JP (1987) Detection of retroperitoneal metastases in early-stage nonseminomatous testicular cancer analysis of different CT criteria. AJR 149: 1187–1190

Wannenmacher M, Pfannmüller-Schurr EL, Bruggmoser G (1988) Adjuvante Strahlentherapie der Seminome im Stadium I. In: Schmoll HJ, Weißbach L (Hrsg) Diagnostik und Therapie von Hodentumoren. Springer, Berlin Heidelberg New York Tokyo, S 152–160

Wilson CB, Young HE, Ott RJ et al. (1995) Imaging metastatic testicular germ cell tumors with 18-FDG positron emission tomography: prospects for detection and management. Eur J Nucl Med 22: 508–513

Zagars GK (1991) Management of stage I seminoma: radiotherapy. In: Horwich A (ed) Testicular cancer: investigation and management. Chapman & Hall, London pp 83–107

5.10 Hodgkin's Disease and Non-Hodgkin's Lymphomas

C. Menzel

This section deals with a heterogeneous group of tumors of the immune system. From both a diagnostic standpoint and an economic perspective, it is important to note not only the comparatively early age at which Hodgkin's disease manifests itself but also the overall increase in incidence of malignant lymphomas, contrasted with the decrease in mortality due to improved therapeutic options.

Lymphomas manifest themselves in lymph nodes or lymphatic tissue of parenchymatous organs. Approximately 90 % of all cases of Hodgkin's disease exhibit initial manifestations in lymph nodes, while only about 60 % of other lymphomas (non-Hodgkin's lymphomas) originate there. Two thirds of these are B-cell lymphomas, and the others are T-cell lymphomas. Various viruses are known to be potential triggers of these diseases along with hereditary factors, which may have an additive effect.

Clinical, differential-diagnostic and also differential-therapeutic approaches to Hodgkin's disease and the other lymphomas differ considerably. We will first present the clinical and therapeutic issues associated with the two disease groups, then discuss the essential factors involved in staging problems for each group, and in conclusion will deal with imaging aspects, which are largely common to the two groups.

5.10.1 Hodgkin's Disease

It is postulated that a typical Hodgkin's disease has a unifocal origin and spreads continuously from that point. In contrast, the involvement of the spleen, an organ without afferent lymph vessels, is attributed to hematogenic tumor cell seeding, a phenomenon that is not in direct agreement with the postulate just cited.

The differential diagnosis of Hodgkin's disease (HD) includes comprehensive differential diagnosis of indeterminate lymphadenopathy. It is especially important to differentiate intrathoracic processes from sarcoidosis or tuberculosis. The primary diagnosis must always be made histologically. It is essential to keep in mind that both the diagnosis itself and further subtyping can involve a certain degree of uncertainty, even in the hands of experienced pathologists, due primarily to the frequent absence of typical tumor cells in the preparation. Reactive lymphadenopathies are also frequently found in association with Hodgkin's disease, and this means that both the samples for histologic analysis and the site of the biopsy play crucial roles.

There are no specific laboratory parameters. The erythrocyte sedimentation rate (ESR) can be useful, especially as a means of following the disease process. The ESR is usually quite elevated, but it often normalizes with good response to therapy and is therefore the basis for follow-up studies. However, we must also keep in mind that this parameter is only of limited value since normalization of the ESR can also occur with persistent viable tumor tissue. The ESR can also remain quite elevated for up to one year after radiation therapy. As for other factors, a slight normocytic and normochromic anemia is frequently associated with a simultaneously reduced serum iron level. Leucocytosis, sometimes pronounced, is also frequently found with Hodgkin's disease, but it must not be confused with chronic myelocytic leukemia. In advanced cases, Hodgkin's disease is often associated with absolute lymphocytopenia. Because of these changes, infections will frequently develop, and they can be significant for functional imaging within the framework of differential diagnosis. The lungs are very often affected (pneumocystis carinii and mycoses).

Accurate staging is essential for therapy planning, particularly for Hodgkin's disease. It is especially important to determine whether the tumor disease is still local or whether an advanced, gen-

Table 5.10.1. Staging of Hodgkin's disease. Substage designations: E for extralymphatic organ involvement, S for spleen involvement, H for liver involvement, A for lack of B symptoms, and B for presence of B symptoms

Stage	Extent of Manifestation
I	One single lymph node group or a single extralymphatic organ is affected.
II	Two (2) or more lymph node groups on the same side of the diaphragm are affected, with or without involvement of extralymphatic organs on the ipsilateral side of the diaphragm.
III	Lymph node groups or extralymphatic organs on both sides of the diaphragm are affected.
IV	Diffuse involvement of extralymphatic organs, with or without additional involvement of associated lymph node groups.

eralized disease process is already involved (Table 5.10.1).

Current staging routine includes a thorough clinical examination followed by a conventional chest X-ray for the purpose of detecting or excluding thoracic or mediastinal lymphomas. If indications of an intrathoracic disease manifestation are found, then a CT scan of the thorax is performed. At present both an abdominal sonogram and an abdominal CT scan are considered obligatory, primarily in order to detect any involvement of the epigastric organs or the retroperitoneal lymph nodes. A bone marrow biopsy is generally required as an adjunct to these techniques.

Once accurate staging has been carried out, approximately three-fourths of all cases of Hodgkin's disease can currently be cured by radiation therapy (linear accelerator) or chemotherapy or a combination of the two. It is known, however, that the primary combination of the two methods does not lead to an immediate improvement in the cure rate (Fig. 5.10.1). Thus the therapy approach can consist of irradiation alone when the stage of spread is limited. Patients who can be treated curatively with irradiation do not need to be subjected to the stresses and risks of chemotherapy. Patients who suffer a relapse can still be treated adequately by chemotherapy without having to fear a worsening of their prognosis, even if they have already undergone radiation therapy

At the present time, chemotherapy based on the COPP or MOPP regimens is the established therapeutic method for Stages III and IV. Six cycles of the therapy can result in complete remission in about 80 % of these advanced cases. If necessary, it is also possible to switch to the non-cross-resistant ABVD regimen or to alternate it with COPP or MOPP on an intermittent basis. For patients with an extended tumor mass, definite clinical symptoms, or extralymphatic organ involvement, however, an initial treatment consisting of a combination of radiation and chemotherapy can also be considered in certain cases – despite the limitations cited above (Hughes-Davies et al. 1997). The effectiveness of combined chemotherapy programs plus irradiation is currently being evaluated in conjunction with the ongoing HD-8 and HD-9 studies.

5.10.2 Malignant Lymphomas – Non-Hodgkin's Lymphomas

This group includes diseases that, like Hodgkin's disease, have their origin in the lymphoreticular tissue but differ significantly from Hodgkin's disease both histologically and as regards various epidemiological and clinical aspects.

Generally non-Hodgkin's lymphomas (NHL) begin with a painless lymphadenopathy that involves one or more lymph node stations but rarely all of them. A hepatosplenal or other localized organ manifestation occurs comparatively frequently. Diagnosis and differential diagnosis are carried out in largely the same way that was described for Hodgkin's disease. However, a careful and thorough histologic analysis is even more critical in this case since therapy for malignant lymphomas depends more on the histologic type than on staging of the disease, unlike therapy for Hodgkin's disease.

Differentiation of non-Hodgkin's lymphomas is based primarily on the malignancy grade of the NHL entities (Tables 5.10.2a,b), regardless of whether the Kiel or the REAL classification is used. Assessments of malignancy are relevant

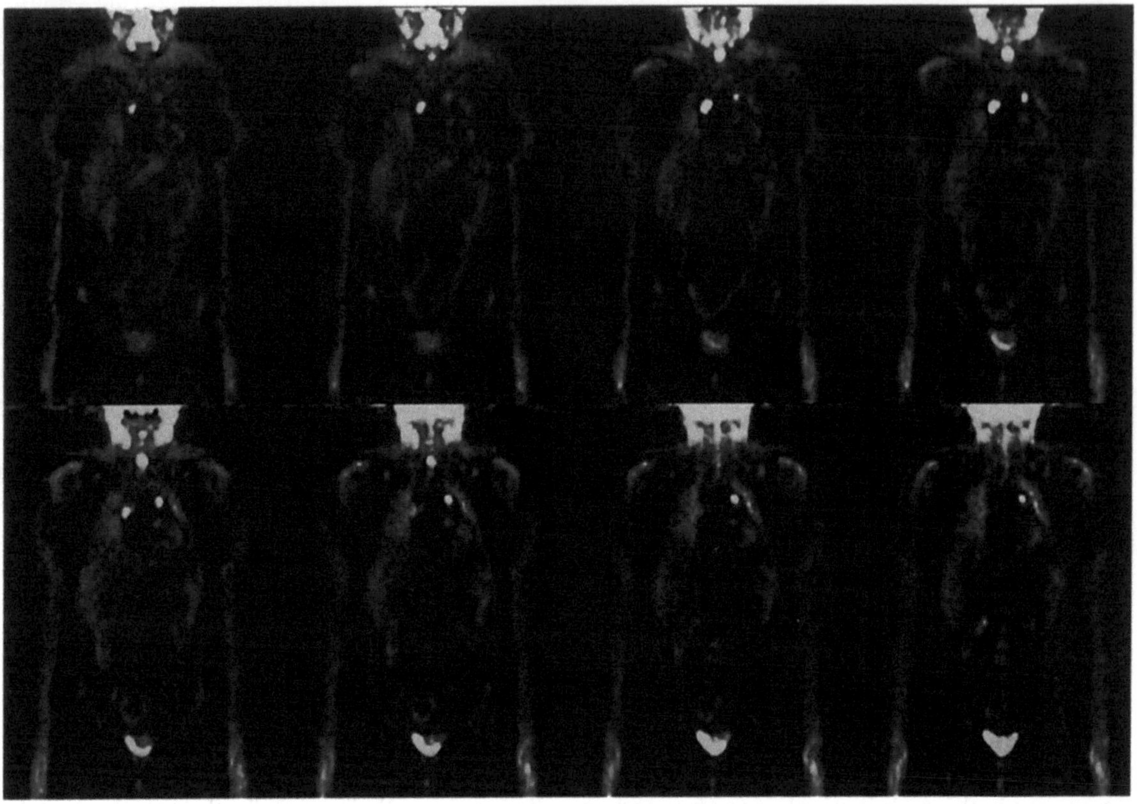

Fig. 5.10.1. Coronal tomograms for a 27 year-old female patient with Hodgkin's disease for final diagnosis after completion of combined radiation and chemotherapy in accordance with the HD9 protocol. There continue to be extended areas of increased glucose metabolism characteristic of malignancy

for possible detectability by PET scans since FDG uptake or glucose utilization seems to be correlated with the malignancy grade (see below). Based on experience acquired with the Kiel classification, it is true on the whole that small-cell (cytic) non-Hodgkin's lymphomas exhibit a comparatively favorable, low-malignancy course of disease, although in the majority of cases there is no curative therapeutic option. Large-cell (blastic) lymphomas, on the other hand, exhibit a higher-grade malignant course. However, they can be cured by chemotherapy, at least in some patients.

For FDG PET applications this means that the patients with the higher-grade malignant NHLs are the relevant patient group, both from a clinical perspective and from the standpoint of tumor biology.

The limitation of immune system functions is generally less pronounced in NHL than in Hodgkin's disease so that intercurrent infections less often pose problems for diagnosis. Pretherapeutic staging focuses on the histologic subtype and the desired therapy for the individual patient and is based on the scheme that was developed for Hodgkin's disease (see also Table 5.10.1). Staging and especially re-staging evaluations in the course of the disease being treated are comparatively less frequent, however, since extralymphatic manifestations occur much more often in malignant lymphomas, and thus in most cases a systemic therapy approach is preferred anyway. More extensive staging – including, if appropriate, exploratory laparotomy – is only required for patients who, after clinical staging, will probably still suffer from a strictly

Table 5.10.2a. Kiel classification of non-Hodgkin's lymphomas (after Stansfield et al. 1988)

B-Cell Lymphomas	T-Cell Lymphomas
B-CLL	CLL, promyelocytic leukemia
Lymphoplasmocytoid or lymphoplasmacytic immunocytoma	Lennert's lymphoma
Centroblastic-centrocytic lymphoma	T-zone lymphoma
Centroblastic lymphoma	Pleomorphic small-cell, medium-cell or large-cell lymphoma
Centrocytic lymphoma	Immunoblastic lymphoma
Large-cell anaplastic lymphoma (CD 30)	Large-cell anaplastic lymphoblastic lymphoma (CD 30+)
Burkitt's lymphoma	Lymphoblastic lymphoma
Lymphoblastic lymphoma	

localized course of disease and who can therefore be considered for isolated radiation therapy.

Since the histologic subtypes of malignant lymphomas permit predictive statements regarding the probable spread of the disease, its reaction to therapeutic intervention, and its prognosis in the majority of cases, knowledge of the subtype is essential for planning the various studies on which staging is based. For example, a Stage III or IV can be determined for some non-Hodgkin's lymphomas in as many as 90 % of all cases by clinical staging and appropriate needle biopsies alone, without any further diagnosis. Treatment of the different NHLs depends very much on the particular subtype and individual factors, and therefore we will not discuss this topic here in greater detail. In each case the staging protocol must be re-evaluated, especially for patients who receive a non-systemic therapy approach. The restaging studies must also be appropriately designed for these patients.

Table 5.10.2b. REAL classification of non-Hodgkin's lymphomas (after Hiddemann 1996)

B-Cell Lineage	T-Cell Lineage
I. Low-grade NHL	
B-cell chronic lymphocytic leukemia	T-cell chronic lymphocytic leukemia
Lymphoplasmacytic lymphoma	Lymphocytic leukemia, T and NK cell types
Hairy cell leukemia	Mycosis fungoides
MALT lymphoma	Sézary syndrome
Follicle center lymphoma, follicular	
II. High-grade to intermediate-grade NHL	
Promyelocytic leukemia	Prolymphocytic leukemia
Plasmocytoma	Peripheral T-cell leukemia
Mantle cell lymphoma	Angioimmunoblastic T-cell lymphoma
	Angiocentric lymphoma
Diffuse large B-cell lymphomas	Intestinal T-cell lymphoma Anaplastic large-cell lymphoma
III. High-grade, very aggressive NHL	
Precursor B-lymphoblastic lymphoma	Precursor T-lymphoblastic lymphoma
Burkitt's lymphoma	Adult T-cell lymphoma (ATLL)
B-cell leukemia Plasma cell leukemia	

Imaging Techniques

In summary, the imaging techniques used for staging must address two critical questions: first, with respect to Hodgkin's disease, the question of staging between Stages II and II, and second, as regards non-Hodgkin's lymphomas, whether a Stage I or a continuously spreading Stage II is present or whether there is already a disseminated higher-grade disease. These two points will determine the difference for the individual patient between a local-surgical or radiation therapy approach and a systemic therapeutic approach dominated by chemotherapy, regardless of whether it is combined with adjunct radiotherapy or not.

Due to the lack of techniques better suited for imaging the entire body, computer tomography (CT) has become established in recent years as the primary imaging method in HD and NHL staging. As a comparatively low-cost, universally available method that can be performed quickly, CT focuses on the morphological correlative of Hodgkin's disease and non-Hodgkin's lymphoma. Nodes are evaluated by CT according to number, size, anatomical location and environmental reaction, among other factors. The groups of diseases under discussion here are especially characterized by the lack of typical or pathognomonic changes. The number and the localization of processes vary substantially. Often there is a variable morphology with respect to node differentiability, surface, and environmental reaction, even as regards single lesions. It is true, however, that pronounced involvement and the presence of large nodes as well as small nodes must be interpreted as an indication of a lymphoma. Large nodes, especially pulmonary nodes, are also found in Wegener's disease and in metastases of various tumors such as malignant melanoma, testicular carcinoma and hypernephroid renal cell carcinoma. On the other hand, if intranodal calcification is found during primary diagnosis, then it should be interpreted in the majority of cases as an indication of benign changes (e.g. tuberculosis or sarcoidosis).

Compared with CT, other techniques have largely played a secondary role, especially those that offer functional whole-body diagnosis. Whole-body scintigraphy with gallium-67 citrate has achieved a certain status in Anglo-American circles. Sensitivities ranging between 70 % and 90 % have been reported for the detection of viable tumor tissue above the diaphragm (McLaughlin et al. 1990). On the other hand, the method's sensitivity drops to about 50 % in the abdominal region. This method has proved to be unsuitable for staging and therapy monitoring, according to other studies (Sandrock et al. 1993).

Table 5.10.3. PET studies

Authors	Hodgkin's Lymphomas (n)	Non-Hodgkin's Lymphomas (n)
Moog et al. (1997)	27	33
Dimitrakopoulou et al. (1995)	20	26
Newman et al. (1994)	5	11
de Wit et al. (1997)	17	17
Hoh et al. (1997)	7	11
Rodriguez et al. (1995)	–	23
Lapela et al. (1995)	–	22

Positron emission tomography or PET, in combination with fluorine-18 as the tracer in ^{18}F-fluorodeoxyglucose (FDG), now available almost universally, is a state of the art technique that is especially well suited for staging in the abdominal region and offers classic whole-body diagnosis. It can also be used for staging and restaging Hodgkin's disease and non-Hodgkin's lymphomas.

It has been shown that FDG uptake in the tumor in NHL is obviously directly correlated with the degree of tumor malignancy (Rodriguez et al. 1995). Lapela et al. (1995) were able to document this in 22 patients with non-Hodgkin's lymphomas after quantification of glucose metabolism (SUV/rMR) in relation to the histologic grade of differentiation of NHLs (Table 5.10.3).

Comparable results were also obtained by Okada et al. (1992), who demonstrated a positive correlation between the proliferative activity of malignant lymphomas and the intratumoral FDG accumulation, while Higashi et al. (1993) described a correlation between FDG accumulation and the number of viable tumor cells. The team of Okada et al. (1994) also reported, on the basis of a long-term study, that the response to therapy and therefore the mean survival time was reduced in patients who initially exhibited a high metabolic rate in PET scans.

FDG PET has been compared with established clinical diagnostic methods, primarily in connection with cervical lymph node staging and findings from the neck region, which is easily accessible both clinically and diagnostically. For example, Benchaou et al. (1996) reported that FDG PET is at least equal to CT in diagnosing malignant lymphomas but that FDG PET offers additional information based on whole-body diagnosis. In the thorax and especially in the abdominal region, FDG PET proved to be superior to CT in staging malignant lymphomas, which was also demonstrated by Thill rt al (1997) who could show that PET- in addition to the demonstration of all CT-Lesions- found almost 25 % more lesions in HD and NHL. Newman et al. (1994), who studied 16 patients, found 49 tumor foci in these regions that were identified equally well by both techniques and 5 additional foci that were only imaged by PET.

Given the fact that FDG PET is comparatively easy to perform and evaluate because of the positive pathologic contrast, the higher sensitivity of this method compared with CT is apparent. This was also confirmed by Knopp et al. (1994) for both tumor detection and N staging in 50 patients with bronchial carcinomas and lymphomas. For untreated lymphomas, a sensitivity of nearly 100 % can be expected. For evaluation of residual viability in masses remaining after therapy, the information provided by FDG PET is superior to that of all alternative methods (Bares et al. 1994). The findings made in the studies cited above correlate well with the results obtained with our own group of patients, which included approximately 40 each with Hodgkin's disease and non-Hodgkin's lymphoma. The PET findings must be interpreted as an image-monomorphic function of the metabolic activity and size of a structure. The small groups of patients in whom the individual disease entities have been imaged to date can be viewed consequently as part of a larger subject group. To this extent the efficiency of the technique is also documented for these indications on the basis of the existing data pool. Potential accumulations in inflammatory processes have only a moderate negative effect on the specificity of the method. Such accumulations generally do not result in false-positive results when the medical history and the clinical data are taken into account (Hübner et al. 1995). Diffuse thymic hyperplasia has also been described as a potential source of false-positive findings (Glatz et al. 1996). More critical, in comparison, is the effect of chemotherapy when the PET scan is performed immediately after chemotherapy. At the present time the data is insufficient for systematically defining the required interval between the completion of chemotherapy and the best time for the PET scan. Data acquired with our own patient group show that it seems to be advisable to wait at least 2–4 weeks between chemotherapy and the FDG PET scan, especially where small lesions are concerned.

To an increasing extent, PET can be considered the method of choice, especially for staging and for eventually replacing invasive staging methods such as laparotomy, but also for persistent masses remaining after therapy and for ruling out a residual or recurrent tumor. This is true even though it is still necessary to expand the data pool cited in the literature. In particular, PET is the method of choice for close monitoring and follow-up of patients undergoing chemotherapy or radiation therapy. Studies of Hodgkin's disease and of medium-grade and higher-grade non-Hodgkin's lymphoma have been central to this effort. Nodular processes represent the primary diagnostic target, whereas the data on issues of diffuse tumor infiltration have so far been limited (Barrington and Carr 1995), and the value of the method for this approach can even be considered questionable.

It is at least equally important, however, that the scan be performed under the best conditions possible. Since systemic administration of steroids is included in the majority of therapy concepts for malignant lymphomas, it is absolutely necessary to consider the current medication and other metabolically relevant information (accompanying diseases such as diabetes mellitus). It is known that steroids can reduce the FDG accumulation in malignant lymphomas (Lewis and Salama 1994; Rosenfeld et al. 1992) and in other malignant tumors (Cremerius et al. 1997) in relation to the surrounding tissue, because of their anti-insulin effect on carbohydrate metabolism.

Since glomerulonephritis occurs relatively frequently in conjunction with malignant lymphomas (Zahner et al. 1997), we must expect that the secondary renal disease will affect the results of functional imaging in some of these patients. Focal physiological activity accumulations in the area of the kidneys and the efferent urinary passages, which can be attributed solely to activity in the urine, must be considered as the potential cause of false-positive results. Since the scanning result is frequently not immediately available, it is advisable – especially if there is a relevant clinical problem at the outset – to take this factor into account by adequately hydrating the patient, administering a diuretic, and extending the tracer accumulation phase accordingly. In individual cases it has also proved useful, in our experience, to repeat the scan over the lower abdomen and the pelvis when these problems are involved. If a dynamic can be detected when comparing the two findings, then a focally malignant process is improbable.

In addition to the established clinical-diagnostic indications, there is a wider application spectrum for FDG PET in the clinical follow-up of established chemotherapy concepts, both with respect to their effectiveness for the individual patient and in clinical research on new therapy concepts. For example, Hoekstra et al. (1993) were already able to detect a drop in the metabolic rate at an early point when the level of chemotherapy was sufficient, whereas there was no significant change among non-responders. Given the considerable cost associated with chemotherapy, early examination of its effectiveness certainly seems desirable, long before volume reduction of the tumor mass is detectable morphologically. Such questions can be answered quickly and probably also cost-effectively for known tumor localization, even with a limited scanning protocol.

In summary, the spectrum of indications for FDG PET in the area of malignant lymphomas includes the staging and re-staging of Hodgkin's disease and especially the nodular variants of non-Hodgkin's lymphoma, the detection or exclusion of residual viability in radiologically persistent residual structures after completion of therapy (de Wit et al. 1997), and – an indication that will be established in the near future – early therapy monitoring of chemotherapy (Barrington and Carr 1995). With regard to the first of these indications we must note that although the specific data pool for malignant lymphomas is still relatively small with respect to the various histologic subtypes, it cannot justifiably be used as a limiting argument – if at all – since FDG's non-specific take-up mechanism and the reliability of FDG PET for all subtypes have already been demonstrated. The last of the indications mentioned above, on the other hand, must be investigated further and verified on the basis of larger studies.

References

Bares R, Altehöfer C, Cremerius U, Handt S, Osieka R, Mittermayer C, Büll U (1994) FDG-PET for metabolic classification of residual lymphoma masses after chemotherapy. J Nucl Med 35: 131 P

Barrington SF, Carr R (1995) Staging of Burkitt's lymphoma and response to treatment monitored by PET scanning. Clin Oncol R Coll Radiol 7: 334–335

Benchaou M, Lehmann W, Slosman DO, Becker M, Lemoine R, Rufenacht D, Donath A (1996) The role of FDG-PET in the preoperative assessment of head and neck cancer. Acta Otolaryngol Stockh 116/2: 332–335

Cremerius U, Bares R, Weis J et al. (1997) Fasting improves discrimination of grade 1 and atypical or malignant meningioma in FDG PET. J Nucl Med 38: 26–30

Dimitrakopoulou-Strauss A, Strauss LS, Goldschmidt H, Lorenz WJ, Maier-Borst W, van Kaick G (1995) Evaluation of tumor metabolism and multidrug resistance in patients with treated malignant lymphomas. Eur J Nucl Med 22/5: 434–442

Glatz S, Kotzerke J, Mogg F, Sandherr M, Heimpel H, Reske SN (1996) Vortäuschung eines mediastinalen Non-Hodgkin-Lymphomrezidives durch diffuse Thymushyperplasie im 18F-FDG-PET. RöFo 165: 309–310

Hiddemann W, Longo DL, Coiffier B et al. (1996) Lymphoma classification – the gap between biology and clinical management is closing. Blood 88: 4085–4089

Higashi K, Clavo A, Wahl RL (1993) Does FDG uptake measure proloferative activity of human cancer cells ? In vitro comparison with DNA flow cytometry and tritiated thymidine uptake. J Nucl Med 34: 414–419

Hoekstra OS, Ossenkoppele GJ, Golding R, van Lingen A, Visser GWM, Teule GJJ, Huijgens PC (1993) Early treatment response in malignant lymphoma as determined by

planar fluorine-18-fluorodeoxyglucose scintigraphy. J Nucl Med 34: 1706–1710
Hoh CK, Glaspy J, Rosen P et al. (1997) Whole body FDG PET imaging for staging of Hodgkin's disease. J Nucl Med 38/3: 343–348
Hübner KF, Buonocore E, Singh SK, Gould HR, Cotten DW (1995) Charaterization of chest masses by FDG positron emission tomography. Clin Nucl Med 20: 293–298
Hughes-Davies L, Tarbell NJ et al. (1997) Stage I A – II B Hodgkin's disease: management and outcome of extensive thoracic involvement. Int J Radiat Oncol Biol Phys 39/2: 361–369
Knopp MV, Bischoff H, Lorenz WJ, van Kaick G (1994) PET imaging of lung tumours and mediastinal lymphoma. Nucl Med Biol 21: 749–757
Lapela M, Leskinen S, Minn HR et al. (1995) Increased glucose metabolism in untreated non-Hodgkin's lymphoma: a study with positron emission tomography and fluorine-18-fluorodeoxyglucose. Blood 86/9: 3522–3527
Lewis PJ, Salama A (1994) Uptake of fluorine-18-fluorodeoxyglucose in Sarcoidosis. J Nucl Med 35/10: 1647–1649
McLaughlin A, Magee MA, Greenough R et al. (1990) Current role of gallium scanning in the management of lymphoma. Eur J Nucl Med 16: 755–771
Moog F, Bangerter M, Diederichs CG et al. (1997) Lymphoma: role of whole-body 2-deoxy-2-[F-18] fluoro-D-glucose (FDG) in nodal staging. Radiology 203/3: 795–800
Newman JS, Francis IR, Kaminski MS, Wahl RL (1994) Imaging of lymphoma with PET with 2-[F-18]-fluoro-2-deoxy-D-glucose: correlation with CT. Radiology 190/1: 111–116
Okada J, Yoshikawa K, Itami M et al. (1992) Positron emission tomography using fluorine-18-fluorodeoxyglucose in malignant lymphoma: a comparison with proliferative activity. J Nucl Med 33/3: 325–329
Okada J, Oonishi H, Yoshikawa K, Imaseki K, Uno K, Itami J, Arimizu N (1994) FDG-PET for the evaluation of tumor viability after anticancer therapy. Ann Nucl Med 8/2: 109–113
Rodriguez M, Rehn S, Ahlström H, Sundström C, Glimelius B (1995) Predicting malignance grade with PET in Non-Hodgkin's lymphoma. J Nucl Med 36: 1790–1796
Rosenfeld SS, Hoffmann JM, Coleman RE, Glantz MJ, Hanson MW, Schild SC (1992) Studies of primary central nervous system lymphoma with fluorine-18 fluorodeoxyglucose positron emission tomography. J Nucl Med 33/4: 532–536
Sandrock D, Lastoria S, Magrath IT, Neumann RD (1993) The role of gallium-67 tumor scintigraphy in patients with small, non cleaved cell lymphoma. Eur J Nucl Med 20: 119–122
Stansfield AG, Diebold J, Noel H et al. (1988) Kiel Classification. Lancet 1: 292–293
de Wit M, Bumann D, Beyer W, Herbst K, Clausen M, Hossfled DK (1997) Whole body positron emission tomography (PET) for diagnosis of residual mass in patients with lymphoma. Ann Oncol 8 [Suppl 1]: 57–60
Zahner J, Bach D, Marms J, Schneider W, Dierckes K, Grabensee B (1997) Glomerulonephritis und malignes Lymphom. Med Klinik 92: 712–719

5.11 PET and Neuro-Imaging: Diagnostic and Therapeutic Value, Current Applications and Future Perspective

J. Reul

5.11.1 Introduction

Despite the fact that today many powerful diagnostic tools have increased the diagnostic value of neuroimaging, most of these instruments are "only" morphologic. Computered Tompgraphy (CT) and Magnetic Resonance Imaging (MRI) are in first line structural diagnostic instruments which – in the hand of an experienced Neuroradiologist – give worthful informations about structural changes and tissue lesions. MRI is a very sensitive tool. However, the specifity is almost lower than the sensitivity. Many lesions have the same appearance and the differentiation of tumours, abscesses, inflammatous processes and necrosis can be very difficult. With small exceptions, MRI and CT cannot give "functional" data or data about metabolism rates. The exception is functional MRI which allows by use of special techniques the acquisition of some kind of functional data (Table 5.11.1).

The advantage of Positron Emission Tomography can be seen in the enormous sensivity for malignant processes and the higher specifity, compared to MRI and other neuroimaging techniques. Table 5.11.2 gives an overview of the actual and possible future indications.

Out of these multiple future indications, the ones which are oncologically of specific interest will be analyzed and discussed more detailled in the following descriptions:

Table 5.11.1. Functional examinations in MRI

– functional MRI (fMRI) by use of BOLD techniques
– Relaxometrie
– Spectroscopy
– Diffusion and Perfusion Imaging

Table 5.11.2. PET indications in Neuroimaging

- Preoperative and pretherapeutic grading of primary CNS tumours
- Differentiation of reactive postoperative changes from rest or recurrent tumour
- Differentiation between radiation necrosis and tumour rest or recurrence
- Differentiation between inflamatous processes and tumour (abscess versus metastasis or glioma)
- Differentiation of gliomas from lymphomas
- Detection and identification of CNS metastases
- Early diagnosis of dementia (especially Alzheimers disease)
- Diagnosis and differential diagnosis of sysemic neurodegegerative diseases (e.g. Multi-System-Atrophia (MSA))
- Diagnostic evaluation of epilepsy including preoperative evaluation
- Diagnostic evaluation of schizophrenia and other psychiatric diseases
- Circulation- and blood flow studies in stroke and atherosclerosis

1. Differentiation and grading of primary CNS tumours
2. Differentiation of reactive postoperative changes from rest or recurrent tumour
3. Differentiation between radiation necrosis and tumour rest or recurrence
4. Differentiation between inflamatous processes and tumour (abscess versus metastasis versus glioma)
5. Differentiation of lymphomas

5.11.2 Diagnostic Neuroimaging and Tumour Classification

The diagnosis of primary CNS tumours is based on the new classification of the WHO (Kleihus et al., Table 5.11.3.). The most frequent brain tumour entity is the glioma. Gliomas are graded from grade I to grade IV. Grade I – the pilocytic astrocytoma – is a special type which is similar to the so called spongioblastoma of the cerebellum. It is seen mostly in younger patients and of dif-

Table 5.11.3. WHO Histological Typing of CNS Tumours

1	**Tumours of Neuroepithelial Tissue**
1.1	**Astrocytic tumours**
1.1.1	Astrocytoma
1.1.1.1	Variants: Fibrillary
1.1.1.2	Protoplasmic
1.1.1.3	Gemistocystic
1.1.2	Anaplastic (malignant) astrocytoma
1.1.3	Glioblastoma
1.1.3.1	Variants: Giant cell glioblastoma
1.1.3.2	Gliosarcoma
1.1.4	Pilocytic astrocytoma
1.1.5	Pleomorphic xanthoastrocytoma
1.1.6	Supependymal giant cell astrocytoma (Tuberous sclerosis)
1.2	**Oligodendroglial tumours**
1.2.1	Oligodendroglioma
1.2.2	Anaplastic (malignant) oligodendroglioma
1.3	**Ependymal tumours**
1.3.1	Ependymoma
1.3.1.1	Variants: Cellular
1.3.1.2	Papillary
1.3.1.3	Clear cell
1.3.2	Anaplastic (malignant) ependymoma
1.3.3	Myoxopapillary ependymoma
1.3.4	Subependymoma
1.4	**Mixed gliomas**
1.4.1	Oligo-astrocytoma
1.4.2	Anaplastic (malignant) oligo-astrocytoma
1.4.3	Others
1.5.	**Choroid plexus tumours**
1.5.1	Choroid plexus papilloma
1.5.2	Choroid plexus carcinoma
1.6	**Neuroepithelial tumours of uncertain origin**
1.6.1	Astroblastoma
1.6.2	Polar spongioblastoma
1.6.3	Gliomatosis cerebri
1.7	**Neuronal and mixed neuronal-glial tumours**
1.7.1	Gangliocytoma
1.7.2	Dysplastic gangliocytoma of cerebellum (Lhermitte-Duclos)
1.7.3	Desmoplastic infantile ganglioglioma
1.7.4	Dysembryoplastic neuroepithelial tumour
1.7.5	Ganglioglioma
1.7.6	Anaplastic (malignant) ganglioglioma
1.7.7	Central neurocytoma
1.7.8	Paraganglioma of the filum terminale
1.7.9	Olfactory neuroblastoma (Aesthesioneuroblastoma)
1.7.9.1	Variant: Olfactory neuroepithelioma
1.8	**Pineal parenchymal tumours**
1.8.1	Pineocytoma
1.8.2	Pineoblastoma
1.8.3	Mixed/transitional pineal tumours
1.9	**Embryonal tumours**
1.9.1	Medulloepithelioma
1.9.2	Neuroblastoma
1.9.2.1	Variant: Ganglioneuroblastoma
1.9.3	Ependymoblastoma

Table 5.11.3. Continued

1.9.4	Primitive neuroectodermal tumours (PNETs)
1.9.4.1	Medulloblastoma
1.9.4.1.1	Variants: Desmoplastic medulloblastoma
1.9.4.1.2	Medullomyoblastoma
1.9.4.1.3	Melanotic medulloblastoma
2	**Tumours of Cranial and Spinal Nerves**
2.1	**Schwannoma (Neurilemmoma, Neurinoma)**
2.1.1	Variants: Cellular
2.1.2	Plexiform
2.1.3	Melanotic
2.2	**Neurofibroma**
2.2.1	Circumscribed (solitary)
2.2.2	Plexiform
2.3	**Malignant peripheral nerve sheath tumour (MPNST) (Neurogenic sarcoma, Anaplastic neurofibroma, "Malignant schwannoma")**
2.3.1	Variants: Epithelioid MPNST with divergent mesenchymal and/or epithelial differentiation
2.3.3	Melanotic
3	**Tumours of the Meninges**
3.1	**Tumours of meningothelial cells**
3.1.1	Meningioma
3.1.1.1	Variants: Meningothelial
3.1.1.2	Fibrous (fibroblastic)
3.1.1.4	Transitional (mixed)
3.1.1.5	Psammomatous
3.1.1.6	Angiomatous
3.1.1.7	Microcystic
3.1.1.8	Secretory
3.1.1.9	Clear cell
3.1.1.10	Lymphoplasmacyte-rich
3.1.1.11	Metaplastic
3.1.2	Atypical meningioma
3.1.3	Papillary meningioma
3.1.4	Anaplastic (malignant)
3.2	**Mesenchymal, non-meningothelial tumours Benign neoplasms**
3.2.1	Osteocartilaginous tumours
3.2.2	Lipoma
3.2.3	Fibrous histiocytoma
3.2.4	Others Malignant neoplasms
3.2.5	Hemangiopericytoma
3.2.6	Chondrosarcoma
3.2.6.1	Variant: Mesenchymal chondrosarcoma
3.2.7	Malignant fibrous histiocytoma
3.2.8	Rhabdomyosarcoma
3.2.9	Meningeal sarcomatosis
3.2.10	Others
3.3	**Primary melanocystic lesions**
3.3.1	Diffuse melanoma
3.3.2	Melanocytoma
3.3.3	Malignant melanoma
3.3.3.1	Variant: Meningeal melanomatosis
3.4	**Tumours of uncertain histogenesis**
3.4.1	Haemangioblastoma (Capillary haemangioblastoma)

Table 5.11.3. Continued

4	**Lymphomas and Haemopoitic Neoplasms**
4.1	Malignant lymphomas
4.2	Plasmacytoma
4.3	Granulocytic sarcoma
4.4	Others
5	**Germ Cell Tumours**
5.1	Germinoma
5.2	Embryonal carcinoma
5.3	Yolk sac tumour (Endodermal sinus tumour)
5.4	Choriocarcinoma
5.5	Teratoma
5.5.1	Immature
5.5.2	Mature
5.5.3	Teratoma with malignant transformation
5.6	Mixed germ cell tumours
6	**Cysts and Tumour-like Lesions**
6.1	Rathke cleft cyst
6.2	Epidermoid cyst
6.3	Dermoid cyst
6.4	Colloid cyst of the third ventricle
6.5	Enterogenous cyst
6.6	Neuroglial cyst
6.7	Granular cell tumour (Choristoma, Pituicytoma)
6.8	Hypothalamic neuronal hamartoma
6.9	Nasal glial heterotopia
6.10	Plasma cell granuloma
7	**Tumours of the Sellar Region**
7.1	Pituitary adenoma
7.2	Pituitary carcinoma
7.3	Craniopharyngioma
7.3.1	Variants: Adamantinomatous
7.3.2	Papillary
8	**Local Extensions from Regional Tumours**
8.1	Paraganglioma (Chemodectoma)
8.2	Chordoma
8.3	Chondroma Chondrosarcoma
8.4	Carcinoma
9	**Metastic Tumours**
10	**Unclassified Tumours**

ferent prognosis than the other gliomas. Beside the glioma and astrocytoma grade II to IV, there can be seen oligodendrogliomas, mixed gliomas (oligoastrocytomas) and rare entities as for example the pleomorphic xanthoastrocytoma and the almost benign entities ganglioglioma, gangliocytoma an neurocytoma.

The diagnosis of a primary (intraaxial) brain tumour in neuroimaging is based on the diagnostic criteria evaluated by the use of cranial CT (CCT) and MRI examinations.

CCT is helpful in the detection of calcifications, e.g. supporting the diagnosis of an oligodendroglioma whereas MRI is the primary tool of diagnostic evaluation today.

For the diffent malignancy grades of gliomas there exist practical neuroradiological criteria to establish the diagnosis and tumour grade:

Grade I: In most cases, the diagnostic identification of a pilocytic astrocytoma is possible: It is based on the age of the patient, the location, the signal behaviour on MRI and the appearance after contrast media adminstration (Fig. 5.11.1).

Grade II: The grade II glioma is typically a well delineated tumour which is hypointense on T1 weighted images and hyperintense on T2 weighted images (Fig. 5.11.2). In some cases it may be difficult to differentiate this tumour from acute ischemic territoral infarction in a stroke patient. Characteristically, the glioma grade II does not enhance upon intravenous administration of contrast media which means that there is no blood-brain-barrier (BBB) -damage, but low vascularisation and low proliferation rate and slow growing. The tumour appearance can remain unchanged for many years.

Grade III: If in a grade II glioma demonstrates contrast enhancement, this means that it is at least a grade III tumour because of focal proliferations and malignant differentiation (Fig. 5.11.3). If there is contrast enhancement, one cannot differentiate between grade III and grade IV. However, small punctual signal increase without signs of necrosis suggests a grade III.

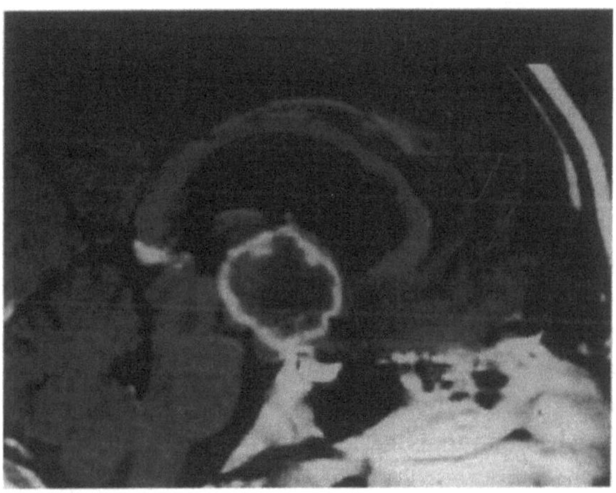

Fig. 5.11.1. The MRI shows an irregualr suprasellar contrast enhancing mass which is typical for a grad I astrocytoma

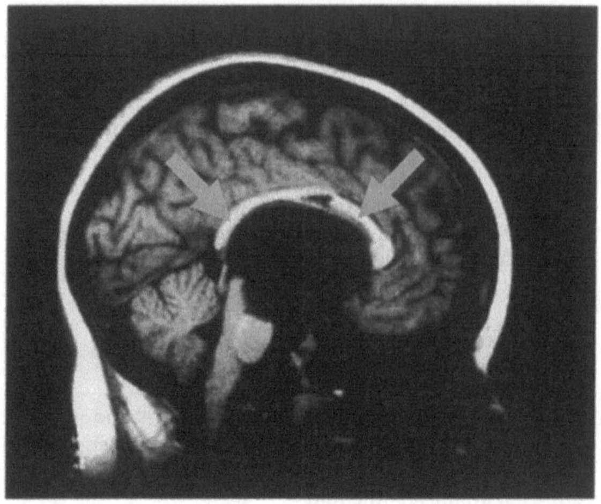

Fig. 5.11.2. The image demonstrates the signal behaviour of an astrocytoma grade II without any contrast enhancement

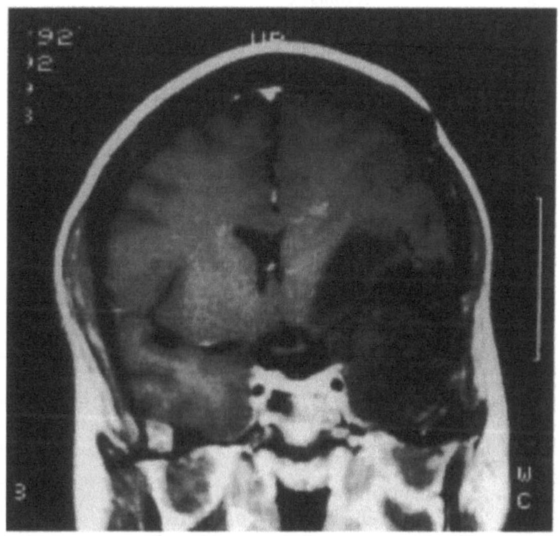

Fig. 5.11.3. The grade III astrocytoma is characterized by a beginning blood brain barrier damage and an increasing mass effect

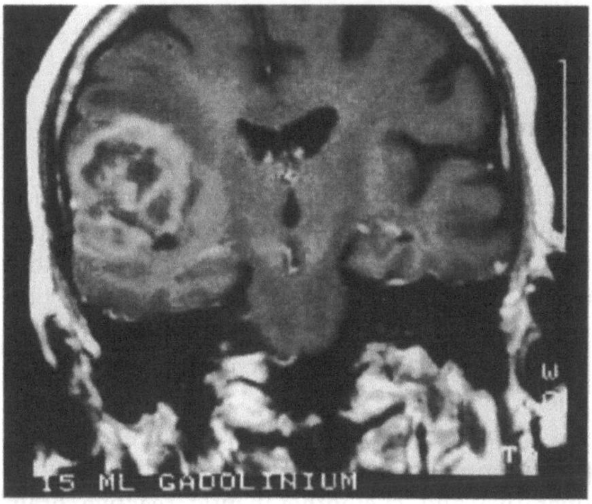

Fig. 5.11.4. The grade IV astrocytoma is a space occupying lesion with marked enhancement

Grade IV: The grade IV glioma, the glioblastoma multiforme, is characterized by marked contrast enhancement in MRI examinations, focal necrosis, intratumoral hemorrhage, peritumoral edema, mass effect and fast growing (Fig. 5.11.4).

Taken together, in many cases the diagnosis can be made based on MRI criteria.

However, problems occur in cases of mixed gliomas, rare cases of low grade or benign astrocytic tumours of grade I and in the follow-up after operation, radiation- and chemotherapy.

5.11.3
Diagnostic Imaging with PET

The Positron Emission Tomography (PET) should be able to anwer the questions MRI cannot give in many cases:

- the grade of malignancy, correlated to the metabolic activity
- the differentiation between operative induced changes, radiation necrosis, and rest or recurrance of tumour.

Typically, after neurosurgical operation of a glioma, MRI demonstrates some contrast enhancement of the normal brain tissue along the resection borders of the tumour. This linear enhancement appears first after 24 to 48 hours after the operation and can be seen for at least three to six months. In individual cases, it persisted up to more than one year.

In the cases where neurosurgical removal of the tumour is followed by adjuvant chemotherapy and radiation-therapy, the resection margins show increased irregular or linear contrast enhancement. After higher radiation doses, focal or diffuse necroses can occur, which exhibit the same appearance as tumour tissue and demonstrate a similar mass effect and perifocal edema.

In such cases the neuorimaging techniques fail to give the correct diagnosis. Even the spectroscopy is not always valid to differentiate malignant tumour tissue from radiation induced necrosis.

The metabolism of primary brain tumours is different from the normal brain tissue. Tumours which tend to develop higher malignancy produce higher rates of lactic acid by nonoxidative glycolysis and utilize higher rates of glucose. This can be used to identify a glioma and to classify the different grades of gliomas. Most authors in the current literature describe the effects of administration of (18F) Fluoro-Deoxy-Glucose (FDG) on the appearance of the tumour in PET. It is shown in the literature that the FDG uptake has a close correlation to the grade of malignancy.

However, some other tumours, for example the pilocytic astrocytoma shows high uptake rates, and acute abscesses can demonstrate a similar metabolic rate than high grade gliomas. Therefore, other techniques and tracers are under evaluation, sometimes used in combination, e.g. the uptake of aminoacids as methionin, or the uptake of ^{201}Thallium. The combined use of ^{201}Thallium-SPECT and ^{11}C-methonine-PET seems to support the delineation of grade II and III from grade IV gliomas whereas in actual studies, FDG was insufficient in the evaluation of the histological grade and in the differentiation between benign and malignant astrocytomas (Sasaki et al., Voges et al.). In contrast, other authors found a close correlation between malignancy rate and FDG uptake.

Some authors (Goldman at al.) descibe a correlation between amino-acid metabolism rate (methionin uptake) and malignancy, however, low grade oligodendrogliomas have markedly higher uptake rates than low grade astrocytomas. The PET differentiation is only possible if other modalities like MRI give additional information on the suspected tumour entity.

If one discusses these findings critically from the neuroradiological point of view, in most cases it is no problem to differentiate a grade II from a grade III or IV glioma by use of MRI. Therefore, these studies are very interesting from the scientific view but may have less implications on the clinical management and therapeutic strategy.

The primary advantage of the PET technique can be seen in

1. The determination of the biopsy location by description of the different metabolism rates in the tumour. This has to be done in close correlation with the MRI findings and requires sophisticated imaging techniques and postprocessing tools for the fusion of MRI and PET data.
2. The follow-up differentiation between postoperative scar formation, tumour recurrance and radiation necrosis.

These points have impact on the therapeutic management as this influences the operation as well as the following chemo- and radiation therapy.

The determination of the biopsy site can be helpful in such cases whitout clear blood brain barrier (BBB) disruption and contrast enhancement in MRI. In most cases malignant tumours exhibit focal enhancement. PET will give additional information in such cases without BBB but other signs of malignant growth.

Radiation necrosis is not correlated with higher cell metabolism. Tumour recurrance will be associated with increased consumption of glucose and higher protein production (aminoacid uptake). Thus, FDG PET demonstrates higher uptake and glucose consumption in cases of malignant tumour recurrance. The specifity is said to be more than 80 %.

5.11.4 Conclusion

In summary, PET is a helpful diagnostic tool in the evaluation of primary brain tumours:

PET using ^{18}FDG and ^{11}C-MET in combination with ^{201}Tl SPECT is a sensitive tool for the delineation of low grade and malignant gliomas and a useful instrument for tumour grading. The best results will be achieved in combination with other modern neuroimaging techniques, especially MRI.

PET in combination with MRI can be used for the diffentiation between radiation necrosis, postoperative and chemotherapeutic reactive brain tissue changes and tumour recurrance.

PET should be applied always in combination with high resolution MRI by use of digital imaging fusion software and 3D- techniques, which requires the close interdisciplinary cooperation between neurosurgeons, neuroradiologists, neurooncologists, radiotherapeuts and nuclear medical experts.

References

Delbeke D, Meyerowitz C, Lapidus RL, Maciunas RJ, Jennings MT, Moots PL, Kessler RM et. al. (1995). Optimal cutoff levels of F-18 fluorodeoxyglucose uptake in the differentiation of low-grade from high-grade brain tumors with PET. Radiology 1995 Apr; 195(1): 47–52

Deshmukh A, Scott JA, Palmer EL, Hochberg FH, Gruber M, Fischman AJ et. al. (1996). Impact of fluorodeoxyglucose positron emission tomography on the clinical management of patients with glioma. Clin Nucl Med Sep; 21(9): 720–5

Goldmann S, Levivier M, Pirotte B, Brucher JM, Wikler D, Damhaut P, Dethy S, Brotchi J, Hildebrand J et. al. (1997). Regional methionine and glucose uptake in high-grade gliomas: a comparative study on PET-guided stereotactic biopsy. J Nucl Med 1997 Sep; 38(9): 1459–62

Goldmann S, Levivier M, Pirotte B, Brucher JM, Wikler D, Damhaut P, Dethy S, Brotchi J, Hildebrand J et. al. (1997). Regional methionine and glucose uptake in high-grade gliomas: a comparative study on PET-guided stereotactic biopsy. J Nucl Med 1997 Sep; 38(9): 1459–62

Gross MW, Weber WA, Feldmann HJ, Bartenstein P, Schwaiger M, Molls M et. al. (1998). The value of F-18-fluorodeoxyglucose PET for the 3-D radiation treatment planning of malignant gliomas. Int J Radiat Oncol Biol Phys Jul 15; 41(5): 989–95

Ishikawa M, Kikuchi H, Nagata I, Yamagata S, Taki W, Yonekura Y, Nishizawa S, Iwasaki Y, Mukai T et. al. (1990).

Glucose consumption and rate constants for 18F-fluorodeoxyglucose in human gliomas. Neurol Med Chir (Tokyo) Jun; 30(6): 377–81
Ishizu K, Nishizawa S, Yonekura Y, Sadato N, Magata Y et al. (1994) J Nucl. Med; 35:1104–1109
Janus TJ, Kim EE, Tilbury R, Bruner JM, Yung WK et. al. (1993). Use of 18F(fluorodeoxyglucose positron emission tomography in patients with primary malignant brain tumors. Ann Neurol May; 33(5): 540–8
Kaschten B, Stevenaert A, Sadzot B, Deprez M, Degueldre C, Del Fiore G, Luxen A, Reznik M (1998). Preoperative evaluation of 54 gliomas by PET with flourine-18-fluorodeoxyglucose and/or carbon-11-methionine. J Nucl Med; 39:778–785.
Kincaid PK, El-Saden SM, Park SH, Goy BW et. al. (1998). Cerebral gangliomas: preoperative grading using FDG-PET and 201T-SPECT. AJNR Am J Neuroradiol, May 19(5): 801–6
Kleihues P, Burger PC, Scheithauer BW (1993). The new WHO classification of brain tumours. Brain Pathology, 3: 255–268
Kuwert T, Bartensteine P, Grünwald F, Herholz K, Larisch R, Sabri O, Biersack H.-J, Moser E, Müller-Gärtner H.-W, Schober O, Schwaiger M, Büll U, Heiss W-D (1998). Klinische Wertigkeit der Positronen-Emissions-Tomographie in der Neuromedizin: Positionspapier zu den Ergebnissen einer interdisziplinären Konsesuskonferenz.
Ogawa T, Inugami A, Hatazawa J, Kanno I, Murakami M, Yasui N, Minura K, Uemura K (1996). Clinical Positron Tomography for brain tumors: comparison of fludeoxyglucose F18 and L-Methyl-11C-methionine. Am J Neuroradiol 17:345–353
Oriuchi N, Tomiyoshi K, Inoue T, Ahmad K, Sarwar M, Tokunaga M, Suzuki H, Watanabe N, Hirano T, Horikoshi STIR-Sequenz; Shibasaki T, Tamura M, Endo K et. al. (1996). Independent thallium-201 accumulation and fluorine-18-fluorodeoxyglucose metabolism in glioma. J Nucl Med Mar; 37(3): 457–62
Roux FE, Ranjeva JP, Boulanoar K, Manelfe C, Sabatier J, Tremoulet M, Berry I et. al. (1997). Motor functional MRI for presurgical evaluation of cerebral tumors. Stereotact Funct Neurosurg; 68(1-4 Pt 1): 106–11
Schulder M, Maldjian JA, Liu WC, Mun IK, Carmel PW et. al. (1997). Functional MRI-guided surgery of intracranial tumors. Stereotact Funct Neurosurg; 68(1–4 Pt 1): 98–105
Sasaki M, Kuwabara Y, Yoashida T, Nakagawa M, Fukumura T, Mihara F, Morioka T, Fukui M, Masuda K (1998). A comparative study of thallium-201 SPET carbon-11 methionine PET and fluorine-18 fluorodeoxyglucose PET for the differentiation of astrocytic tumours. Eur J Nucl Med; 25: 1261–1269
Tamura M, Shibasaki T, Zama A, Kurihara H, Horikoshi STIR-Sequenz, Ono N, Oriuchi N, Hirano T et. al. (1998). Assessment of malignancy of glioma by positron emission tomography with 18F-fluorodeoxyglucose and single photon emission computed tomography with thallium-201 chloride. Neuroradiology Apr; 40(4): 210–5
Voges J, Herholz K, Holzer T, Wurker M, Bauer B, Pietrzyk U, Treuer H, Schroder R, Strum V, Heiss WD et. al. (1997). 11C-methionine and 18F-2-fluorodeoxyglucose positron emission tomography: a tool for diagnosis of cerebral glioma and monotoring after brachytherapy with 125I seeds. Stereotact Funct Neurosurg; 69(1-4 Pt 2): 129–35

5.12 Miscellaneous Tumors

H.-J. Biersack, P. Willkomm, R. An, and J. Ruhlmann

In this chapter we will discuss a number of tumor types for which there are already clinical data available. However, the value of PET for these tumors must still be evaluated based on larger numbers of patients. This does not apply to brain tumors, however; the German PET consensus conference has already established indications for this type of tumor.

5.12.1 Brain Tumors

Diagnosis and differential diagnosis of brain tumors is the domain of CT and MRI. However, it has been found in recent years that PET can provide important information about grading and differential diagnosis of scar vs. recurrent tumor (Fig. 5.12.1). PET makes it possible to evaluate kinetics or chemical processes on the cellular level with a "biological resolution" that the morphological and radiological imaging methods (CT and MRI) cannot offer. The grading and detection of vital tumor tissue after irradiation or surgery is a particular area of application. Delbecke et al. (1995) examined 58 patients with brain tumors and reported a sensitivity of 94 % and a specificity of 77 % with respect to grading. After therapy the residual tumor can be imaged and distinguished from necrosis. Kim et al. (1992) reported a sensitivity of 80 % and a specificity of 94 % for this indication. Mogard et al. (1994) obtained similarly good results, but for a smaller group of patients.

5.12.2 Musculoskeletal Tumors

In 1991 Adler et al. published initial results regarding non-invasive grading of musculoskeletal tumors using PET. Highly malignant tumors had a significantly higher FDG uptake than benign or low-grade malignant tumors (Fig. 5.12.2). These authors set the cut-off point at 1.6 (tumor/healthy) for differentiating highly malignant from slightly malignant lesions. Kern et al. (1988) described similarly good results, whereas Griffeth et al. (1992) did not find a very good correlation with grading in 20 patients with malignant and benign tumors.

5.12.3 Prostate Cancer

The five-year survival rate for patients with prostate cancer increased from 50 % in the 1960s to 70 % in the 1980s as the result of improved therapeutic methods. Primary prognostic factors are the clinical stage and differentiation of the tumor, whereas tumor size, regional lymph node involvement, liver metastases and response to therapy are of lesser importance. Nonetheless, positive paraaortic lymph node metastases are associated with a significantly reduced disease-free survival rate (30 vs. 70–86 %). A total of approximately 150 patients with prostate cancer have been studied, including our own patients (Bares et al. 1994; Bender et al. 1997; Hoh et al. 1996; Laubenbacher et al. 1995; Reinhardt et al. 1995; Shreve et al. 1995; Yeh et al. 1995). In all cases a moderate concentration of FDG in the primary tumor or in lymph node metastases and also in bone metastases was observed. Differential diagnosis of recurrent tumor vs. scar was limited. Conventional bone scintigraphy exhibited better results than PET, especially in the case of detected bone metastases. These results have been confirmed in 23 of our own cases.

Fig. 5.12.1.
Malignant brain stem tumor

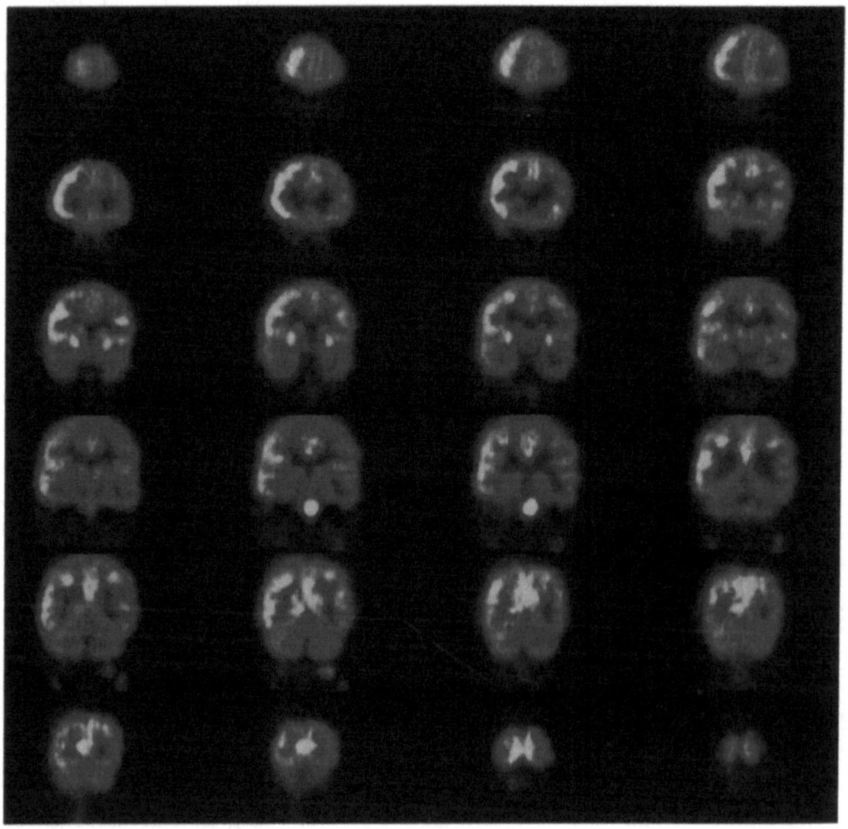

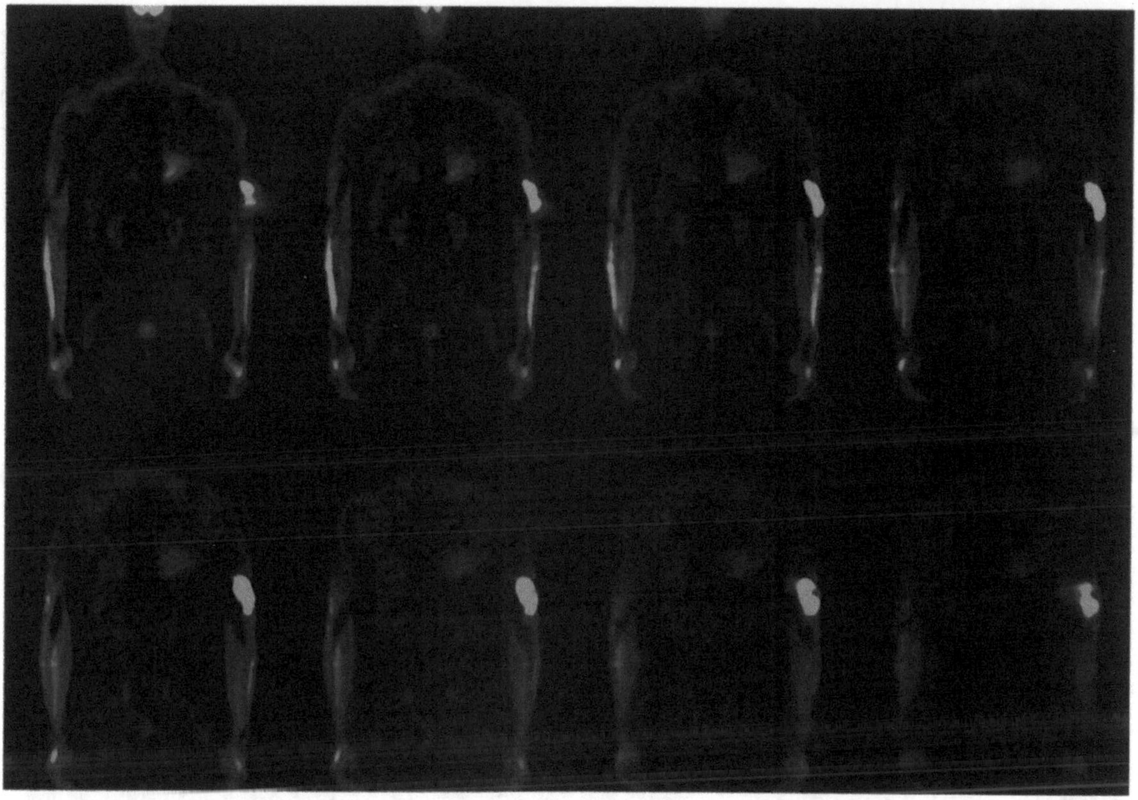

Fig. 5.12.2. Soft tissue sarcoma of the left upper arm

5.12.4 Bladder Cancer

Ninety percent of bladder cancers are papillary carcinomas, 6–8 % are squamous cell carcinomas, and only 2 % are adenocarcinomas. An important prognostic factor is the degree of invasion of the muscularis. Unfortunately, bladder tumors often metastasize before any symptoms appear. Most patients are "understaged" when conventional modalities are used. The PET results published to date involve fewer than 100 patients (Bachor et al. 1995; Kocher et al. 1995; Kosuda et al. 1996). All studies have demonstrated relatively high sensitivity and specificity, and differentiation between tumor and scar was possible. PET also detected lymph node involvement in two studies. Sensitivity for PET ranged between 86 % and 100 %, according to Kocher et al. (1995), while specificity was between 63 % and 100 %.

5.12.5 Kidney Tumors

Only 4 studies have been published to date dealing with PET and kidney tumors. They cover a total of fewer than 60 patients. However, FDG PET exhibited a sensitivity of between 80 and 90 % and a specificity ranging from 70 to 90 %. The response to therapy was also checked in a study done by Hoh et al. (1996). These researchers found a good correlation between PET findings and response both with regard to progressive vs. stable disease and complete vs. partial response. In every case PET proved to be superior to conventional diagnostic modalities.

5.12.6 Esophageal Cancer

Flanagan et al. (1997) used PET to study a total of 36 patients suffering from cancer of the esophagus. In each case the tumor exhibited elevated FDG uptake (Fig. 5.12.3). Twenty-nine patients underwent a curative esophagus operation, and PET diagnosed lymph node involvement correctly in 76 % of these cases, whereas CT provided a correct diagnosis in only 45 % of the cases. Seven patients were subjected to an endoscopic tissue ex-

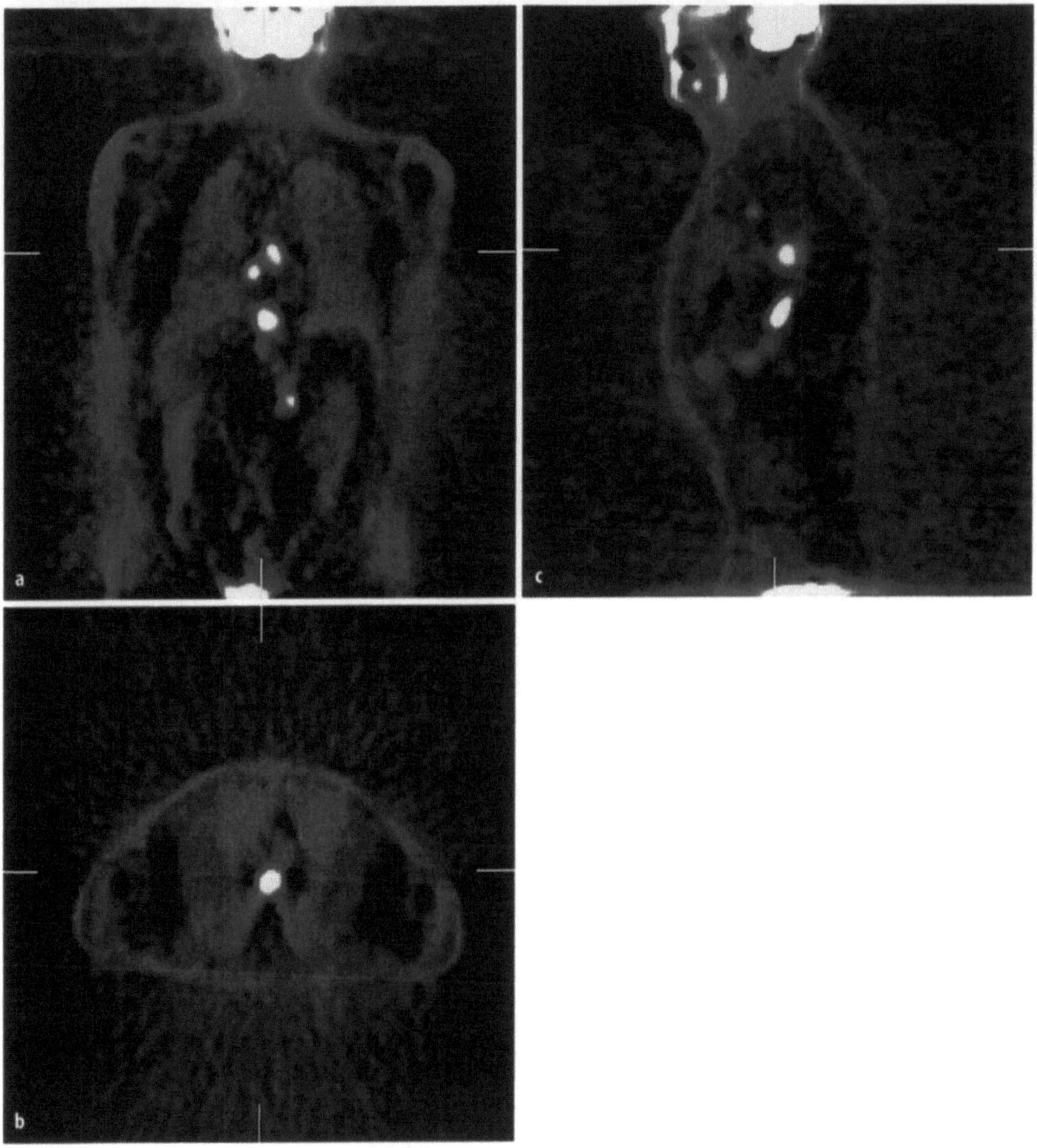

Fig. 5.12.3. Esophageal carcinoma with multiple lymph node metastases

amination only. PET indicated metastases in 5 of these cases, which made it possible to dispense with surgery.

5.12.7 Gastric Cancer

Cronin et al. (1997) published results for a large series of patients, including data for 57 cases of cancer of the stomach or the esophagus. However, no precise data were presented. Aside from this, only experimental data (xenografts of human gastric carcinomas) have been published.

5.12.8 Liver Cancer

Torizuka et al. (1994) were the first to report results for patients with hepatocellular carcinoma. In all cases the PET scan was performed before and after catheter embolization of the metastases. It was the first time that a distinction was made between three different types of tumors: tumors with elevated FDG uptake (n = 19, Fig. 5.12.4), tumors with the same FDG uptake as the liver (n = 7, Fig. 5.12.5), and tumors with a reduced glucose uptake or a complete lack of uptake (n = 6).

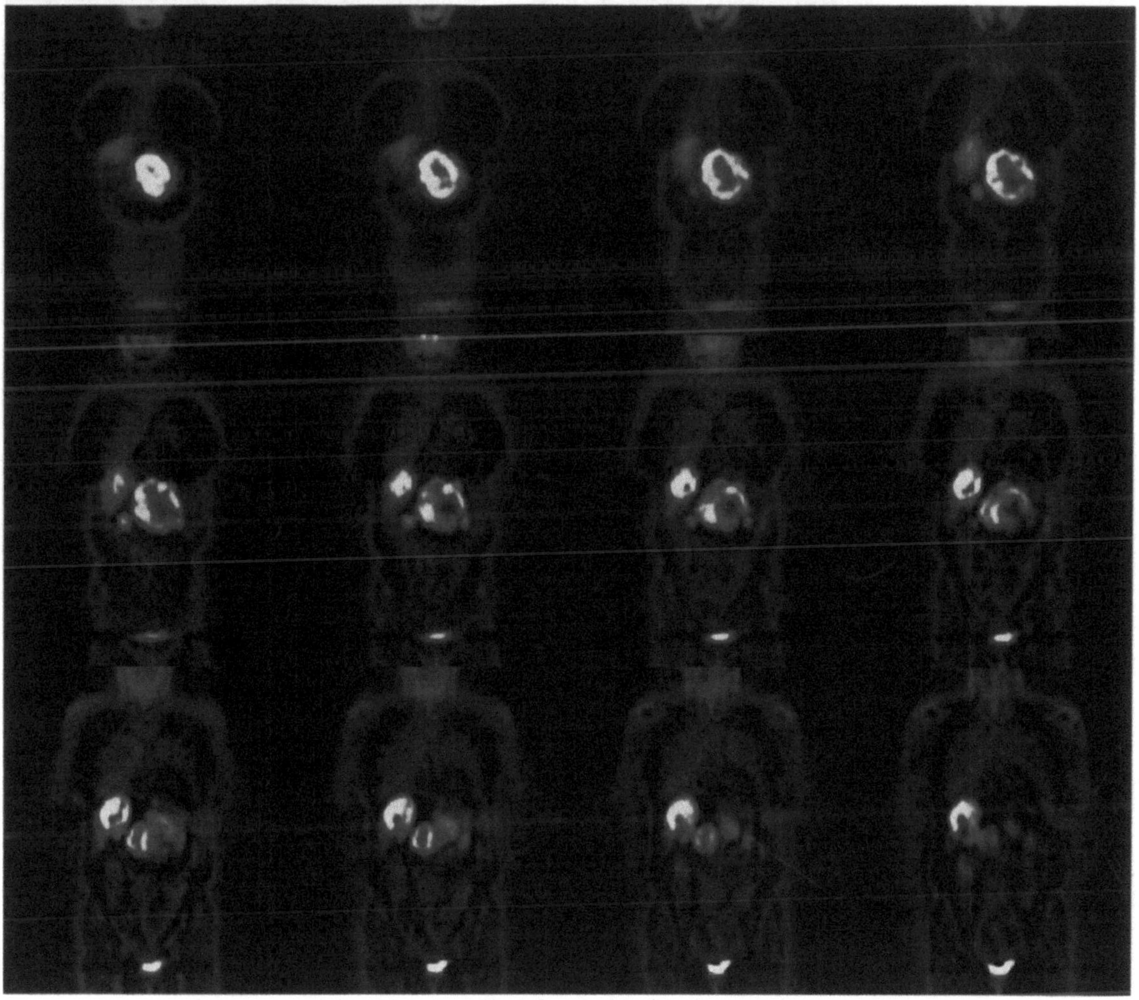

Fig. 5.12.4. Hepatocellular carcinoma: elevated glucose uptake

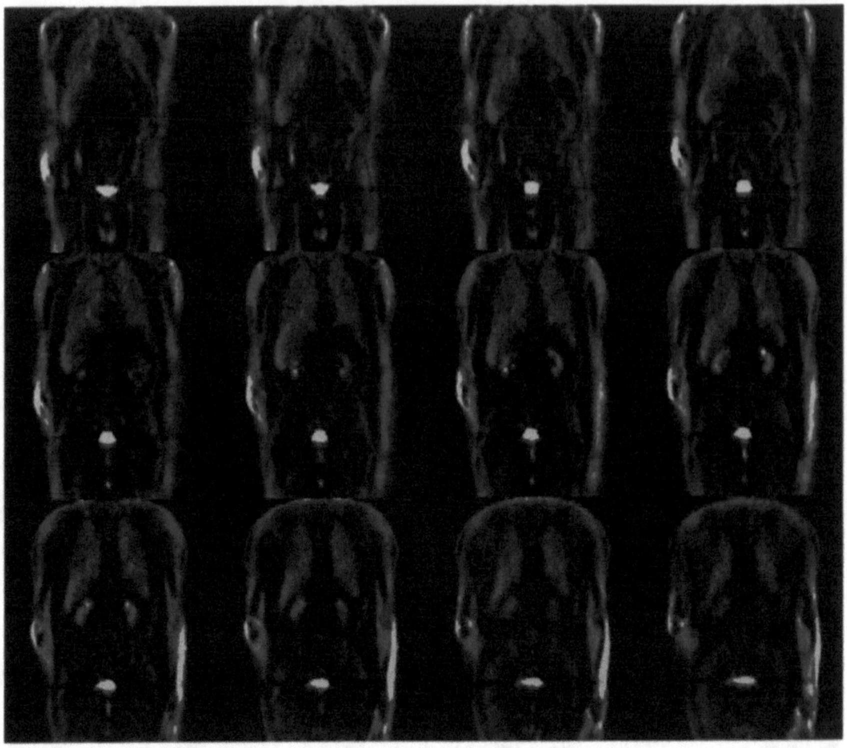

Fig. 5.12.5. Hepatocellular carcinoma: glucose uptake as in normal liver tissue

It was found that chemoembolization was always successful in cases where more than 90 % necrotic tissue was detected. In these cases the FDG uptake was also reduced. In another study by Enomoto et al. (1991) the tumor could not be correctly distinguished from the liver in 50 % of the cases involving hepatocellular carcinoma (n = 23). However, k-values were used for further differentiation. Dimitrakopoulou-Strauss et al. (1996) arrive at similar results.

References

Adler LP, Blair HF, Makley JT et al. (1991) Noninvasive grading of musculoskeletal tumors using PET. J Nucl Med 32: 1508–1512

Bachor R, Kocher F, Gropengiesser F et al. (1995) Positron emission tomograpy. Introduction of a new procedure in diagnosis of urologic tumors and initial clinical results. Urol Arch 34: 138–142

Bares R, Effert P, Handt S et al. (1994) Metabolic classification of untreated prostate cancer by use of FDG-PET. J Nucl Med 35: 230P

Bender H, Schomburg A, Albers P et al. (1997) Possible role of FDG-PET in the evaluation of urologic malignancies. Anticancer Res 17: 1655–1660

Cronin V, Galantowicz P, Nabi HA (1997) Development of oncology protocol using fluorine-18-FDG: one center's experience. J Nucl Med Technol 25: 66–69

Delbecke D, Meyerowitz C, Lapidus RL et al. (1995) Optimal cutoff levels of F-18 fluorodexyglucose uptake in the differentiation of low-grade from high grade brain tumors with PET. Radiology 195: 47–52

Dimitrakopoulou-Strauss A, Gutzler F, Strauss LG et al. (1996) PET-Studien mit C-11-Athanol bei der intratumoralen Therapie von hepatozellularen Karzinomen. Radiologe 36: 744–749

Enomoto K, Fukunaga T, Okazumi S et al. (1991) Can fluorodeoxyglucose-positron emission tomography evaluate the functional differentiation of hepatocellular carcinoma. Kaku-Igaku 28: 1353–1356

Flanagan FL, Dehdashti F, Siegel BA et al. (1997) Staging of esophageal cancer with 18F-fluorodexyglucose positron emission tomography. Am J Roentgenol 168: 417–424

Griffeth LK, Dehdashti F, McGuire AH et al. (1992) PET evaluation of soft-tissue masses with fluorine-18-fluoro-2-deoxy-d-glucose. Radiology 182: 185–194

Hoh CK, Rosen PJ, Belldegrun A et al. (1996) Quantitative and whole body FDG PET in the evaluation of suramine

therapy in patients with metastatic prostate cancer. J Nucl Med 37: 267P
Hoh CK, Figlin RA, Belldegrum A et al. (1996) Evaluation of renal cell carcinoma with whole body FDG PET. J Nucl Med 37: 141P
Kern KA, Brunetti A, Norton JA et al. (1988) Metabolic imaging of human extremity musculoskeletal tumors by PET. J Nucl Med 29: 181–186
Kim E, Chung SK, Hayne TP et al. (1992) Differentiation of residual or recurrent tumors from post-treatment changes with F-18 FDG PET. Radiographics 12: 269–279
Kocher F, Bachor R, Stollfuss JC et al. (1995) Positron-emission-tomography of urinary bladder carcinoma. Eur J Nucl Med 20: 888
Kosuda S, Grossman HB, Kison PV et al. (1996) Preliminary FDG-PET study in patients with bladder cancer. J Nucl Med 37: 260P
Laubenbacher C, Hofer C, Avril N et al. (1995) F-18 FDG PET for differentiation of local recurrent prostatic cancer and scar. J Nucl Med 36: 198 P
Miyauchi T, Brown RS, Grossman HB et al. (1996) Correlation between visualization of primary renal cancer by FDG-PET and histopthological findings. J Nucl Med 37: 64 P
Mogard J, Kihlstrom L, Ericson K et al. (1994) Recurrent tumor vs radiation effects after gamma knife radiosurgery of intracerebral metastases: diagnosis with PET-FDG. J Comput Assist Tomogr 18: 177–181
Reinhardt M, Mueller-Matheis V, Larisch R et al. (1995) Time activity analysis improves specificity of FDG-PET in staging of pelvic lymph node metastases. Eur J Nucl Med 22: 803
Shreve P, Gross MD, Wahl RL (1995) Detection of prostate cancer metastases with FDG. J Nucl Med 36: 189P
Torizuka T, Tamaki N, Inokuma T et al. (1994) Value of fluorine-18-FDG-PET to monitor hepatocellular carcinoma after interventional therapy. J Nucl Med 35: 1965–1969
Yeh SDJ, Imbriaco M, Garza D et al. (1995) Twenty percent of hormone resistant prostate cancer are detected by PET-FDG whole body scanning. J Nucl Med 36: 198 P

CHAPTER 6

Cancer Screening with Whole-Body FDG PET

S. Yasuda, M. Ide, and A. Shohtsu

In general, whole-body positron emission tomography (PET) with ^{18}F-fluorodeoxyglucose (FDG) is used for individuals with medical indications. We have been using whole-body PET for cancer screening in a large number of *asymptomatic* individuals (Yasuda et al. 1997b, Ide et al. 1996). A wide variety of cancers have been detected in resectable stages. We have also observed PET-negative cancers and PET-positive benign lesions. Understanding the images obtained in such cases helps in preventing misinterpretation of PET images. In the following section we report on our 3-year experience with whole-body PET for cancer screening in individuals *without* symptoms of disease.

6.1 Background

Transmission scanning was not included in our PET screening program. This saves time. In an earlier study of patients with various cancers, we compared attenuation-corrected images with non-attenuation-corrected images with respect to cancer detection (Yasuda et al. 1996b). A total of 106 lesions in 32 patients were analyzed, and 104 out of 106 lesions (98.1 %) were recognizable on uncorrected images as well as corrected images. On uncorrected images, the boundary between the lung and the liver was not distinct. In lesions located near the body surface, intensity was enhanced in directions tangential to the body surface. Because of the elliptical cross section of the body, the anteroposterior dimension appears longer on uncorrected images. If attenuation correction using filtered back-projection algorithms for image reconstruction is not performed, image artifacts can result due to high activity in the myocardium, renal pelvis, and bladder. In spite of these image distortions, lesion contrast was not diminished (Fig. 6.1).

It was demonstrated quantitatively that on uncorrected images anteroposterior tumor dimensions were significantly longer and left-to-right tumor dimensions were significantly smaller than on corrected images (Zasadny et al. 1996). Although lesion-to-background ratios decrease in the lung and soft tissue without attenuation correction, these ratios increase in the liver, mediastinum, and gut (Biersack et al. 1997). On the basis of clinical studies and phantom experiments, Bengel et al. (1997) demonstrated that focal hypermetabolism is more readily discernible on uncorrected images. PET imaging without transmission scanning is definitely of practical use with respect to lesion detectability.

6.2 Cancer Screening with Whole-Body FDG PET

6.2.1 Subjects and Methods

Our institution is a medical health club located in Yamanashi, Japan. Our cancer screening program includes whole-body PET in conjunction with conventional screening modalities. With 3 PET scanners in operation (ECAT EXACT47 scanners manufactured by Siemens/CTI, Knoxville, TN), a maximum of 24 whole-body PET studies can be performed per day. In 1997, for example, 1290 whole-body PET studies were performed.

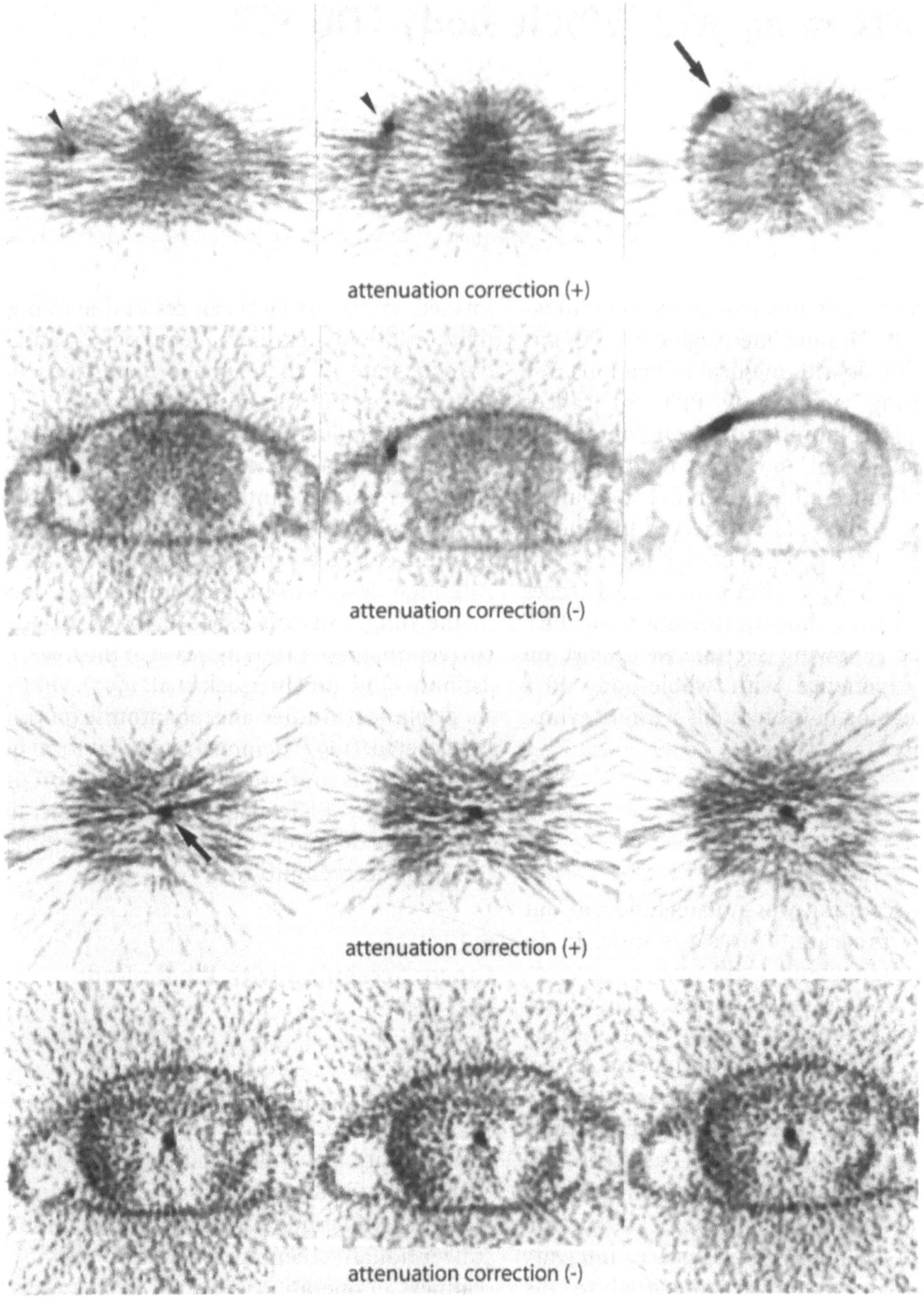

a

b

Fig. 6.1. a Three selected transaxial images from a patient with right breast cancer and axillary nodal involvement. The primary (*arrow*) and two metastatic nodes (*arrow heads*) are well visualized on both images. **b** Three consecutive transaxial images from a patient with advanced esophageal cancer with celiac node metastasis. The metastatic celiac node is well visualized (*arrow*). The lesion-to-background contrast in high on both images

Under our current protocol, all subjects fast for at least 6 hours before FDG injection. Water intake is encouraged to dilute the urinary concentration of FDG. Coffee intake is also allowed to reduce myocardial FDG uptake, although the effect is not evident. We use a dose of 260 MBq FDG. Resting is encouraged during the uptake period to prevent FDG uptake in the muscles, especially the skeletal, oculomotor, and laryngeal muscles. After an uptake period of 45 to 60 minutes, the subjects are encouraged to void. To minimize bladder activity, emission scanning (7 minutes for each bed position) starts from the pelvis and moves upward to the maxilla. Gray-scale hard copy images of transaxial slices are printed out and interpreted visually; images of coronal and sagittal slices are also made available.

6.2.2 Results

During a 3-year period (from September 1994 to August 1997), 2114 club members (1365 men and 749 women; mean age 52 years) underwent cancer screening; the total number of examinations was 3093. Cancers were detected in 30 subjects. The detection rates were therefore 1.4 % (30 of 2114 subjects) and 1.0 % (30 of 3093 examinations). PET findings were true-positive for 16 cancers (Table 6.1, Figures 6.2–6.4) and false-negative for 14 cancers (Table 6.2).

The true-positive patients underwent surgery, with the exception of one lymphoma patient. Microscopic metastatic foci were observed in a dis-

Table 6.1. PET-positive cancers

Diagnosis	No. of Patients	Tumor Size
Lung cancer	5	1–2.4 cm
Colorectal cancer	3	3.5–6 cm
Breast cancer	3	1.3–2 cm
Thyroid cancer	2	1 cm, 3 cm
Gastric cancer	1	3.5 cm
Renal cancer	1	4 cm
Malignant lymphoma	1	

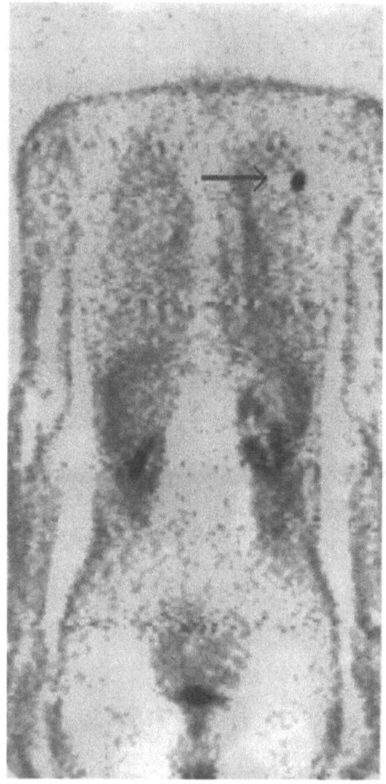

Fig. 6.2. Lung cancer (66 year-old man): 1 cm papillary adenocarcinoma (Stage I)

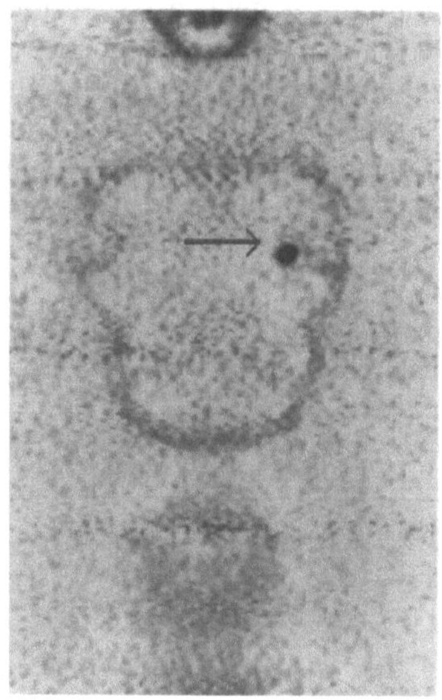

Fig. 6.3. Breast cancer (48 year-old woman): 1.3 cm invasive ductal carcinoma (Stage I)

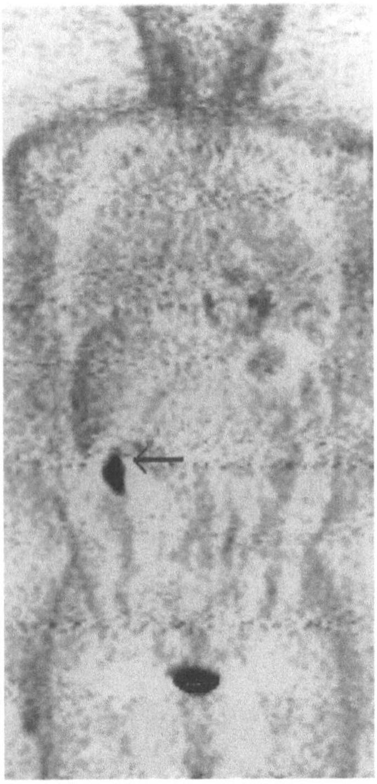

Fig. 6.4. Colon cancer (45 year-old man): 3.5 cm differentiated adenocarcinoma (Dukes A)

sected lymph node in one patient with breast cancer, but lymph node metastasis was not observed in any other patient. All lung cancers were pathological Stage I. Of the PET-negative cancers, 8 of the 14 (57 %) were of urologic origin. There were 3 false-negative lung cancers: an 8 mm tubular adenocarcinoma, a 1.2 cm bronchoalveolar adenocarcinoma, and a 1.5 cm bronchoalveolar adenocarcinoma. These were also negative with chest radiography. Two hepatomas, 1.5 cm and 1.6 cm in diameter, were negative with PET and positive with ultrasonography. One scirrhous-type breast cancer (1.5 cm) was negative with PET and positive with ultrasonography.

Table 6.2. PET-negative cancers (*PSA* prostate-specific antigen, *US* ultrasonography, *CT* computer tomography, *PE* physical examination)

Diagnosis	No. of Patients	Clinical Stage or Tumor Size	Method of Detection
Prostate cancer	4	Stage II–IV	PSA
Renal cancer	3	1.5–8.5 cm	US
Lung cancer	3	0.8–1.5 cm	CT
Hepatoma	2	1.5 cm, 1.6 cm	US
Breast cancer	1	1,5 cm	PE, US
Bladder cancer	1	3 cm	US

A substantial number of benign lesions were detected with PET (Table 6.3). Unnecessary surgery was performed in one case of chronic thyroiditis encountered early in our study (Yasuda et al. 1997c). The result of ultrasonographic diagnosis in this case was thyroid tumor. Three subjects with benign pulmonary lesions (one 1 cm tuberculoma and two 1 cm organized pneumonias), for whom PET and CT scans were inconclusive, had to undergo surgery before definite diagnoses could be obtained. High FDG uptake was noted in other benign lesions such as colonic adenoma (Yasuda et al. 1998c), Warthin's tumor (Horiuchi et al. 1998), thyroid adenoma, sarcoidosis (Yasuda et al. 1996a), chronic maxillary sinusitis, and lymphadenitis.

Table 6.3. PET-positive benign lesions diagnosed through biopsy or surgery

Diagnosis	Procedure	No. of Patients	Tumor Size
Colonic adenoma	Endoskopic polypectomy	10	1.2–3 cm
Warthin's tumor	Surgery	4	1.5–2.6 cm
Thyroid adenoma	Aspiration cytology, surgery	4	1–2,3 cm
Organized pneumonia	(Thoracoscopic) surgery	2	1 cm
Tuberculoma	Thoracoscopic surgery	1	1 cm
Sarcoidosis	Mediastinoscopy and biopsy	1	
Chronic sinusitis	Surgery	1	
Lymphadenitis	Aspiration cytology	2	
Chronic thyroiditis	Surgery	1	

6.2.3 Cancer Screening

Cancer is still a major cause of death. The efficacy of cancer screening to date has been confirmed by the fecal occult blood test for colorectal cancer (Hardcastle et al. 1996) and by mammography for breast cancer in women in their fifth decade (Taubes 1997). In addition, several studies are underway to determine the efficacy of screening for prostate cancer, lung cancer, and ovarian cancer (Kramer et al. 1994). Current screening methods target single organs or a few organs independently. Furthermore, these mass screening programs do not target low-prevalence cancers, primarily because of cost-benefit considerations.

Whole-body PET can be used to survey the entire body seamlessly; the targets are not confined to single organs. Ovarian cancer, pancreatic cancer, and lymphoma can be targeted, although there is still no evidence that PET can be used to detect these cancers in resectable stages in asymptomatic individuals. However, when cancer detection by a single examination is considered, PET proves to be superior to other screening methods. Cancers of many types can be detected in resectable stages.

Cancer screening raises issues of cost and risk. PET examination does entail a substantial cost. At our center the members themselves pay the cost of the examination. In order to win widespread acceptance, screening methods must be not only of high quality but also inexpensive. Because of the short half life of FDG, the radiation dose to the individual is low. It can be further reduced if the patient voids at the proper times (Mejia et al. 1991).

PET-Negative Cancers

PET-negative cancers were identified in our series of studies and were tentatively categorized as belonging to one of four groups on the basis of our observations:

1. urologic cancers,
2. cancers of low cell density,
3. small-sized cancers,
4. hypometabolic cancers.

All 4 prostate cancers were PET-negative in our PET screening, and they were all detected by measurement of prostate-specific antigen levels in the serum. Although urinary excretion of FDG may hamper the detection of urologic cancers, there may be another reason for the false-negative results in the case of urologic cancers. For example, the positive rate was less than 50 % in our study of 19 patients with renal cancer (unpublished results). Low tumor cellularity, such as in signet ring cell cancers or mucinous cancers, may result in low FDG accumulation. The spatial resolution of our PET scanner is approximately 6 mm, and partial-volume effects decrease the sensitivity in tumors smaller than twice that resolution.

In any event, endoscopy is superior to PET for detecting superficial lesions, especially in the esophagus and stomach. Furthermore, hypometabolic cancers exist. A 1.5 cm bronchoalveolar carcinoma of the lung was PET-negative in our study. Bronchoalveolar cancers of certain histologic types show the most favorable prognosis (Noguchi et al. 1995). How glucose metabolism relates to biological malignancy is not well known. These limitations must be recognized in PET screening.

Benign Lesions with High FDG Uptake

It has been thought that FDG PET is not suitable for unselected screening because of the likelihood of false positives (Rigo et al. 1996). Our study is the first to deal with a large number of asymptomatic persons. Although false-positive lesions were occasionally discovered, these subclinical lesions were thought to warrant further clinical examination or follow-up. Early in our study we found that diffuse thyroidal FDG uptake was not uncommon in otherwise healthy women and that it was a sign of subclinical chronic thyroiditis or Hashimoto's thyroiditis (Hasuda et al. 1997a; Fig. 6.5 – 6.11).

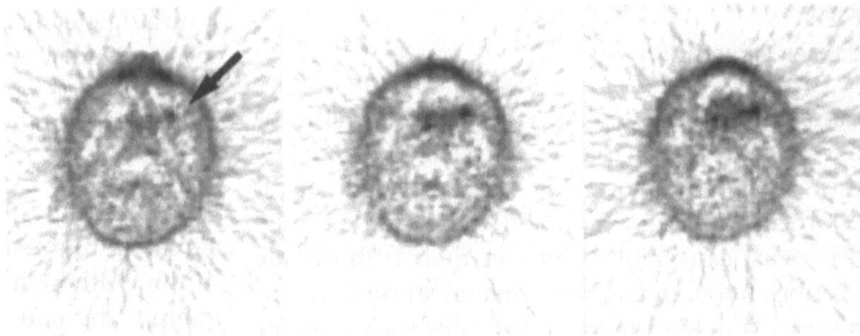

Fig. 6.5.
Gingivitis (60 year-old man). It is not uncommon to see focal FDG accumulation in the gingiva. This subject had a toothache, and gingivitis caused by dental caries was noted. Granulomas may accumulate a high level of FDG in this region

Physiological FDG Accumulation

Physiologically increased FDG uptake is occasionally noted in PET screening. FDG accumulation can be observed in the uterus during menstruation (Yasuda et al. 1997a). High FDG uptake can be observed in lactating mammary glands (Binns et al. 1997). Increased FDG uptake may be observed in skeletal muscles after exercise (Yasuda et al. 1998b). FDG appears to accumulate in laryngeal muscles in proportion to contractile activity during speech (Kostakoglu et al. 1996). Although patients' eyes are closed during the period of FDG uptake, this does not prevent FDG accumulation in the oculomotor muscles.

Intense FDG uptake was observed occasionally in the myocardium as well as in the bowel. Image artifacts caused by intense myocardial FDG accu-

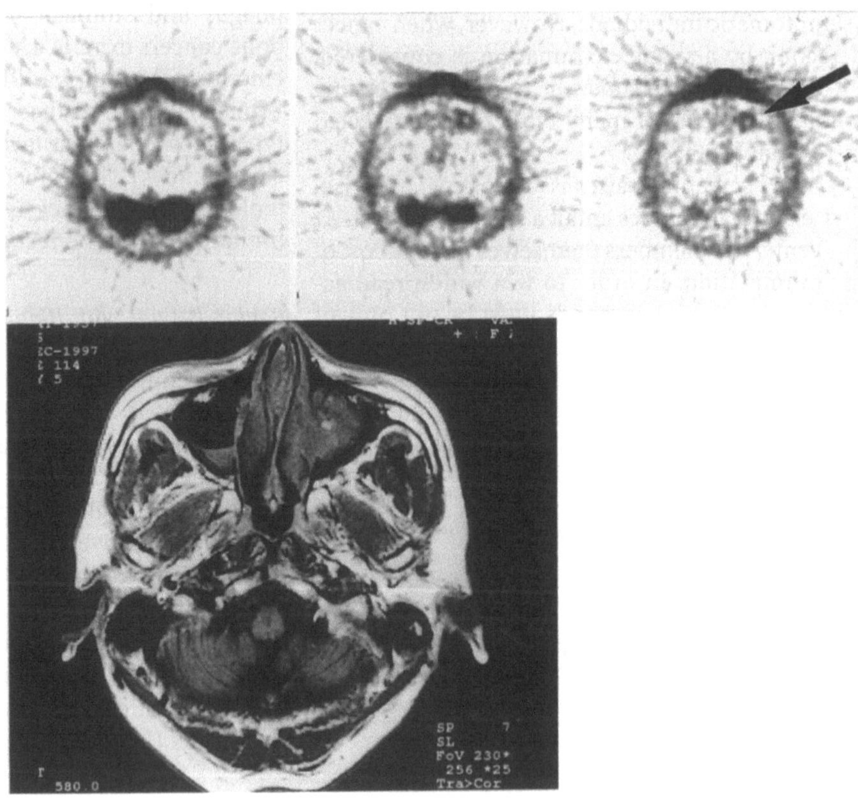

Fig. 6.6.
Maxillary sinusitis (60 year-old man). Unilateral maxillary FDG accumulation is not rare. FDG tends to accumulate along the sinus wall. Disappearance of FDG accumulation was confirmed in one subject after erythromycin treatment lasting 3 months

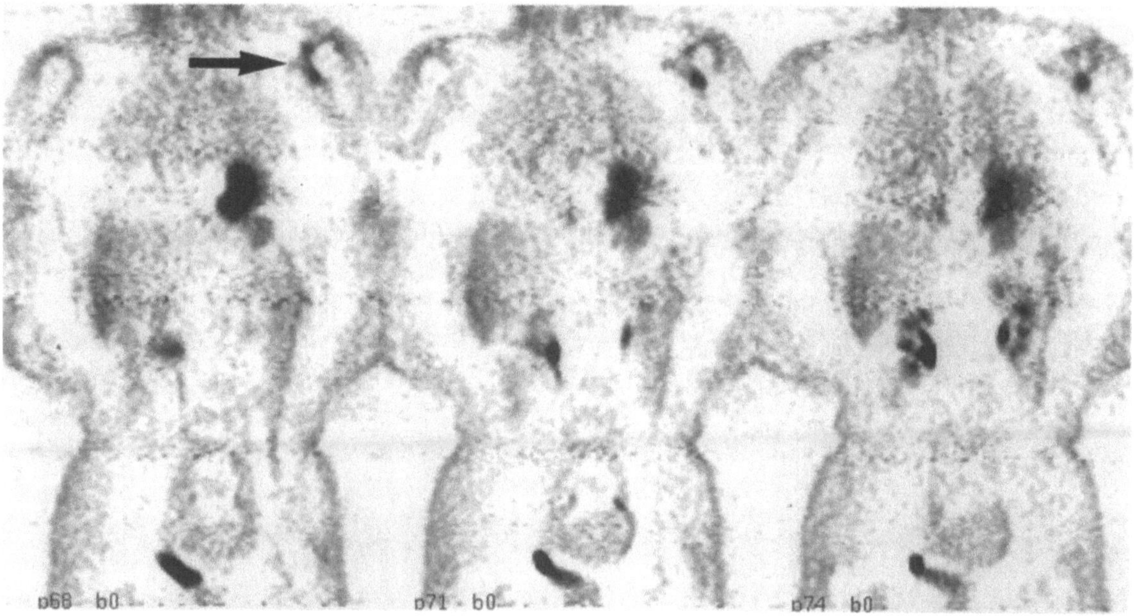

Fig. 6.7. Periarthritis of the shoulder (60 year-old woman). Arch-shaped FDG accumulation along the shoulder joints is strongly suggestive of periarthritis of the shoulder. There may be a correlation between the intensity of FDG uptake and clinical symptoms (pain and restriction of movement). FDG accumulation in this area is not uncommon in PET screening

Fig. 6.8.
Contusion of the chest (41 year old man). The subject had injured his chest skiing 17 days before. Faint FDG accumulation was observed at the chest wall on PET images. Chest radiography (postcroanterior projection) performed at the same time was negative. The pain had already disappeared. Although confirmation was not obtained, rib fractures were suspected

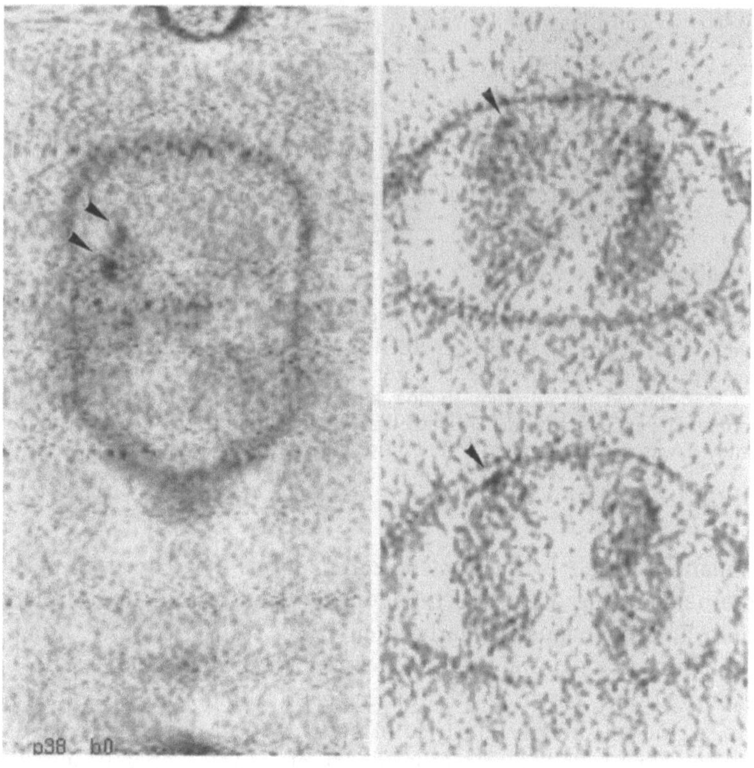

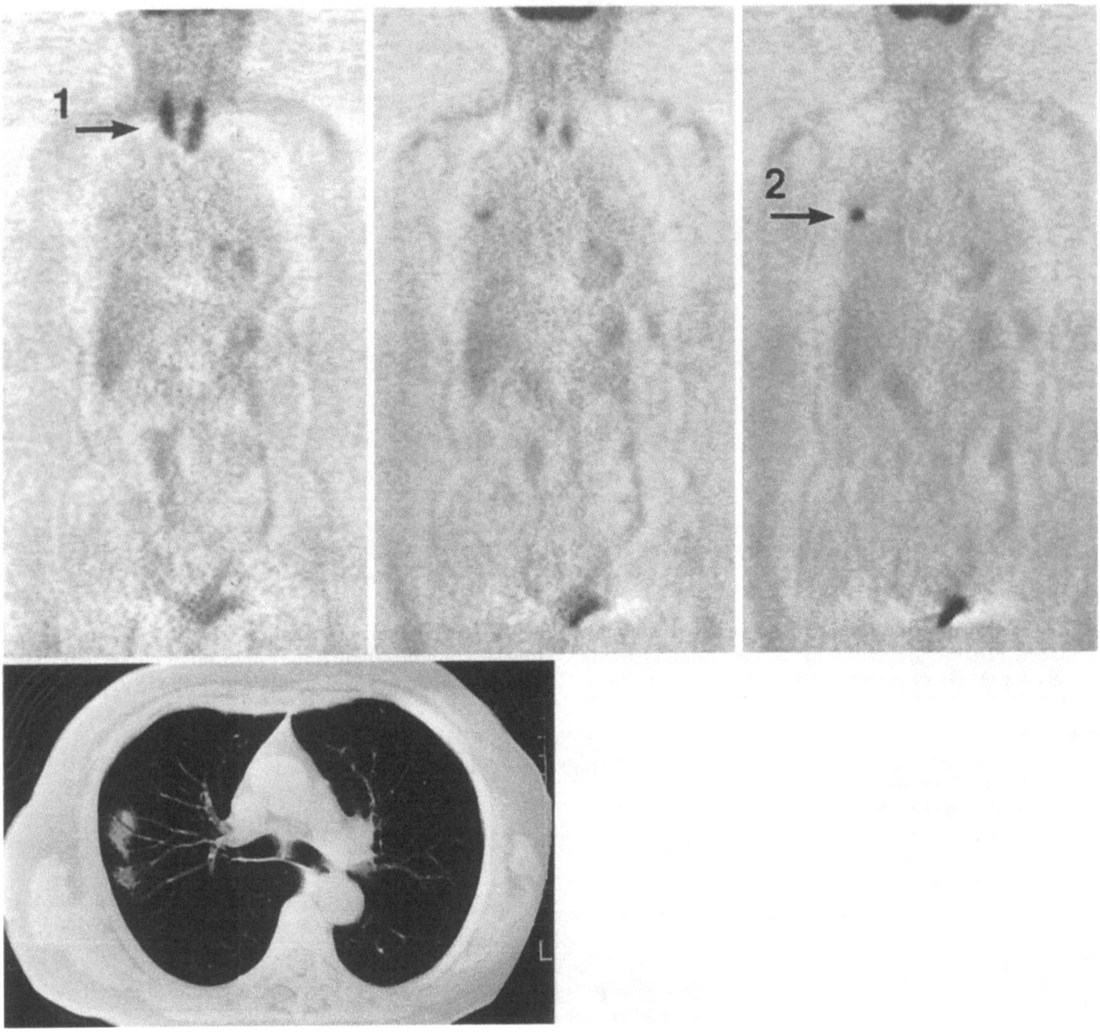

Fig. 6.9. Bronchopneumonia and chronic thyroiditis (64 year-old woman). High FDG uptake was observed in the lung and the thyroid gland on three selected coronal images. A chest CT scan showed an infiltration shadow suggestive of pneumonia. The anti-microsomal antibody titer was high. In our study it was not uncommon to find diffuse thyroidal FDG uptake in female subjects. The cause is thought to be chronic thyroiditis. Diffuse thyroidal FDG uptake persisted for 3 years in this woman. High FDG uptake is occasionally observed in pneumonia in PET screening. In such cases it is necessary to perform a spiral CT scan of the chest simultaneously

mulations result in incomplete examinations of the neighboring organs such as lungs, mediastinum, and esophagus. Similarly, intense FDG accumulations in the bowel result in incomplete bowel examinations. We tried administering Intralipid (10 %, 100 ml) intravenously in 10 patients to increase serum FFA levels (Nuutila et al. 1992). However, we did not observe significant reduction of myocardial FDG uptake as compared with a control group. We also tried administering scopolamine butylbromide (Buscopan) intravenously in 10 patients in order to reduce bowel peristalsis. But in this case as well, we did not observe any significant reduction in bowel FDG

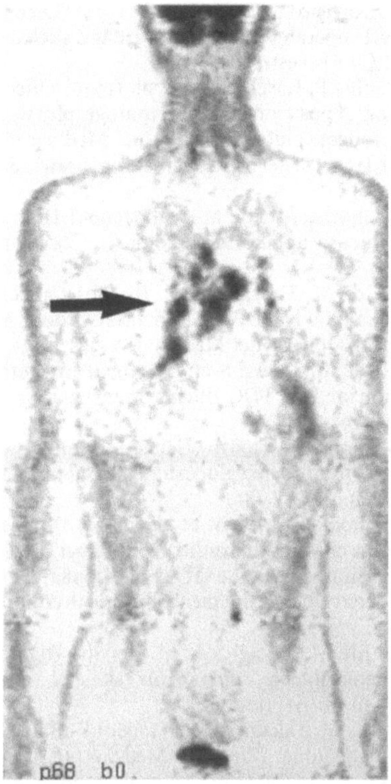

Fig. 6.10. Sarcoidosis (75 year-old man). Tissue diagnosis was obtained by mediastinoscopy and biopsy. This subject has been followed for 4 years, without medication, and no remarkable changes have been observed. Although this is a typical case of sarcoidosis, multiple FDG accumulation is occasionally observed in lymph nodes of the lung hilum in healthy subjects. The etiology is unknown

uptake when compared with a control group. Further studies are required in order to find a way to reduce FDG uptake in the myocardium and bowel.

6.3 Conclusions

Because of the prevalence of PET-negative cancers, PET cannot be used as an alternative to all other conventional methods. However, PET is sensitive for detecting hypermetabolic sites. As regards cancer detection by means of a single examination, PET is superior to other methods. Although benign lesions exhibiting hypermetabolism were detected, they were worthy of clinical attention. False-positive interpretations can be avoided by recognizing potential sites and characteristics of benign lesions. Our experience over 3 years showed that PET can be used to detect a wide variety of cancers in resectable stages in asymptomatic individuals. Further study should be initiated in order to determine how glucose metabolism relates to biological malignancy. And further technological advances will likely increase the usefulness and significance of PET for cancer screening.

Fig. 6.11.
Colonic adenoma (74 year-old man). High FDG uptake is observed in a 1.1 cm adenoma of the ascending colon. Tissue diagnosis was obtained by colonoscopic polypectomy. Focal FDG accumulation in this subject was recognizable retrospectively on PET images taken 15 months before

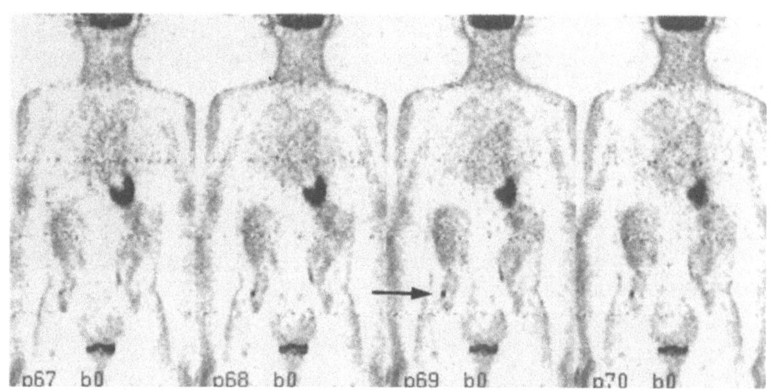

References

Bengel FM, Ziegler SI, Avril N et al. (1997) Whole-body positron emission tomography in clinical oncology: comparison between attenuation-corrected and uncorrected images. Eur J Nucl Med 24: 1091–1098

Biersack HJ, Bender H, Ruhlmann J et al. (1997) FDG-PET in clinical oncology. Review on evaluation of results of a private clinical PET center. In: Freeman LM (ed) Nuclear medicine annual. Lippincott-Raven, Philadelphia, pp 1–29

Binns D, Hicks RJ (1997) Pattern of F-18 FDG uptake and excretion in the lactating breast. 9th ICP Conference. Poster abstract, p3Eur J Nucl Med 23: 1677–1679

Hardcastle JD, Chamberlain JO, Robinson MHE et al. (1996) Randomised controlled trial of faecal-occult-blood screening for colorectal cancer. Lancet 348: 1472–1477

Horiuchi M, Yasuda S, Shothsu A et al. (1998). Four cases of Warthin's tumor of the parotid gland detected with FDG PET. Ann Nucl Med 12: 47–50

Ide M, Suzuki Y (1996) A window on Japan: medical health club with clinical PET

Kostakoglu L, Wong JCH, Barrington SF et al. (1996) Speech-related visualization of laryngeal muscles with fluorine-18-FDG. J Nucl Med 37: 1771–1773

Kramer BS, Gohagan J. Prorok PC 1(994) NIH consensus 1994: Screening. Gynecol Oncol 55: 20–21

Mejia AA, Nakamura T, Itoh M et al. (1991) Estimation of absorbed dose in humans due to intravenous administration of fluorine-18-fluorodeoxyglucose in PET studies. J Nucl Med 32: 699–706

Noguchi M, Morikawa A, Kawasaki M et al. (1995) Small adenocarcinoma of the lung. Histologic characteristics and prognosis. Cancer 75: 2844–2852

Nuutila P, Koivisto A, Knuuti J et al. (1992) Glucose-free fatty acid cycle operates in human heart and skeletal muscle in vivo. J Clin Invest 89: 1767–74

Rigo P, Paulus P, Kaschten BJ et al. (1996) Oncological application of positron emission tomography with fluorine-18 fluorodeoxyglucose. Eur J Nucl Med 23: 1641–1674

Taubes G (1997) The breast-screening brawl. Science 275: 1056–1059

Yasuda S, Shothsu A, Ide M et al. (1996a) High fluorine-18 deoxyglucose uptake in sarcoidosis. Clin Nucl Med 21: 983–984

Yasuda S, Ide M, Takagi S et al. (1996b) Cancer detection with whole-body FDG PET images without attenuation correction. Jpn J Nucl Med 33: 367–373

Yasuda S, Ide M, Takagi S et al. (1997a) Intrauterine accumulation of F-18 FDG during menstruation. Clin Nucl Med 22: 793–794

Yasuda S, Shohtsu A (1997b) Cancer screening with whole-body 18F-fluorodeoxyglucose positron-emission tomography. Lancet 359: 1819

Yasuda S, Shohtsu A, Ide M et al. (1997c) Diffuse F-18 FDG uptake in chronic thyroiditis. Clin Nucl Med 22: 341

Yasuda S, Shothsu A, Ide M et al. (1998a) Diffuse 18-F-fluorodeoxyglucose uptake in chronic thyroiditis. Radiology 207: 775–778

Yasuda S, Ide M, Takagi S et al. (1998b) High fluorine-18 fluorodeoxyglucose uptake in skeletal muscle. Clin Nucl Med 23: 111–112

Yasuda S, Ide M, Takagi S et al. (1998c) F-18 FDG uptake in colonic adenoma. Clin Nucl Med 23: 99–100

Zasadny KR, Kison PV, Quint LE et al. (1996) Untreated lung cancer: quantification of systemic distortion of tumor size and shape on non-attenuation-corrected 2-(fluorine-18)fluoro-2-deoxy-D-glucose PET scans. Radiology 201: 873–876

CHAPTER 7

PET and Radiotherapy

Val J. Lowe

7.1 Introduction

In the late 1800's radioactivity and x-rays were discovered. The uses of radioactive treatment developed over the subsequent years and in the early 1900's some of the standard radiotherapy principles were devised. Experimentation led to the law of Bergonie and Tribondeau which states that radiosensitivity is highest in tissues with a high mitotic index. Other scientists from this time described the dependence of radiation response to oxygen. Further advancement in radiation production equipment and computer assisted treatment planning then occurred. This brought us the radiotherapy practice of today that can provide the generation of controlled radiation doses and radiation delivery to precise tissue areas that optimizes desired radiation dosing.

Radiotherapy cellular toxicity results from a combination of direct and indirect action. Radiotherapy can directly ionize the DNA molecule and lead to DNA strand breaks which, when multiple, can result in cell death. Radiation also has an indirect effect by creating free radicals of which the most important is likely the hydroxyl radical. Free radicals may then damage DNA or other important targets of cellular reproduction. Experts believe that roughly two thirds of total radiotherapy toxicity can be attributed to the actions of free radical (1).

Assessing the effects of radiation therapy can be a difficult endeavor. Some aspects of radiotherapeutic assessment could not be assessed in humans prior to the advent of PET. The following sections will deal with the use of PET in aiding the planning and assessment of radiation therapy.

7.2 PET Before Radiation Therapy

PET scans before, during and after treatment may each provide information that is useful for managing patients undergoing radiation therapy. In patients with locally advanced cancer, FDG-PET imaging performed before radiation therapy can be a valuable tool. It can assist in radiation therapy planning by aiding to focus radiation ports to precise areas of tumor activity.

One group has described an evaluation of the possible effect of PET in altering radiation treatment plans. This group performed a retrospective assessment of whether PET would have changed treatment regions. A qualitative assessment was performed to determine whether abnormal thoracic PET activity was present in areas regarded as normal by diagnostic imaging. Additionally, adequacy of coverage of each patient's abnormal PET activity by the actual radiation field was assessed. Of 15 patients analyzed, 26.7 % (four patients) would have had their radiotherapy volume influenced by PET findings (2).

Hughes and coworkers are using PET in the dosing design for stereotactic implantation of iodine-125 seeds for the palliative treatment of recurrent malignant gliomas (3). This groups describes using 3-dimensional models of PET and anatomic imaging to aid in dosing design.

Treatment planning with PET will likely require substantial image manipulation and compatibility with existing 3-dimensional planning computers. It is our good fortune that computer development seems to be keeping pace with these demands. The advantage for patients is that PET can assist in radiation therapy planning preventing both irradiation of uninvolved areas and omission of regions of active tumor from radiation ports.

7.3 PET During Radiation Therapy

Further work needs to be done to evaluate the use of PET during radiation therapy as data is very sparse. Some data suggests that radiotherapy may induce early acute inflammatory hypermetabolism that can be confused with tumor hypermetabolism. As well, some investigators have concluded that an early decrease in FDG uptake did not necessarily indicate a good prognosis. Hautzel showed in a single patient that after only 6 Gy the metabolic level in cancer can increase and then subsequently decrease (4).

In sarcomas treated with combined radiotherapy and hyperthermia, well-defined central regions of absent uptake, with reduction of peripheral uptake, developed on FDG PET 1–3 weeks after initiating therapy(5). Immediately after completion of radiation therapy, PET demonstrated continued uptake, albeit less in some cases than in the pretreatment tumor, in the periphery of the tumor. This FDG accumulation was found to correlate pathologically with the formation of a fibrous pseudocapsule rather than residual disease(5). In cases were tumor kill was over 90 %, such residual hypermetabolism was seen but was usually at some reduced level from the pretreatment PET.

Brun and coworkers looked at the implications of PET in the early weeks of therapy. They concluded that a rapid reduction from a high metabolic level may imply a higher likelihood of response (6)

7.4 Reoxygenation and PET

Reoxygenation is the process by which tumor cells that were once hypoxic, regain access to oxygen due to shrinkage of tumor secondary to therapy. Animal models have demonstrated that reoxygenation occurs a different rates with different tumors. Because oxygen is needed for the production of free radicals, reoxygenation is an essential factor for optimal tumor kill (1). Fractionated radiation therapy takes advantage of reoxygenation for more complete tumor kill. An initial dose will sterilize only the oxygenated cells, but, with a subsequent dose, cells that were once hypoxic that have become reoxygenated will be susceptible. There are no radiation therapy studies of this effect in humans but PET can offer a method to evaluate tumor hypoxia and reoxygenation in humans.

PET imaging of [F-18]fluoromisonidazole (FMISO) uptake allows noninvasive assessment of tumor hypoxia. Increased uptake is seen where cell hypoxia is present due to bioreduction and deposition of the agent but FMISO is rapidly removed from well-oxygenated areas. Koh and colleagues used FMISO to assess tumors undergoing fractionated therapy and concluded that although there is a general tendency toward improved oxygenation in human tumors during fractionated radiotherapy, these changes were unpredictable and insufficient to overcome the negative effects of existing pretreatment hypoxia(7). They suggested that trials including pretreatment hypoxia assessments with PET would be advised to further test fractionated therapy protocols.

Minn and coworkers have also described the visualization of hypoxia with the metabolic tracers 2-[5,6-3H]fluoro-2-deoxy-D-glucose ([3H]FDG), L-[methyl-3H] methionine ([3H]MET), and L-[1-3H]leucine ([3H]LEU) (8). This group showed that [3H]FDG accumulation is increased in hypoxic squamous cell cancer. They saw a decrease in acid-precipitable [3H]LEU uptake in hypoxia that may indicate a decline in protein synthesis, while unchanged [3H]MET uptake may reflect unaffected amino acid transport.

Further study of this type of assessment by PET may lead to improved radiation therapy planning. Fractionated radiation regimens would be more effective on tumors that are able to reoxygenate more quickly and can demonstrate reductions in tumor hypoxic fractions as radiation therapy is ongoing.

7.5 PET Imaging After Completion of Radiation Therapy

Radiotherapy response had been traditionally associated with reduction in tumor size. Complete response is generally felt to be the only standard for indicating tumor control. A partial response is considered to be a radiotherapeutic failure in most cases. The definition of complete response can be problematic as complete disappearance of the tumor may only occur rarely and more commonly residual tissue, whether it be scar or residual tumor, can remain.

PET has been used to assess the therapeutic response to radiation therapy. FDG-PET can identify changes in glucose uptake after treatment and may prove to be a better indicator of a favorable response to therapy. However, it may be important to differentiate between a decrease in FDG uptake and the complete absence of FDG uptake. Some investigators have concluded that a simple decrease in FDG uptake does not necessarily indicate a good prognosis (9). Rather, it has been suggested that a decrease in FDG uptake may only indicate a partial response due to destruction of cells sensitive to the therapy while other resistant cells continue to be metabolically active. This is consistent with current thinking by radiotherapists of a partial response.

Post-treatment normalization of FDG uptake, on the other hand, appears to be a good prognostic sign. One study by Hebert and coworkers has demonstrated that negative PET findings after radiation therapy, even in the presence of non-specific radiographic changes, are an indicator of a good response (10). Hebert noted that all of their patients with negative PET findings were alive at 2 years after treatment whereas 50 % of patients with residual hypermetabolism, albeit reduced, had expired within that same 2 year period. Other investigators have used this logic to justify further treatment of asymptomatic individuals whose PET scans demonstrate residual hypermetabolism after an initial course of therapy. Frank and colleagues treated 5 such asymptomatic patients in their study based solely on residual hypermetabolism and all were alive at 3 years. (11).

Head and neck cancer reports have resulted in similar findings. Lindholm and others described C11 methionine PET imaging as it relates to treatment response (12). They showed that reduced methionine uptake after therapy was more likely to indicate response. Minn and coworkers described the reduction in FDG uptake in patients imaged after radiation therapy and prior to surgery. A complete histological response was verified in none of 9 cases with a post-irradiation SUV larger than 3.1, whereas 7 of the 10 cases with a SUV of 3.1 or smaller had complete response. This was a statistically significant finding (p 0.003) (13).

7.6 Diagnosing Recurrent Disease with PET

Diagnosis of recurrent cancer is another potential use of FDG-PET after radiation therapy. Radiologic changes such as scarring and necrosis which occur after radiotherapy may obscure the identification of recurrent tumor unless significant volume changes occur over time. The interpretation of recurrence is often not made until the disease progresses to the point of marked enlargement of questionable abnormalities. Unfortunately, a tissue biopsy that is negative for tumor in such situations is suspect due to the inherent difficulty in identifying and accurately sampling the areas of viable tumor in the midst of scar. A PET evaluation of tumor recurrence can potentially assist in this determination.

For example, patients who have chest radiographic findings suspicious for tumor recurrence can be accurately characterized by FDG-PET. Benign, nonspecific pleural thickening is another example of post-treatment changes which may be difficult to differentiate from recurrent disease. Pleural biopsy itself may be relatively unreliable when performed percutaneously. PET imaging can differentiate recurrent tumor from radiation inducing benign pleural thickening (14). Patz and coworkers (15) demonstrated a very high accuracy of PET in distinguishing recurrent disease from benign treatment effects when patients were scanned after therapy. The report of Inoue and coworkers (16) yielded similar results. Greven, in a nonblinded, prospective, single institution study, assessed 18 patients after radiation therapy and found a 100 % sensitivity and a 92 % specificity for detection of residual or recurrent head and neck cancer (17).

7.7 Timing of PET After Radiation Therapy

Normal tissues can manifest radiotherapy toxicity to different degrees. Some tissue will demonstrate toxicity in a few days. These tissues are bone marrow, gonads, lymph nodes, salivary glands, gastrointestinal tract, larynx, and skin. Other tissues demonstrate radiation damage in weeks to months and some examples are lung, liver, kidney, spinal cord and brain. Because of these effects, significantly increased FDG uptake can be seen in selected soft tissue regions that are irradiated. Data suggests that radiotherapy may induce early acute inflammatory hypermetabolism on PET that is likely related to healing of tissues damaged by radiation. This effect will likely depend on the radiosensitivity of the normal tissues being irradiated.

In chest radiotherapy, increased FDG uptake in the chest wall correlates with clinical evidence of radiation damage. Increased FDG accumulation in normal chest wall tissue can be statistically significant at least 12–16 months after treatment. The standardized uptake ratio (SUR) of this radiation related uptake is generally less than what is found in recurrent tumor (SUR<2.5) (18). Nevertheless, FDG uptake from radiation effects can in a few cases be in a range that is worrisome for malignancy. This study showed that normal tissue activity inflammatory responses are maximum at about 6 months but can be seen for at least a year (Figure 1).

The study by Jones et al suggests that immediately following radiation a hypermetabolic pseudocapsule can be seen that may appear to falsely represent tumor (5). And still, Greven and coworkers showed that within one month of radiation it is to a small degree more likely to see negative PET scans in people with some residual disease. They also found that a 4 month PET assessment did not demonstrate any false negatives (17). (Figures 2,3)

A fair compromise may be to recommend PET imaging 4–6 months after completion of radiation if possible. This would allow for assessment of early recurrence and probably give high accuracy of treatment assessment. If inflammatory hypermetabolism is confusing, a follow-up scan may be required to see if the activity diminishes over time. If one is forced to image earlier due to clinical necessity, particular attention should be paid

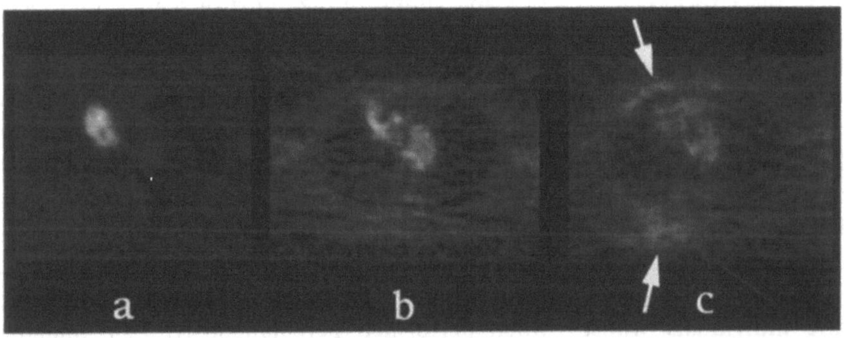

Fig. 7.1 a–c. Axial FDG PET images of a patient with right lung cancer before (**a**), 1 month after (**b**) and 6 months after (**c**) radiation therapy with 73.6 Gy. Mild chest wall inflammatory hypermetabolism is seen on the six month scan in radiation port locations (*arrows*). The tumor activity continues to decrease over the period but is only less intense than blood pool activity (negative for disease) at 6 months. The patient was free of disease one year later

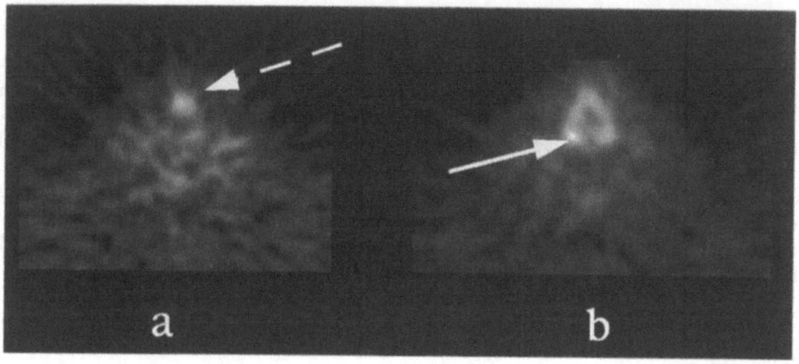

Fig. 7.2 a, b. Axial FDG PET images of a patient with T1 larynx cancer (broken arrow) before (**a**) and 1 month after (**b**) radiation therapy with 68 Gy. Hypermetabolism in the arytenoid cartilage regions is intense on the post therapy scan because they are very radiation sensitive (solid arrow). Additional uptake more anteriorly in the vocal cords due to inflammation or muscle activity makes interpretation difficult in this one month post-therapy scan. The patient was disease free 2 years later

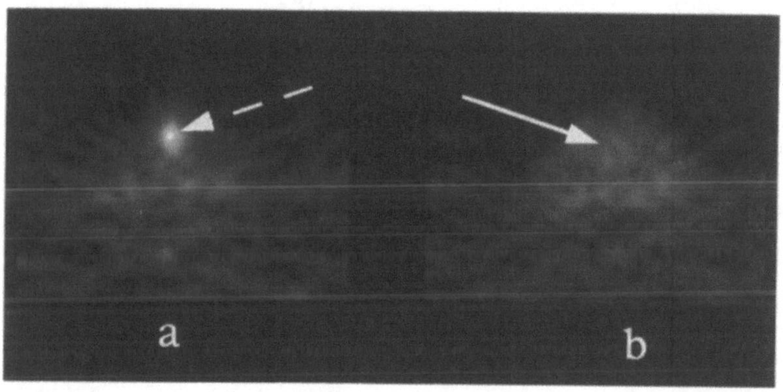

Fig. 7.3 a, b. Axial FDG PET images of a patient with T2 larynx cancer (broken arrow) before (a) and 4 months after (b) radiation therapy with 70 Gy. No intense post-therapy uptake is seen although mild uptake is present in the vocal cord region (*arrow*). This post-therapy scan is confidently negative. The patient was disease free 2 years later

to the patterns of any hypermetabolism present in hopes of distinguishing inflammation from residual disease. Clinicians should realize that even with a negative PET scan early after therapy, it is advisable to perform an additional follow-up scan in 4–6 months.

7.8 Summary

PET imaging can aid in radiation therapy planning and in the assessment of residual or recurrent disease. Areas of ongoing research that hold promise for additional uses of PET include early assessment of radiation effects and assessment of tumor hypoxia.

References

Brun E, Ohlsson T, Erlandsson K, et al. Early prediction of treatment outcome in head and neck cancer with 2-18FDG PET. Acta Oncologica 1997; 36: 741–7

Frank A, Lefkowitz D, Jaeger S, et al. Decision logic for retreatment of asymptomatic lung cancer recurrence based on positron emission tomography findings. Inter J Radiat Oncol Biol Physics 1995; 32: 1495–512.

Greven KM, Williams D3, Keyes JJ, et al. Positron emission tomography of patients with head and neck carcinoma before and after high dose irradiation [see comments]. Cancer 1994; 74: 1355–9

Hall EJ, Cox JD. Physical and biologic basis of radiation therapy. In: Cox JD, ed. Moss' Radiation Oncology. St. Louis: Mosby-Year Book, Inc, 1994: 3–66

Hautzel H, Muller GH. Early changes in fluorine-18-FDG uptake during radiotherapy. J Nuc Med 1997; 38: 1384–6

Hebert ME, Lowe VJ, Hoffman JM, Patz EF, Anscher MS. Positron emission tomography in the pretreatment evaluation and follow-up of non-small cell lung cancer patients treated with radiotherapy: preliminary findings. Amer J Clin Oncol 1996; 19: 416–21

Hughes SW, Sofat A, Kitchen ND, et al. Computer planning of stereotactic iodine-125 seed brachytherapy for recurrent malignant gliomas. Brit J Radiology 1995; 68: 175–81

Ichiya Y, Kuwabara Y, Otsuka M, et al. Assessment of response to cancer therapy using fluorine-18-fluorodeoxyglucose and positron emission tomography. J Nucl Med 1991; 32: 1655–60

Inoue T, Kim EE, Komaki R, et al. Detecting recurrent or residual lung cancer with FDG-PET. J Nucl Med 1995; 36: 788–93

Jones DN, McCowage GB, Sostman HD, et al. Monitoring of neoadjuvant therapy response of soft-tissue and musculoskeletal sarcoma using fluorine-18–FDG PET. J Nucl Med 1996; 37: 1438–44

Kiffer JD, Berlangieri SU, Scott AM, et al. The contribution of 18F-fluoro-2-deoxy-glucose positron emission tomographic imaging toradiotherapy planning in lung cancer. Lung Cancer 1998; 19: 167–77

Koh WJ, Bergman KS, Rasey JS, et al. Evaluation of oxygenation status during fractionated radiotherapy in human nonsmall cell lung cancers using [F-18]fluoromisonidazole positron emission tomography. Inter J Radiat Oncol Biol Physics 1995; 33: 391–8

Lindholm P, Leskinen KS, Grenman R, et al. Evaluation of response to radiotherapy in head and neck cancer by positron emission tomography and [11C]methionine. Inter J Radiat Oncol Biol Physics 1995; 32: 787–94

Lowe VJ, Hebert ME, Anscher MS, Coleman RE. Chest Wall FDG Accumulation in Serial FDG-PET Images in Patients Being Treated for Bronchogenic Carcinoma with Radiation. Clin Positron Imag 1998; 1: 185–192

Lowe VJ, Patz EF, Harris L, et al. FDG-PET evaluation of pleural abnormalities. J Nucl Med 1994; 35: 229P

Minn H, Clavo AC, Wahl RL. Influence of hypoxia on tracer accumulation in squamous-cell carcinoma: in vitro evaluation for PET imaging. Nuc Med Biol 1996; 23: 941–6

Minn H, Lapela M, Klemi PJ, et al. Prediction of survival with fluorine-18-fluoro-deoxyglucose and PET in head and neck cancer. J Nucl Med 1997; 38: 1907–11

Patz EJ, Lowe VJ, Hoffman JM, Paine SS, Harris LK, Goodman PC. Persistent or recurrent bronchogenic carcinoma: detection with PET and 2-[F-18]-2-deoxy-D-glucose. Radiology 1994; 191: 379–82.

CHAPTER 8

Cost Effectiveness of PET in Oncology*

P. E. Valk

The cost effectiveness of a diagnostic or therapeutic procedure is most commonly expressed in terms of cost effectiveness ratio:

Cost Effectiveness Ratio = Net Cost Increase/Net Effectiveness Increase

This is expressed in dollars per quality-adjusted life-year. Two clinically positive outcomes are possible: effectiveness increases and cost decreases or effectiveness and cost increase. For a diagnostic modality, effect on survival is difficult to evaluate, since this outcome is dominated by the therapeutic procedures that follow the diagnosis. In the present evaluation, we assumed that increased sensitivity resulting in decreased surgery for non-resectable tumor, and increased specificity resulting in fewer operations for non-malignant lesions, would produce an equal or better clinical outcome, and did not attempt to quantify effectiveness. It therefore remained to evaluate the diagnostic accuracy of PET, and to determine the effect of PET findings on cost of patient management.

For determination of cost, in the United States today, only Medicare reimbursement rate has universal significance, and is not affected by managed-care contracts. Accordingly, we used Medicare reimbursement rates to determine cost of surgical and diagnostic procedures. During the time of the study, there was no Medicare reimbursement for PET, and we used instead the average reimbursement rate at the Northern California PET Imaging Center during this period, which proved to be 1,800 per whole-body FDG study.

In order to evaluate clinical efficacy, we need to determine the accuracy of PET in terms of sensitivity and specificity for a particular clinical indication, and the impact of PET findings on patient management, both diagnostic and therapeutic. When this work started in 1992, oncologic PET was largely a hypothetical field. Anecdotal reports of PET findings in various tumors had been published, but there were no data on sensitivity and specificity, and management studies had not been done. It was, therefore, necessary to commence our evaluation by looking at these factors.

8.1 Diagnosis and Staging of Non-Small Cell Lung Cancer

The only area of oncology where clinical efficacy of PET had already been determined was the diagnosis of solitary pulmonary nodules. Analysis of published studies by the Institute for Clinical PET in 1994 showed that a total of 237 patients had been reported from five different institutions. Sensitivity for cancer detection was 96 %, and specificity was 90 %. Since PET was accurate for diagnosis of non-small cell lung cancer, it seemed that it should also be accurate for staging. We therefore undertook a prospective comparison of PET and CT in staging non-small cell lung cancer, and eventually accrued 103 tumors in 99 patients (1).

Mediastinal PET and CT findings were compared to results of surgical staging in 76 patients. PET and CT results that indicated possible distant metastases were compared to biopsy results and results of clinical and imaging follow-up. Sensitivity and specificity for diagnosis of mediastinal

---

* Lecture at a PET-conference in Leipzig (Germany), September 1997.

metastatic disease were 83 % and 94 % for PET and 63 % and 73 % for CT, respectively. PET showed previously unsuspected distant metastases in 11 patients (11 %) with no false-positive results. Normal PET findings were obtained at distant sites of CT abnormality in 19 patients (19 %). In one of these cases, a negative PET finding involving a small nodule in the opposite lung proved to be incorrect. In the remaining 18 patients, clinical progress and follow-up imaging showed no evidence of metastasis.

Since PET was clearly more accurate than CT in staging, we next undertook an evaluation of the effect of PET findings on patient management. This was done by reviewing the treatment records of 72 patients that had been referred for PET imaging over a two-year period from a single thoracic surgical practice, in order to determine the effect of PET on treatment decisions. Thirty-eight patients were initially referred for diagnosis of indeterminate pulmonary nodules. Twenty of these proved to be malignant, and 18 were found to be benign. Thirty-four patients were referred for staging of known lung cancer, so that the total number of staging studies was 54. The following impact on patient management was determined: Thoracotomy for tumor resection was avoided in six patients by demonstrating non-resectable tumor that had not been detected by conventional staging procedures. In the 18 patients with benign lung nodules, it was determined that diagnostic thoracotomy would have been undertaken in eight, if a negative PET result had not been available. Follow-up of these patients indicated that none of the PET findings in this group proved to be false negative. In 11 patients with CT evidence of enlarged mediastinal lymph nodes, mediastinoscopy was avoided by demonstration of absence of mediastinal metastases by PET. Finally, 15 CT-guided fine-needle biopsy procedures were avoided (10 lung, three adrenal, two liver) by demonstrating that abnormalities detected on CT were benign on PET imaging. Altogether, the availability of PET findings had an effect on diagnostic or therapeutic patient management in 38 cases. We evaluated the cost of procedures avoided on the basis of Medicare reimbursement rates, and this proved to be $ 292,000. The most important savings, of course, were in diagnostic and tumor-resection thoracotomies. The cost of PET studies in the entire group of 72 patients, based on an average reimbursement rate of $ 1800 was $ 130,000. From this, we deducted the cost of an abdominal CT study and a bone scan in the 54 patients who underwent staging, thereby reducing the net cost of PET to $ 98,000. The saving per patient was $ 2,690.

8.2 Staging of Recurrent Colorectal Cancer

Colorectal cancer is one of the few tumors where surgical resection is commonly employed for treatment of recurrent disease. However, surgical results are limited by the low accuracy of CT for initial detection and for detection of non-resectable disease. At surgery, 25–50 % of patients with solitary liver lesions on CT are found to have non-resectable tumor, and a five-year survival rate in remaining patients is only 25 %. For these reasons, it appeared likely that the high sensitivity and specificity of PET for tumor metabolism could improve selection of patients for surgery, resulting in fewer resections in patients with non-resectable tumor.

Accordingly, shortly after the center opened, we also commenced an evaluation of PET in recurrent colorectal cancer. (2). PET detected 96/100 patients (96 %) and 146/156 anatomic sites (94 %) with recurrence, whereas CT detected 78/100 patients (78 %) and 105/156 anatomic sites (68 %). PET was false positive in three patients and at five sites, whereas CT was false positive in six patients and at 18 sites. For both technologies, sensitivity varied by anatomic site of recurrence. PET sensitivity was 97 % in the pelvis and 96 % in the liver, but only 85 % in the abdomen and retroperitoneum. For CT, sensitivity was highest in the liver at 84 %, lower in the pelvis at 66 % and lowest of all in the abdomen and retroperitoneum at 50 %.

Because of the importance of accurate pre-operative staging in patients with apparently localized recurrence, we undertook a post-PET follow-up of 76 patients who had been imaged specifically for pre-operative evaluation. In these patients, PET showed tumor that was apparently resectable in 46 patients (61 %) and non-resectable in 25 (33 %). No evidence of recurrence was found at the site of CT abnormality in five patients (6 %). In terms of management impact, in 25 patients tumor resection was avoided by diagnosis of non-resectable recurrence, and in five patients exploratory laparotomy was avoided by exclusion of recurrence. From published surgical results (3), it was determined that non-resectable tumor is found at surgery in approximately 50 % of patients with hepatic recurrence. These patients undergo laparotomy without hepatic resection, and the numbers of procedures avoided were adjusted accordingly. Surgical procedures were avoided in 30/76 patients (39 %) including hepatic resection in 7 patients, laparotomy in 21 patients and thoracotomy in 2 patients.

The total cost of surgical procedures avoided was $ 438,000. Cost of PET imaging was $ 137,000. If the cost of two avoided CT imaging procedures per patient were deducted from this, the net cost of PET would be $ 76,000. The per patient savings was $ 3,960 when PET was used as an additional imaging procedure and $ 4,750 when PET was used to replace CT imaging.

8.3 Staging of Metastatic Melanoma

Commencing in 1993, we undertook a prospective evaluation of PET in metastatic melanoma by comparing PET to CT in final diagnosis in 36 patients (4). In this group, PET detected 43/45 tumor sites (96 %), compared to 21/38 tumor sites (55 %) for CT. PET had one false-positive site, which was at a site of recent surgery, whereas CT had 13 false-positive sites.

To evaluate the impact of PET findings on patient management, we reviewed the post-PET treatment records of 68 patients, 48 patients who had been studied at Northern California PET Imaging Center and 20 at the Stanford PET Center in Palo Alto, CA (5). Thirty-five of these patients had clinical or imaging evidence of probable recurrent tumor, and were being studied specifically for pre-operative evaluation. In this subgroup, PET findings indicated that resectable tumor was present in 20 patients (57 %). In eight patients (23 %), unsuspected tumor of non-resectable extent was demonstrated, and in seven patients (20 %), no tumor was detected at the site of abnormality.

These findings had the following impact on surgical patient management: Surgery was avoided by diagnosis of non-resectable tumor in eight patients, and was avoided by exclusion of tumor in seven patients. In three other patients tumor resection was initiated by demonstrating resectability in patients whose tumor was thought to be non-resectable on the basis of conventional staging. Altogether, surgical procedures were avoided in 15/35 pre-operative patients (43 %). These included lung resection in six patients, lymph node resection in four patients, hepatic resection in two patients and laparotomy in three patients.

The total cost of these avoided surgical procedures was $ 216,000. The cost of PET imaging in the subgroup of 35 pre-operative patients was $ 63,000. When PET was considered as replacing two CT imaging procedures per patient, the net cost was reduced to $ 35,000. The cost savings per patient was $ 4,371 when PET was used as an additional procedure and $ 5,200 when PET replaced CT.

These cost findings are summarized in Table 1, where it is assumed that PET replaces an abdominal CT scan and a bone scan in staging lung cancer, and replaces two CT scans in staging recurrent colorectal cancer and metastatic melanoma. When PET is used as an additional diagnostic procedure, without replacing other forms of imaging, the savings will be reduced by $ 600 and $ 800 per patient respectively.

In cost-analysis terms, the improvement in patient management that results from more accurate

Table 8.1. Net cost savings resulting from use of PET

	NSCLC (SPN & Staging)	Colorectal Cancer (Pre-op.)	Melanoma (Pre-op.)
No. of Patients	72	76	35
Cost of Procedures Avoided	$ 292,000	$ 438,000	$ 216,000
Net Cost of PET	$ 98,000	$ 76,000	$ 35,000
Net Savings/ Cost Ratio	3.0	5.8	6.2
Net Savings per Patient	$ 2,690	$ 4,750	$ 5,200

diagnosis, combined with reduced management cost, means that PET is dominant over conventional procedures for these indications. Pre-operative staging of patients with colorectal cancer or metastatic melanoma, who are thought to have resectable recurrence on the basis of conventional staging procedures, is the most cost-effective application of PET that we have so far evaluated. Cost savings in patients with indeterminate pulmonary nodules and primary non-small cell lung cancer are smaller per patient, but affect a much larger total patient population.

We have also demonstrated the clinical efficacy of PET in recurrent head and neck cancer (6) and Hodgkin's disease (7), and clinical efficacy has also been demonstrated in staging non-Hodgkin's lymphoma, staging esophageal cancer, diagnosis of recurrent breast cancer and ovarian cancer, and detection of non-functioning thyroid metastases. Cost evaluation of these applications of PET has not been reported to date, but further cost-effective uses can be expected in these and other tumors.

References

Abella-Columna E, Manolidis S, Isaacs RS, Pounds TR, Donald PJ, Valk PE (1997). Staging recurrent head and neck cancer by whole-body FDG PET imaging. J Nucl Med 38:155P

Abella-Columna E, Valk PE, Pounds TR, Wolkov HB, Liebenhaut MH, Haseman MK, Lutrin CL (1996). Staging Hodgkin's disease by whole-body PET-FDG imaging. J Nucl Med 37:139P

Pounds TR, Valk PE, Spitler L, Haseman MK, Myers RW, Lutrin CL (1995). Whole-body PET-FDG imaging in diagnosis of metastatic melanoma: Comparison to CT. J Nucl Med 36:116P

Steele GJ, Bleday R, Mayer RJ, Lindblad A, Petrelli N, Weaver D. (1991). A prospective evaluation of hepatic resection for colorectal carcinoma metastases to the liver: Gastrointestinal tumor study group protocol 6584. J Clin Oncol 1991;9:1105–1112

Valk PE, Abella-Columna E, Tesar RD, Pounds TR, Haseman MK, Myers RW (1996). Diagnostic accuracy and cost-effectiveness of whole-body PET-FDG imaging in recurrent colorectal cancer. J Nucl Med 37:132P

Valk PE, Pounds TR, Hopkins DM, Haseman MK, Hofer GA, Greiss HB, Myers RA, Lutrin CL (1995). Staging non-small-cell lung cancer by whole-body PET imaging. Ann Thor Surg 60:1573–1582

Valk PE, Segall GM, Johnson DL, Pounds TR, Tesar RD, Jadvar H, Abella-Columna E. (1997). Cost-effectiveness of whole-body FDG PET imaging in metastatic melanoma. J Nucl Med 38:90P

Subject Index

U

V

Y

MIX
Papier aus verantwortungsvollen Quellen
Paper from responsible sources
FSC® C105338

If you have any concerns about our products,
you can contact us on
ProductSafety@springernature.com

In case Publisher is established outside the EU,
the EU authorized representative is:
Springer Nature Customer Service Center GmbH
Europaplatz 3, 69115 Heidelberg, Germany

Printed by Libri Plureos GmbH
in Hamburg, Germany